NATIONAL ACADEMIES
Sciences
Engineering
Medicine

NATIONAL ACADEMIES PRESS
Washington, DC

The Future Pediatric Subspecialty Physician Workforce

Meeting the Needs of Infants, Children, and Adolescents

Committee on the Pediatric Subspecialty Workforce and Its Impact on Child Health and Well-Being

Board on Health Care Services
Health and Medicine Division

Board on Children, Youth, and Families
Division of Behavioral and Social Sciences and Education

Consensus Study Report

NATIONAL ACADEMIES PRESS 500 Fifth Street, NW, Washington, DC 20001

This activity was supported by contracts between the National Academy of Sciences and the American Academy of Pediatrics, the American Board of Pediatrics, the Association of Medical School Pediatric Department Chairs, The Annie E. Casey Foundation, the Children's Hospital Association, the Council of Pediatric Subspecialties, the National Institute of Child Health and Human Development, and the Robert Wood Johnson Foundation. Any opinions, findings, conclusions, or recommendations expressed in this publication do not necessarily reflect the views of any organization or agency that provided support for the project.

International Standard Book Number-13: 978-0-309-70840-1
International Standard Book Number-10: 0-309-70840-0
Digital Object Identifier: https://doi.org/10.17226/27207

This publication is available from the National Academies Press, 500 Fifth Street, NW, Keck 360, Washington, DC 20001; (800) 624-6242 or (202) 334-3313; http://www.nap.edu.

Copyright 2023 by the National Academy of Sciences. National Academies of Sciences, Engineering, and Medicine and National Academies Press and the graphical logos for each are all trademarks of the National Academy of Sciences. All rights reserved.

Printed in the United States of America.

Suggested citation: National Academies of Sciences, Engineering, and Medicine. 2023. *The future pediatric subspecialty physician workforce: Meeting the needs of infants, children, and adolescents.* Washington, DC: The National Academies Press. https://doi.org/10.17226/27207.

The **National Academy of Sciences** was established in 1863 by an Act of Congress, signed by President Lincoln, as a private, nongovernmental institution to advise the nation on issues related to science and technology. Members are elected by their peers for outstanding contributions to research. Dr. Marcia McNutt is president.

The **National Academy of Engineering** was established in 1964 under the charter of the National Academy of Sciences to bring the practices of engineering to advising the nation. Members are elected by their peers for extraordinary contributions to engineering. Dr. John L. Anderson is president.

The **National Academy of Medicine** (formerly the Institute of Medicine) was established in 1970 under the charter of the National Academy of Sciences to advise the nation on medical and health issues. Members are elected by their peers for distinguished contributions to medicine and health. Dr. Victor J. Dzau is president.

The three Academies work together as the **National Academies of Sciences, Engineering, and Medicine** to provide independent, objective analysis and advice to the nation and conduct other activities to solve complex problems and inform public policy decisions. The National Academies also encourage education and research, recognize outstanding contributions to knowledge, and increase public understanding in matters of science, engineering, and medicine.

Learn more about the National Academies of Sciences, Engineering, and Medicine at **www.nationalacademies.org**.

Consensus Study Reports published by the National Academies of Sciences, Engineering, and Medicine document the evidence-based consensus on the study's statement of task by an authoring committee of experts. Reports typically include findings, conclusions, and recommendations based on information gathered by the committee and the committee's deliberations. Each report has been subjected to a rigorous and independent peer-review process and it represents the position of the National Academies on the statement of task.

Proceedings published by the National Academies of Sciences, Engineering, and Medicine chronicle the presentations and discussions at a workshop, symposium, or other event convened by the National Academies. The statements and opinions contained in proceedings are those of the participants and are not endorsed by other participants, the planning committee, or the National Academies.

Rapid Expert Consultations published by the National Academies of Sciences, Engineering, and Medicine are authored by subject-matter experts on narrowly focused topics that can be supported by a body of evidence. The discussions contained in rapid expert consultations are considered those of the authors and do not contain policy recommendations. Rapid expert consultations are reviewed by the institution before release.

For information about other products and activities of the National Academies, please visit www.nationalacademies.org/about/whatwedo.

COMMITTEE ON THE PEDIATRIC SUBSPECIALTY WORKFORCE AND ITS IMPACT IN CHILD HEALTH AND WELL-BEING

FREDERICK P. RIVARA (*Chair*), Seattle Children's Guild Association Endowed Chair in Pediatric Outcomes Research; Vice Chair and Professor, Department of Pediatrics; Adjunct Professor, Department of Epidemiology, University of Washington

KELLY J. BETTS, Assistant Dean/Assistant Professor, University of Nebraska Medical Center, College of Nursing West Nebraska Division; Primary Care Pediatric Nurse Practitioner, Community Action Health Clinic, Gering, Nebraska

KENDALL M. CAMPBELL, Professor and Chair, Department of Family Medicine, University of Texas Medical Branch

KECIA N. CARROLL, Chief, Division of General Pediatrics, Professor of Pediatrics, Environmental Medicine and Public Health, The Icahn School of Medicine at Mount Sinai

CANDICE CHEN, Associate Professor, Fitzhugh Mullan Institute for Health Workforce Equity, Milken Institute School of Public Health, The George Washington University

CHRISTOPHER B. FORREST, Professor of Pediatrics, Applied Clinical Research Center, Children's Hospital of Philadelphia, Perelman School of Medicine at the University of Pennsylvania

ELENA FUENTES-AFFLICK, Professor of Pediatrics and Vice Dean, Zuckerburg San Francisco General Hospital, University of California, San Francisco

RACHEL L. GARFIELD, Executive Director, Vermont Child Health Improvement Program; Associate Professor, Department of Pediatrics, Larner College of Medicine at the University of Vermont

KRISTIN HITTLE GIGLI, Assistant Professor, Graduate Nursing University of Texas at Arlington; Pediatric Nurse Practitioner, Pediatric Intensive Care Unit, University of Texas Southwestern Medical Center, Children's Health

JAVIER A. GONZALEZ DEL REY, Professor of Clinical Pediatrics, Division of Pediatric Emergency Medicine, Cincinnati Children's Hospital Medical Center; Associate Chair for Education and Director, Cincinnati Children's Pediatric Education Center; Designated Institutional Official, University of Cincinnati College of Medicine

SHAFALI SPURLING JESTE, Las Madrinas Chair and Chief, Division of Neurology, Children's Hospital Los Angeles, Professor of Pediatrics and Neurology, USC Keck School of Medicine

OPHIR D. KLEIN, Executive Director, Cedars-Sinai Guerin Children's; Vice Dean for Children's Services, David and Meredith Kaplan Distinguished Chair in Children's Health, Professor of Pediatrics, Cedars-Sinai Medical Center; Adjunct Professor of Orofacial Sciences and Pediatrics, University of California San Francisco

VICTORIA FAY NORWOOD, Robert J. Roberts Professor of Pediatrics, Division of Pediatric Nephrology, University of Virginia School of Medicine, and Children's Hospital

ELIANA M. PERRIN, Bloomberg Distinguished Professor of Primary Care, Department of Pediatrics—School of Medicine, School of Nursing, Johns Hopkins University

SAMIR S. SHAH, Vice Chair, Clinical Affairs and Education, Cincinnati Children's Hospital Medical Center; James M. Ewell Professor, Department of Pediatrics, University of Cincinnati College of Medicine

CHRISTOPHER J. STILLE, Professor and Section Head, General Academic Pediatrics, and Stephen Berman, M.D. Endowed Chair in General Pediatrics, University of Colorado School of Medicine

BONNIE T. ZIMA, Professor-in-Residence, Child and Adolescent Psychiatry, Vice Chair for Faculty Development, Associate Chair for Academic Affairs, UCLA-Semel Institute for Neurosciences and Human Behaviors; UCLA Center for Health Services and Society

National Academy of Medicine (NAM) Fellow

JULIEANNE P. SEES, Associate Professor of Pediatrics and Orthopaedic Surgery, Midwestern University; Chair, Department of Affiliates, American Osteopathic Association; Director, American Osteopathic Academy of Orthopaedics

Study Staff

TRACY A. LUSTIG, Study Director
RUTH COOPER, Associate Program Officer
ISAAC SUH, Research Associate (*starting August 2022*)
NIKITA VARMAN, Research Associate (*through June 2022*)
ADAEZE OKOROAJUZIE, Senior Program Assistant (*starting January 2023*)
TOCHI OGBU-MBADIUGHA, Senior Program Assistant (*through November 2022*)
ARZOO TAYYEB, Finance Business Partner (*through April 2023*)
JULIE WILTSHIRE, Senior Finance Business Partner (*starting April 2023*)
JULIE SCHUCK, Senior Program Officer, Board on Children, Youth, and Families
NATACHA BLAIN, Senior Board Director, Board on Children, Youth, and Families
SHARYL J. NASS, Senior Director, Board on Health Care Services

Reviewers

This Consensus Study Report was reviewed in draft form by individuals chosen for their diverse perspectives and technical expertise. The purpose of this independent review is to provide candid and critical comments that will assist the National Academies of Sciences, Engineering, and Medicine in making each published report as sound as possible and to ensure that it meets the institutional standards for quality, objectivity, evidence, and responsiveness to the study charge. The review comments and draft manuscript remain confidential to protect the integrity of the deliberative process.

We thank the following individuals for their review of this report:

RICHARD D. ALBA, City University of New York, Graduate Center
BETH N. BOLICK, Rush University College of Nursing
GARY L. FREED, University of Michigan
ALISON A. GALBRAITH, Boston Medical Center and Boston
　University Chobanian & Avedisian School of Medicine
BRUCE HERMAN, University of Utah
LAUREN S. HUGHES, University of Colorado Anschutz Medical
　Campus
LUCKY JAIN, Emory & Children's Healthcare of Atlanta
KEILA N. LOPEZ, Texas Children's Hospital & Baylor College of
　Medicine
KRISTIN RAY, University of Pittsburgh School of Medicine
ANDY SCHNEIDER, Georgetown University McCourt School of
　Public Policy
DIANA M. V. SHAW, University of Hawaii

SCOTT SHIPMAN, Creighton University
ANDREA SPENCER, Ann & Robert Lurie Children's Hospital of Chicago
FRANKLIN TRIMM, Frederick P. Whiddon College of Medicine at the University of South Alabama
CHARLENE WONG, Duke University and North Carolina Department of Health and Human Services

Although the reviewers listed above provided many constructive comments and suggestions, they were not asked to endorse the conclusions or recommendations of this report nor did they see the final draft before its release. The review of this report was overseen by **PATRICK H. DELEON**, Uniformed Services University, and **SHARI BARKIN**, Virginia Commonwealth University. They were responsible for making certain that an independent examination of this report was carried out in accordance with the standards of the National Academies and that all review comments were carefully considered. Responsibility for the final content rests entirely with the authoring committee and the National Academies.

Acknowledgments

The study committee and the Health and Medicine Division (HMD) project staff take this opportunity to recognize and thank the many individuals who shared their time and expertise to support the committee's work and to inform deliberations.

This committee appreciates the sponsors of this study for their generous financial support: the American Academy of Pediatrics, the American Board of Pediatrics, The Annie E. Casey Foundation, the Association of Medical School Pediatric Department Chairs, the Children's Hospital Association, the Council of Pediatric Subspecialties, the National Institute of Child Health and Human Development, and the Robert Wood Johnson Foundation. The contents provided do not necessarily represent the official views of the sponsors.

The committee benefitted greatly from discussions with individuals who made presentations during the committee's open sessions:

Ileana Barron, Parent Perspective
Hunter Beck, PKIDS Patient and Family Partners
Louis Bell, Children's Hospital of Philadelphia
Tami D. Benton, Children's Hospital of Philadelphia
Ericka Boone, National Institutes of Health
April Buchanan, Council on Medical Student Education in Pediatrics
Eva Catenaccio, Children's Hospital of Philadelphia
Sandy Chung, American Academy of Pediatrics

Denice Cora-Bramble, Children's National Hospital
Scott Cyrus, Burrell College of Osteopathic Medicine
Stephanie Davis, University of North Carolina's Children's Hospital
Laura Degnon, AMSPDC Workforce Initiative
Sherin U. Devaskar, Association of Medical School Pediatric Department Chairs
Matthew Di Guglielmo, Nemours Children's Health
Gary Freed, University of Michigan
Reem M. Ghandour, Health Resources and Services Administration
Rohan Hazra, National Institute of Child Health and Human Development
Clarissa Hoover, Family Voices
Robert Hostoffer, Case Western Reserve University
Maya S. Iyer, Nationwide Children's Hospital
Steven Kairys, Hackensack Meridian School of Medicine
Christian Lawson, Improve Care Now
Mary Leonard, Stanford University
Lauren K. Leslie, American Board of Pediatrics
Joanna Lewis, Advocate Children's Hospital – Park Ridge
Alex Li, L.A. Care
Stephanie Lovinsky-Desir, Columbia University
Furman McDonald, American Board of Internal Medicine
Michael Melfe, American Board of Internal Medicine
Louis J. Muglia, Burroughs Wellcome Fund
Colin Orr, University of North Carolina, Chapel Hill
Sallie Permar, Weill Cornell Medicine
Kristin Ray, University of Pittsburgh
Sara Rosenbaum, George Washington University
LaToshia Rouse, Birth Sisters Doula Services
Scott Shipman, Creighton University
Harold Simon, Emory University
Joseph St. Geme, Association of Medical School Pediatric Department Chairs
Bob Tamburro, National Institute of Child Health and Human Development
Bob Vinci, AMSPDC Workforce Initiative
Mark Wietecha, Children's Hospital Association
Xavier Williams, University of North Carolina's Children's Hospital
Sue Woods, American Board of Pediatrics
Charlene Wong, Duke University School of Medicine
Hal Yee, Jr., Los Angeles County Department of Health Services

The committee is thankful for the team at Carelon Research, including Lauren Parlett, Katherine Harris, Claire Bocage, Roopalini Bakthavachalam, and Madhavi Sunkara, who produced a commissioned analysis of pediatric subspecialty use among a commercial health plan population.

The committee also thanks researchers who contributed to two other analyses submitted to this committee. They include Mitchell Maltenfort and Andrea Allen at the Children's Hospital of Philadelphia who contributed to an analysis of PEDSnet data of children at academic pediatric medical centers, and Qian Luo at The George Washington University who contributed to an analysis of data from the Transformed Medicaid Statistical Information System.

Deep appreciation goes to staff at the National Academies of Sciences, Engineering, and Medicine for their efforts and support in the report process, especially to Elizabeth Ferre, Erin Fox, Joe Goodman, Anne Marie Houppert, Christopher Lao-Scott, Megan Lowry, Amber McLaughlin, Rachael Nance, Shaakira Parker, Marguerite Romatelli, Leslie Sim, Roberta Wedge, Anesia Wilks, and Taryn Young. The committee also gives special thanks to Tasha Bigelow, Mark Goodin, and Laura Penny, copyeditors.

Finally, the committee thanks the many patients, families, residents, fellows, and practicing clinicians who shared their perspectives and experiences.

Contents

PREFACE   xvii

ACRONYMS AND ABBREVIATIONS   xxi

SUMMARY   1

1 INTRODUCTION   19
Study Origin and Statement of Task, 20
Definitions and Terminology, 20
Study Context, 23
Study Focus, 27
Previous Work of the National Academies, 32
Study Approach, 33
References, 36

**2 CHILDREN'S HEALTH CARE NEEDS AND ACCESS
TO SUBSPECIALTY CARE**   41
Framework, 42
Demand and Need, 43
Access to Subspecialty Care, 50
Use of Subspecialty Care, 63
Outcomes of Subspecialty Care, 63
Key Findings and Conclusions, 66
Recommendation, 67
References, 68

3 PEDIATRIC SUBSPECIALTY USE DATA ANALYSES   81
Methods, 82
Results, 85
What These Data Mean, 95
Key Findings and Conclusions, 98
Reference, 100

4 THE PEDIATRIC HEALTH CARE WORKFORCE LANDSCAPE   101
The Pathway to Becoming a Pediatric Subspecialty Physician, 101
General Pediatricians, 105
Pediatric Subspecialty Fellows, 107
Actively Practicing Pediatric Subspecialty Physicians, 114
Modeling the Future Subspecialty Workforce, 119
Primary Care Clinicians, 120
Mental Health, Behavioral Health, and Social Care Professionals, 132
Other Related Health Professionals, 136
Key Findings and Conclusions, 137
Recommendation, 139
References, 139

5 INFLUENCES ON THE CAREER PATH OF A PEDIATRIC SUBSPECIALTY PHYSICIAN   151
Exposure to Pediatrics, 153
Education and Training Model, 156
Coaching, Mentorship, and Role-Modeling, 164
Financing of Graduate Medical Education, 166
Educational Debt and Earning Potential, 172
Influences on Lifestyle, 179
Workforce Planning and Recruitment Efforts, 181
Retention, 185
Key Findings and Conclusions, 188
Recommendations, 191
References, 193

6 TRENDS IN THE PEDIATRIC–SCIENTIST WORKFORCE   203
The Importance of Pediatric Research, 204
Unique Challenges of Pediatric Research, 207
The Pediatric Physician–Scientist Workforce, 210
Challenges to the Physician–Scientist Workforce and Interventions to Support Pediatric Researchers, 218

The Pediatric Research Funding Landscape: Adequacy
   and Distribution, 232
Key Findings and Conclusions, 241
Recommendations, 244
References, 246

7 INNOVATIONS AT THE PRIMARY-SPECIALTY CARE
   INTERFACE   261
   Collaboration and Coordination Between Pediatric Primary
      and Specialty Care, 262
   Challenges of Consultation, Referral, and Co-management, 267
   Promising Primary–Specialty Care Models, 270
   Investing in Pediatric Primary Care to Improve the
      Primary-Specialty Care Interface, 294
   Key Findings and Conclusions, 295
   Recommendations, 296
   References, 298

8 FINANCING CHILDREN'S HEALTH CARE   313
   Financing and Coverage of Children's Subspecialty Care, 314
   Payment Rates for Children's Subspecialty Care, 319
   Compensation for Pediatric Medical Subspecialty
      Physicians, 324
   How Financing and Payment Tie to Provider Salaries, Practice
      Decisions, and Access to Care, 331
   Key Findings and Conclusions, 336
   Recommendations, 337
   References, 338

APPENDIX
A COMMITTEE MEMBER, FELLOW, AND
   STAFF BIOGRAPHIES   347

Preface

The health of children has dramatically changed in the last 2–3 decades. Mortality rates for children have decreased, although children still die at much higher rates in the United States compared to those in other high-income countries. While the number of children in the United States has not appreciably increased over the last 20 years, the sociodemographic composition and the physical, mental, and behavioral health of the pediatric population has shifted. The miracle of immunizations has virtually eradicated infections such as measles, bacterial meningitis, varicella, pertussis, and many other diseases that once filled hospitals, but their places are now taken by children with a large variety of chronic, and often lifelong, illnesses. The rate of teen suicide has increased, reflecting the large burden of pediatric mental health problems that have been highlighted by the COVID-19 pandemic. Many children live in families that are stressed by poverty, language barriers, and interpersonal and structural racism, creating challenges for parents and health care providers to meet their needs.

The United States does not have a pediatric health care "system." We have health care organizations that have grown organically to meet the needs of our patients. They have attempted to use the continuing, tremendous advances in science to improve the health outcomes of children they serve. One of the main ways this has occurred has been in focusing on pediatric subspecialists to deliver the majority of care to the ever increasingly complicated acutely and chronically ill children in the population. This has often resulted in relegating primary care practitioners to providing preventive and acute illness care, and being referrers to subspecialists, with a lack of partnership between the two groups in caring for these children.

The effect of this evolution has been to create enormous strains in health care organizations. The demand for pediatric services has led to large growth in pediatric departments in U.S. medical schools and other multi-specialty groups to meet the demand. But this has often been unsuccessful, resulting in barriers to care that do not meet the Institute of Medicine criteria for high-quality care as being safe, timely, efficient, equitable, effective, and patient centered. Since children constitute the largest group in America living in poverty, they are the largest group in which their health care is insured by Medicaid. Following the development of the Children's Health Insurance Program (CHIP) in the 1990s, the Affordable Care Act and Medicaid expansion, and other changes, uninsured rates dropped overall so that very few children in the United States are uninsured (recognizing some geographic variation). While Medicaid provides good coverage for children, reimbursement to hospitals and clinicians is inadequate to cover the costs of care, resulting in further strains on pediatric health care organizations. Access to pediatric subspecialty care is threatened, in part, by relatively low salaries, which in turn reflect low Medicaid/CHIP reimbursement rates for all types of care and reimbursement methodologies, and a limited supply of new entrants into the workforce, particularly in the non-procedurally based pediatric subspecialties. The financial realities of college and medical school debt coupled with the high cost of living in many of the cities in which academic medical centers are located, and the relatively low salaries for many specialists, necessitate a variety of mechanisms to overcome financial disincentives.

The academic "triple threat" (clinician, researcher, teacher) is dead—if it ever truly existed. Academic medical centers cannot fulfill their missions of clinical care, education, and research without a workforce that is composed of faculty who are individually differentiated in the skills and effort in each of these three areas. Access to subspecialty care is further threatened by the complexification of subspecialty medicine, which like much of health care, has become more time intensive. In addition, most pediatric subspecialists work for large health systems, decreasing physicians' sense of control and contributing to burnout and a desire to cut back on clinical time to reduce attendant stress. The burnout of many pediatricians combined with the dissatisfaction of families with long wait times for specialist appointments beg for new models of care that reset the relationship between pediatric specialists and primary care providers, making them more *partners* in care of children with chronic diseases. The pandemic has shown us how rapidly new technology such as telehealth can be implemented and widely adopted. Indeed, many organizations did in 2 weeks what they had previously spent 2 years discussing. Finally, continued advances in child and adult health require continued scientific discovery, but the system for producing and nurturing pediatric physician–scientists has been inadequate, particularly at the beginning of their careers. Overall, increasing the number of pediatric subspecialists alone is not the answer. The situation requires a more comprehensive approach that addresses all of these factors.

The committee is grateful to our sponsors for, first of all, appreciating the current crisis and then coming together to support this work. We hope that the information gathered in this report and the recommendations of the committee will be used to bring about substantial change to the systems that determine the health care of the most vulnerable children who are entrusted to us for their care. The needs of children today are not the same as the needs of children 50 or 75 years ago. The systems that provide them care need to evolve to meet these demands.

Frederick P. Rivara, M.D., M.P.H., *Chair*
Committee on the Pediatric Subspecialty Workforce
and Its Impact on Child Health and Well-Being

Acronyms and Abbreviations

AAFP	American Academy of Family Practitioners
AAMC	Association of American Medical Colleges
AANP	American Association of Nurse Practitioners
AAP	American Academy of Pediatrics
ABP	American Board of Pediatrics
ABPN	American Board of Psychiatry and Neurology
ACA	Affordable Care Act
ACCR	American Chiropractic College of Radiology
ACGME	Accreditation Council for Graduate Medical Education
ACO	accountable care organization
ADHD	attention deficit hyperactivity disorder
AHEC	area health education center
AHRQ	Agency for Healthcare Research and Quality
AMA	American Medical Association
AMBS	American Board of Medical Specialties
AMG	American medical graduate
AML	acute myeloid leukemia
AOA	American Osteopathic Association
AOBP	American Osteopathic Board of Pediatricians
APRN	advanced practice registered nurse
ASO	administrative services only
BOS	Bureau of Osteopathic Specialties
BPCA	Best Pharmaceuticals for Children Act

CAMPP	Consortium of Accelerated Medical Pathway Programs
CAP	child and adolescent psychiatry
CBO	Congressional Budget Office
CDC	Centers for Disease Control and Prevention
CHA	Children's Hospital Association
CHC	community health center
CHGME	Children's Hospital Graduate Medical Education program
CHIP	Children's Health Insurance Program
CKD	chronic kidney disease
CMMI	Capability Maturity Model Integration
CMS	Centers for Medicare and Medicaid Services
COE	centers of excellence
CORE	Coordinating Optimal Referral Experiences
CRS	Congressional Research Service
CSHCN	children with special health care needs
CYSHCN	children and youth with special health care needs
DEIA	diversity, equity, inclusion, accessibility
DO	doctor of osteopathic medicine
DSRIP	Delivery System Reform Incentive Payment Program
E/M	evaluation and management
EPA	entrustable professional activity
EPSDT	early and periodic screening, diagnosis, and treatment
FDA	Federal Drug Administration
FFS	fee-for-service
FMAP	Federal Medical Assistance Percentage
FOPE	Future of Pediatric Education
FOPE II	Future of Pediatric Education II
FSMB	Federation of State Medical Boards
GAO	Government Accountability Office
GME	graduate medical education
HCOP	Health Careers Opportunity Program
HCUP	Healthcare Cost and Utilization Project
HHS	Department of Health and Human Services
HiSTEP	High School Scientific Training and Enrichment Program
HRSA	Health Resources and Services Administration
IAP	Innovation Acceleration Program
IHI	Institute for Healthcare Improvement

IMG	international medical graduates
InCK	Integrated Care for Kids
INMED	Indians into Medicine Program
IOM	Institute of Medicine
IPPS	Inpatient Prospective Payment System
IVIG	intravenous immunoglobin
IWPR	Institute of Women's Policy Research
LCME	Liaison Committee on Medical Education
MACPAC	Medicaid and CHIP Payment and Access Commission
MCHB	Maternal and Child Health Bureau
MCO	managed care organization
MCPAP	Massachusetts Child Psychiatry Access Project
MedPAC	Medicare Payment Advisory Commission
MEPPS	Medical Expenditure Panel Survey
MOC	maintenance of certification
MS1	first-year medical student
MSQ	Matriculating Student Questionnaire
NAM	National Academy of Medicine
NASEM	National Academies of Sciences, Engineering, and Medicine
NCBDDD	National Center on Birth Defects and Developmental Disabilities
NCIPC	National Center for Injury Prevention and Control
NCIRD	National Center for Immunization and Respiratory Diseases
NCQA	National Committee for Quality Assurance
NEHRS	National Electronic Health Records Survey
NES	non-English speaking
NHSC	National Health Service Corps
NICHD	National Institute of Child Health and Development
NICU	neonatal intensive care unit
NIH	National Institutes of Health
NP	nurse practitioner
NRC	National Research Council
NRMP	National Resident Matching Program
PA	physician assistant
PACT	Pediatricians Accelerate Childhood Therapies
PCCM	primary care case management
PCMH	patient-centered medical homes
PCORI	Patient Centered Outcomes Research Institute
PCP	primary care providers

PGY	postgraduate year
PICU	pediatric intensive care unit
PREA	Pediatric Research Equity Act
OASH	Office of the Assistant Secretary for Health
OECD	Organization for Economic Co-operation and Development
OHDSI	Observational Health Data Sciences and Informatics
ONC	Office of the National Coordinator for Health Information Technology
QBS	quality bonus system
R01	research project grants
RACE	Research to Accelerate Cures and Equity for Children
RBRVS	resource-based relative value scale
RCT	randomized controlled trials
RVU	relative value units
SAMHSA	Substance Abuse and Mental Health Services Administration
SCHIP	State Children's Health Insurance Program
SCTC	Subspeciality Clinical Training and Certification
SEPA	Science Education Partnership Award
SHCN	special heath care needs
SIM	State Innovation Model
STEM	science, technology, engineering, and math
TAGGS	Tracking Accountability in Government Grants System
THCGME	Teaching Health Center Graduate Medical Education program
T-MSIS	Transformed Medicaid Statistical Information System
URiM	underrepresented in medicine
VBP	value-based purchasing
WHO	World Health Organization

Summary

The health of today's children sets the foundation for the future health of the nation. When children require preventive care or experience illness, injury, or a limitation in their functioning, a wide variety of health professionals provide expert care to maintain and promote their health and well-being. Pediatric subspecialists (physicians who typically complete a pediatric residency and then receive additional fellowship training in discrete areas) are critical to ensuring state-of-the-science care and pursuing research to improve prevention, diagnosis, and treatment for children. Pediatric subspecialists augment the care provided by primary care clinicians, such as general pediatricians, advanced practice providers (e.g., advanced practice registered nurses, physician assistants), and family medicine physicians by caring for children who require technical procedures or have health conditions that occur too infrequently for primary care clinicians to gain and maintain up-to-date clinical knowledge. For many children, pediatric subspecialty care is essential to their survival and a flourishing life. Approximately 10–20 percent of U.S. children visit a pediatric subspecialist each year. However, there are substantial disincentives to pursuing a career as a pediatric subspecialist—in both the clinical and research settings. These challenges are often heightened for individuals from groups underrepresented in medicine (URiM). Notably, there has been very little change in the proportion of URiM pediatric residents and fellows over the past several decades, and the pediatric workforce does not reflect the growing diversity of the pediatric population.

Tremendous advances in pediatric care have resulted in an increased number of children living with chronic health conditions or surviving illnesses that previously would have meant a poor quality of life, a shortened life span, or even death during childhood, leading to a pediatric population with new and complex challenges. These changing health care needs and increasing care complexity—combined with perceived shortages of primary care clinicians, pediatric subspecialists, and pediatric physician–scientists and changing practice patterns—have raised concerns about the current and future availability of pediatric subspecialty care and research and the potential ramifications for child health and well-being. In 2022, the National Academies of Sciences, Engineering, and Medicine (National Academies), with support from a coalition of sponsors, formed the Committee on the Pediatric Subspecialty Workforce and Its Impact on Child Health and Well-Being to recommend strategies and actions to ensure an adequate pediatric subspecialty physician workforce to support broad access to high-quality subspecialty care and a robust research portfolio to advance the health and health care of infants, children, and adolescents.[1]

STUDY FOCUS AND CONTEXT

The committee recognizes the important contribution of many different types of clinicians toward the care of children; however, based on the statement of task and discussions with study sponsors, this report focuses on the medical subspecialty physician workforce. The committee particularly focused on the 15 medical subspecialties certified by the American Board of Pediatrics (ABP) (see Table S-1). These represent the bulk of pediatric subspecialty physicians and share common pathways for education and training; furthermore, many of these subspecialties experience significant challenges in recruitment and retention. When appropriate and relevant, the committee also considered other pediatric subspecialty physicians. As a secondary focus, the committee discussed the interaction and collaboration between pediatric medical subspecialty physicians and primary care clinicians because these types of physicians commonly collaborate with each other on patient management. Other members of the health care workforce—including pediatric surgical subspecialists, adult-trained subspecialists who provide some care for children, and child and adolescent psychiatrists, among others—are also involved in the care of infants, children, and adolescents but not a primary focus for this report.

The committee recognized that advanced practice providers are increasingly used to provide both inpatient and outpatient pediatric subspecialty care and an important part of the pediatric workforce, especially in children's hospitals. However, their training and certification is separate from that of pediatric physicians and therefore not a primary focus in this

---

[1] The complete statement of task is presented in Chapter 1 of this report.

TABLE S-1 Primary and Secondary Focus of Report

Focus	Grouping	Examples
Primary Focus	American Board of Pediatrics (ABP)–Certified Pediatric Medical Subspecialty Physicians (Clinicians and Researchers)	• Adolescent Medicine • Child Abuse Pediatrics • Developmental-Behavioral Pediatrics • Neonatal-Perinatal Medicine • Pediatric Cardiology • Pediatric Critical Care Medicine • Pediatric Emergency Medicine • Pediatric Endocrinology • Pediatric Gastroenterology • Pediatric Hematology/Oncology • Pediatric Hospital Medicine • Pediatric Infectious Diseases • Pediatric Nephrology • Pediatric Pulmonology • Pediatric Rheumatology
	Other Pediatric Medical Subspecialty Physicians (Clinicians and Researchers)	• American Osteopathic Board of Pediatrics–certified subspecialties • ABP co-sponsored subspecialties (certified by another board of the American Board of Medical Specialties [ABMS]) • ABP nonstandard pathways and combined training programs* • Subspecialties certified by other ABMS boards without collaboration of ABP (e.g., pediatric dermatology) • Emerging medical subspecialties (e.g., obesity)
Secondary Focus	Primary–Subspecialty Care Interface	Interaction of subspecialists with primary care clinicians, including the following: • General Pediatricians • Advanced Practice Providers (e.g., Advanced Practice Registered Nurses, Physician Assistants) • Family Medicine Physicians

NOTES: *Although the ABP recognizes a combined training program for child and adolescent psychiatry, very few physicians choose this pathway, so it is not included as part of the committee's primary focus. See Chapter 1 for a fuller description of the range of pediatric subspecialty physicians.

report. The committee is also aware that scientists conducting research on conditions that occur in the pediatric age group represent a diverse group of individuals. Following the charge, the committee's focus for research was on the recruitment, training, funding, and retention of pediatric physician–scientists.

The committee's task was not to redesign the overall health system of pediatric care delivery, including transitions to adult care, but rather to focus on equitable access to pediatric subspecialty care. Furthermore, the committee recognizes the importance of high-quality primary care as a foundation for high-quality subspecialty care. Although the committee did examine some new models of subspecialist–primary care clinician interaction for patient care, the 2021 National Academies report *Implementing High-Quality Primary Care: Rebuilding the Foundation of Health Care* specifically addresses strategies to improve primary care broadly, including the use of interprofessional teams, and the committee considered its work to build upon that study. The committee also recognizes a study in progress at the National Academies that is charged to address "innovations that can be implemented in the health care system to improve the health and wellbeing of children and youth," including workforce development and team-based care.[2]

CHALLENGES IN ENSURING AN ADEQUATE PEDIATRIC SUBSPECIALTY WORKFORCE

Whether patients obtain subspecialty care, and the timeliness of that care, depends on a complex mix of patient, family, clinician, health system, and societal influences. Some of the major influences include demand for subspecialty care, referral patterns, organization of services, geography, and health care financing. Furthermore, the adequacy of the workforce itself is also affected by children's changing health care needs, how well primary care clinicians and subspecialists are prepared to address those needs, the number of subspecialists, the influences on an individual's decision to pursue subspecialty training, how subspecialists interact with the larger health care workforce, and how pediatric subspecialists are reimbursed.

Access to Care

A high-quality health care workforce needs to be organized and prepared to ensure adequate access to care for both common and uncommon

---

[2] For more information, see https://www.nationalacademies.org/our-work/improving-the-health-and-wellbeing-of-children-and-youth-through-health-care-system-transformation (accessed July 7, 2023).

acute and chronic health problems. Patients and families may consult with their primary care clinician about the need for referral to a subspecialist or directly seek subspecialty care (self-referral). Subspecialists can also create additional demand through extensive follow-up of patients more appropriately followed by primary care clinicians and cross-referring to other subspecialists. Judicious use of referrals can improve access to needed subspecialty care, but unnecessary or uncoordinated subspecialty care may lead to overuse of these services and thus prolonged wait times for appointments.

Type of insurance (i.e., Medicaid, Children's Health Insurance Program [CHIP], commercial/private), insurance status (insured versus uninsured), and families' out-of-pocket costs can affect whether patients can access subspecialty care and with what frequency. For example, although children enrolled in Medicaid/CHIP have higher use rates of medical subspecialty care (as compared with those who are commercially insured), evidence shows that these children experience more challenges in obtaining new appointments. Other cultural and economic factors contribute to disparities in timely access to subspecialty care, including language barriers and opportunity costs (e.g., ability to take time off work). Furthermore, many adolescents with chronic conditions experience fragmented care as they transition from pediatric to adult subspecialty care.

Geographic barriers to pediatric subspecialty care vary by region and type of subspecialist. Patients and families may experience difficulty in accessing subspecialists because of long travel times or a lack of transportation. Factors contributing to such regionalization include the larger percentage of children living in urban areas (versus rural), the inability to support a practice in some locations because of the lower prevalence of many disorders, and certain technologies being more available in larger, centralized care centers. In addition, a subspecialist who is interested in teaching and research is likely to have limited opportunities to pursue these interests outside of an urban academic center. More than half of ABP-certified pediatric subspecialists work primarily in medical school or university settings, and most report some form of academic faculty appointment. Some, but not all, of these geographic barriers can be lessened via telehealth and other innovations, such as outreach clinics.

Education and Training Model

Although the most common health conditions that affect children today are acute and recurrent illnesses, a growing proportion of children have long-term medical and behavioral health conditions. Chronic pediatric conditions traditionally have been stratified as physical or mental. However, over the past decades, there has been greater awareness of the holistic nature of health and the common co-occurrence of physical and mental health conditions. Finally, new illnesses may still emerge that will require related changes in education and training.

However, the model of education and training has not evolved substantially in response to the changing context of society and medical practice, including pediatric patients' health needs and practice patterns. In particular, the model of education and training for pediatric medical subspecialists has limited flexibility in the design and length of fellowship; nearly all ABP-certified fellowships require 3 years of training, including a minimum of 12 months of clinical training and 12 months of scholarly activity (e.g., research). Although all subspecialty fellows are required to participate in scholarly activity, nearly half of practicing subspecialists report not being involved in any research activities, and very few spend a substantive percentage of their time on research. Furthermore, although ABP provides a limited number of alternate, streamlined pathways for trainees who are committed to careers in research, similar pathways do not exist for trainees who are committed to careers in clinical practice.

Influences on Pursuing a Career in a Pediatric Subspecialty

Many factors can influence the choice to pursue subspecialty training, including:

- Exposure to the complete array of board-certified pediatric subspecialties and subspecialists (e.g., before medical school, during medical school, during residency);
- The presence of role models from subspecialty fields, particularly for URiM trainees (which may be scarce owing to the small numbers of subspecialists);
- The length of fellowship training;
- The requirement for scholarly activity during fellowship;
- The debt burden of education and training;
- Relatively lower salaries, particularly for some pediatric medical subspecialties compared with general pediatricians in outpatient practice and adult medical subspecialists; and
- Lifestyle factors (e.g., work–life balance, job satisfaction, burnout).

As a result of lower salaries and longer training, many pediatric subspecialists face a high debt burden, which can discourage pediatricians from pursuing careers in lower-paid subspecialties. The retention of pediatric subspecialists is also important; longevity may be predicted by personal or professional factors, such as concerns surrounding financial considerations (e.g., educational debt and compensation) and clinician burnout, well-being, and job satisfaction.

Challenges exist in ensuring the adequacy of both the clinical and pediatric physician–scientist research workforces. Pediatric research is the cornerstone of evidence-based care delivery, and advances in pediatric research are central to improving the lives of children. However, specific challenges for pediatric research include a paucity of subspecialty-specific workforce data; lack of a robust mentorship environment, particularly for early career investigators; financial considerations that affect trainees' decisions to pursue research; lack of dedicated research time; competing clinical responsibilities; and inadequate research funding.

The Primary Care–Subspecialty Interface

In high-functioning health systems, primary care clinicians and pediatric subspecialists work collaboratively at the interface of primary and specialty care to provide the appropriate level and full spectrum of care for children with complex and atypical acute and chronic disorders. However, there are widespread inefficiencies and variability in the connections between primary care and subspecialty care. Communication and coordination between primary care clinicians and physician subspecialists is frequently absent or fragmented, leaving parents as the main link between them. Productivity demands on primary care clinicians may prompt some to refer patients even though the condition could have been managed entirely in primary care with additional time or resources. Additionally, primary care clinicians often refer patients for short-term consultation for advice on diagnosis or management, but the subspecialist takes over the care for the referred problem. There is virtually no evidence base to guide decision making on the frequency and timing of return subspecialty visits versus transition care back to a primary care clinician, resulting in wide primary care and subspecialist practice variation. Allowing adequate time and reimbursement and preparing primary care clinicians to provide some part of the care they might otherwise refer to a subspecialist would allow subspecialists to focus on the more severe, complex, or rare cases or procedure-based care that primary care cannot best deliver.

Several promising evidence-based models can increase access to pediatric subspecialty care and support the judicious use of all members of interprofessional pediatric care teams without necessarily changing the number of subspecialists. Innovations include integrating primary and subspecialty care (e.g., integrated behavioral health and primary care, embedding generalists into subspecialty clinics and vice versa, active co-management, development of a pediatrician's skills to manage more complex care, referral and treatment guidelines), using telehealth (e.g., electronic consults [e-consults], telementoring), facilitating access through nurse-led models of care, and financing innovations to support primary–specialty care collaborations.

However, the implementation and scaling of these models face several barriers, including a lack of payment mechanisms; limitations of practice due to state-based regulations (including for telehealth); and a lack of education and training in team-based care, making appropriate referrals, and the use of more innovative care models and modalities.

Financing Children's Health

Medicaid covers 35 percent of children overall and a substantially higher share of the children with complex medical needs treated by pediatric subspecialists. Comparisons of Medicaid and Medicare fee schedules generally find Medicaid rates to be substantially lower, with some variation across states, specialties, or services. Additionally, productivity-based fee schedules (i.e., relative value units [RVUs]) provide greater levels of remuneration for procedure-based subspecialties and undervalue the increased time needs per clinical interaction, increased pre- and post-service time, and higher practice expenses for most subspecialty care, particularly pediatric subspecialty care. The exact methods through which pediatric subspecialists' salaries are set are subject to complex formulas that vary by institution, but expected revenue is a major factor. The large percentage of children covered by Medicaid, especially those cared for by subspecialists, coupled with low payment rates, adversely affects reimbursement. This results in lower salaries for many pediatric subspecialties compared with internal medicine subspecialty counterparts; particularly in medical subspecialties, this can influence the career decisions of trainees pursuing pediatrics and pediatric subspecialty training.

VISION, GOALS, AND RECOMMENDATIONS[3]

Ideally, the subspecialty workforce would be adjusted in both numbers and skills to fully meet children's subspecialty care needs. Attracting physicians to pursue training in many of the pediatric medical subspecialties has been problematic, and a variety of mechanisms will be needed to generate and maintain a diverse array of subspecialists. However, a larger workforce alone will not solve the problems of meeting children's subspecialty health care needs. Rather, intentional efforts are needed to recruit and retain subspecialists in specific areas of clinical care in combination with judicious use of all members of the health care team in effective models of team-based care.

---

[3] The committee's recommendations are numbered according to the chapter of the main report in which they appear. Thus, Recommendation 2-1 is the first recommendation in Chapter 2.

In its evaluation of the available data, the committee concluded that the need for interventions to support and optimize the pediatric subspecialty workforce varies substantially and dynamically across subspecialties over time. Some subspecialties receive many fellowship applicants, but others have a dearth. The anticipated earnings vary by subspecialty, and individuals who train in critical care and other procedure-based subspecialties have incomes that are far above those for nonprocedural pediatric subspecialists. The number and proportion of extramurally funded physician–scientists vary substantially by pediatric subspecialty. Waiting times to access care also vary among pediatric subspecialists, from days for some to months for others, and by geographic location. Despite few URiM pediatric subspecialists, some fields have been more successful in advancing diversity. Given these variables, the groups referenced as "high-priority subspecialties" in the ensuing recommendations will differ by specific context and may change over time. Thus, this report does not employ a single definition for "high-priority."

A Vision of a High-Quality Pediatric Subspecialty Workforce

To achieve the goal of a high-quality pediatric subspecialty workforce for clinical care and research, the committee envisions an accessible and efficient health system that enables all children to receive the appropriate type and amount of primary and specialty care whenever they need it. Such a system would value high-quality care for all children, with care that embodies the six elements for quality defined by the Institute of Medicine[4]: safety, timeliness, effectiveness, efficiency, equity, and patient-centeredness. High-quality pediatric subspecialty care is *safe* when the referral, or lack of referral, does not result in harm. It is *timely* when diagnosis and treatment alleviate anxiety and symptoms as quickly as feasible and avoid delays that exacerbate symptoms or functional limitations attributable to the disease or its course. It is *effective* when patient and family questions and concerns are addressed fully and it produces the best possible health outcomes. It is *efficient* when the diagnostic and treatment journey does not create unneeded testing or treatments or delays in delivery of appropriate services. It is *equitable* when the access to necessary knowledge and the use of appropriate treatment is provided according to patient need rather than social determinants of health. It is *patient- and family-centered* when

---

[4] As of March 2016, the Health and Medicine Division of the National Academies of Sciences, Engineering, and Medicine (National Academies) continues the consensus studies and convening activities previously carried out by the Institute of Medicine (IOM). The IOM name is used to refer to reports issued prior to July 2015.

patients, families, and clinicians are considered partners in determining the goals of care and shared decision making is incorporated when appropriate.

High-quality pediatric subspecialty care requires a well-supported, superbly trained, and appropriately used primary care, subspecialty, and physician–scientist workforce achieved through effective education and training, well-designed care models, and continued attention to the changing health care and economic landscapes. In addition, all clinicians need to be able to provide care that aligns with the full extent of their education and training and receive appropriate reimbursement for their administrative and clinical work. Increased opportunities are needed to implement innovative delivery system models and health care technologies, and flexible training pathways are needed in response to the changing medical and behavioral health needs of infants, children, and adolescents.

The committee developed four goals with associated recommendations to help achieve its vision of a high-quality pediatric subspecialty workforce with a robust research portfolio to advance the health and health care of infants, children, and adolescents:

1. Promote collaboration and the effective use of services between pediatric primary care clinicians and subspecialty physicians;
2. Reduce financial and payment disincentives;
3. Enhance education, training, recruitment, and retention; and
4. Support the pediatric physician–scientist pathway.

The committee re-emphasizes the importance of high-quality primary care for achieving high-quality subspecialty care. Although the following recommendations are focused on improving the delivery of subspecialty care, many will also help to support primary care clinicians.

Goal 1: Promote Collaboration and the Effective Use of Services Between Pediatric Primary Care Clinicians and Subspecialty Physicians

Improved monitoring of children's changing health care needs and demands, the status of their access to needed care, disparities, and trends in workforce composition are all essential to inform future workforce planning efforts. Understanding these trends will help determine the appropriate education and training needed to prepare the pediatric workforce to work collaboratively toward meeting children's health care needs and which subspecialties should be prioritized for different interventions or programs (e.g., loan repayment) and inform innovative models of care to improve access. Therefore, the committee provides the following recommendation:

RECOMMENDATION 2-1 The Agency for Healthcare Research and Quality should submit a biennial report to the Secretary of the Department of Health and Human Services summarizing the changing demands and needs for pediatric primary and subspecialty care, status of access to that care, and disparities in receipt of those services. This report should include information on the pediatric generalist and subspecialist workforce broadly (including data on clinicians from backgrounds underrepresented in medicine).

Pediatric subspecialists need to focus on their essential role in the care of children with complex, severe, and rare disorders or requiring technical procedures, while collaborating with primary care clinicians. However, in general, both groups of clinicians are not optimally trained about their role and responsibilities in the referral process. Many children with common and lower-complexity or -severity diagnoses referred to subspecialists could be managed by primary care clinicians either alone (with appropriate time, financial resources, and training) or through active, collaborative co-management with the subspecialist. In addition, the COVID-19 pandemic has shown how rapidly technology, such as telehealth, can be implemented and widely adopted. The use of new technologies and methods of care can increase patient access; improve care coordination; strengthen the role of the primary care clinician; and allow subspecialists the time to provide inpatient and outpatient care in a manner that is feasible, fulfilling, and financially sustainable and best for children. However, barriers in payment and regulation prevent the full implementation and scaling of current evidence-based models of team-based care. Finally, innovative models of care are needed to reset the relationship between pediatric subspecialty physicians and primary care clinicians, making them greater *partners* in care of children. Enhanced communication at the interface of primary and subspecialty care is essential within these models. Therefore, the committee provides the following recommendations:

RECOMMENDATION 7-1 American Academy of Pediatrics, the Council of Pediatric Subspecialties, and other pediatric professional societies should collaboratively develop, disseminate, and implement testing, management, and referral guidelines for health conditions commonly managed by subspecialists. This should include when to consult, when to co-manage, and what the appropriate follow-up roles are for both the primary care clinician and the subspecialist.

RECOMMENDATION 7-2 Public and private health insurance payers should adequately reimburse evidence-based care delivery models that improve interprofessional, integrated, team-based care to enhance

access to pediatric subspecialty care. These models include but are not limited to
- E-consults (with payment for both the referring and the receiving clinician);
- Telehealth visits (both within and across state lines); and
- Integrated care teams that support mental and physical primary and specialty health care clinicians and include advanced practice providers, social workers, and care coordinators.

RECOMMENDATION 7-3 The Centers for Medicare & Medicaid Services (in conjunction with state Medicaid agencies), private foundations, and health systems should sponsor the development, implementation, and evaluation of innovations (including new models of care delivery and reimbursement) in the primary–specialty care interface and the pediatric subspecialty referral and care coordination processes.

Goal 2: Reduce Financial and Payment Disincentives

Expansions in insurance coverage over the past decades, including via CHIP, expanded Medicaid eligibility for children, and the Affordable Care Act, have successfully removed the barrier of uninsurance for most U.S. children. However, the typically lower rates of Medicaid reimbursement for many of the children that pediatric medical subspecialists treat, coupled with low RVU-based payment rates, contribute to their comparatively lower salaries. As noted, these challenges are especially prominent for pediatric subspecialists because of the relatively higher percentage of patients covered by Medicaid. The federal government has used Medicaid financing to achieve broad policy goals through the program, but low Medicaid payments represent a significant underinvestment by federal and state governments in children's health. Finally, the committee notes that the Pediatric Specialty Loan Repayment Program was authorized at $30 million per year but has not yet been fully funded at this level. Overall, the financial realities of educational debt (particularly for students from URiM and/or economically disadvantaged backgrounds), along with the relatively low salaries and added time demands for some training pathways, require considering ways to remove financial disincentives to entering and staying in pediatric subspecialty careers. Therefore, the committee provides the following recommendations:

RECOMMENDATION 8-1 To invest in children's health and address the factors that contribute to limited access to pediatric subspecialty care, Congress should allocate additional federal funding to increase payment for pediatric services.

- Within 5 years, Congress should provide federal funds to states to increase Medicaid payment rates for pediatric services to achieve or exceed parity with Medicare payment rates.

These federal funds should be provided to all states, and the federally funded payment increases should be mandatory. The committee recognizes that this recommendation may be difficult to implement immediately, but it should be phased in as soon as possible. The committee also recognizes that states can increase payments for pediatric services themselves, but many states have not done so on their own, which is why federal action is necessary.

RECOMMENDATION 8-2 CMS should prioritize attention to pediatric services in assigning relative value units that accurately reflect the time and resource use for pediatric subspecialty care.

RECOMMENDATION 5-4 Congress should increase funding for the Pediatric Specialty Loan Repayment Program to $30 million as originally authorized. The Health Resources and Services Administration should focus on loan repayment for high-priority pediatric medical subspecialties as well as subspecialists from underrepresented in medicine and/or economically disadvantaged backgrounds.

Goal 3: Enhance Education, Training, Recruitment, and Retention

The preparation of the subspecialty workforce has not evolved to fully meet the demands of the 21st century's population of infants, children, and adolescents, with limited ability to change education and training models quickly in response to emerging challenges. The committee notes that the biennial report called for in Recommendation 2-1 could be used to help inform adjustments in curricula to meet these evolving needs. Furthermore, the model of education and training for pediatric medical subspecialists includes a single model for most graduates with a focus on creating subspecialists who demonstrate competency in all aspects of academic careers, including clinical care, research, and education. However, pediatric subspecialty care would benefit from a workforce that is differentiated in skills and effort in each of these three areas. Increased flexibility in fellowship design and length could encourage more residents to pursue careers in a pediatric subspecialty by allowing them to tailor their training in accordance with their career goals. The design of residency and fellowship training programs also faces barriers from the structure of Medicare-funded graduate medical education (GME) and Children's Hospitals GME (CHGME) program funding. Pediatric training programs increasingly depend on discretionary

CHGME funding that may limit the number of slots, and Medicare-funded GME in general does not place any institutional requirements on types of clinicians. Finally, recruitment and training needs to evolve to enhance the number of URiM clinicians in the pediatric subspecialty workforce to mirror the diversity of the children and families it serves. Therefore, the committee provides the following recommendations:

> RECOMMENDATION 4-1 The Association of Medical School Pediatric Department Chairs should periodically convene representatives from the American Board of Pediatrics, the Accreditation Council for Graduate Medical Education, all pediatric professional societies, and major pediatric education and training organizations (including, but not limited to, child and adolescent psychiatry, family medicine, and advanced practice providers) to review and adjust educational and training curricula (e.g., continuing education, standardized pediatric subspecialty training, and specialty recognition and certification) for pediatric residents and fellows. The goal of these convenings is to ensure that residency and fellowship programs are preparing a workforce that can address the evolving physical and mental health needs of the pediatric population.

> RECOMMENDATION 5-1 The American Board of Pediatrics, the American Osteopathic Board of Pediatrics, and the Accreditation Council for Graduate Medical Education should develop, implement, and evaluate distinct fellowship training pathways, including a 2-year option for those who aspire to a career with a primary focus on clinical care.

The committee emphasizes multiple novel pathways should be considered and that a pathway focused on clinical training, for example, does not mean that the trainees will receive no academic training or experience in research principles. Rather, distinct pathways would allow for tailoring training programs for specific career goals, as already exist for the alternative pathways for research.

> RECOMMENDATION 5-2 Congress should reform graduate medical education (GME) formulas and programs, including Medicare GME and Children's Hospital GME, to ensure equitable and sufficient support for pediatric GME. Funding should be distributed to address priority pediatric workforce needs, such as increased inclusion of clinicians from underrepresented in medicine backgrounds, high-priority

subspecialties, geographic shortages, and enhanced training for new models of care.

RECOMMENDATION 5-3 Pediatric department chairs, medical school deans, and health systems should develop, implement, and publicly report on plans and outcomes to attract, support, and retain students, residents, fellows, and faculty from underrepresented in medicine backgrounds in pediatric subspecialties.
- These plans should include efforts to further the development and growth of recruitment programs for pre-college URiM students and initiatives to make learning and working environments more inclusive at all levels of the subspecialist career pathway.
- The responsible individuals and entities above should publicly report annual metrics on the demographics of their pediatric subspecialty workforce.

Goal 4: Support the Pediatric Physician–Scientist Pathway

Advances in child health require a highly skilled research workforce in which all disciplines pursue improved outcomes. For the purposes of this report, the committee focused on the role of the pediatric subspecialty physician–scientists who are crucial in research to improve subspecialty care and related health and organizational outcomes. Training this workforce cannot be fully accomplished during the 12 months of scholarly activity required within a 3-year overall fellowship. Rather, physician–scientists need extended training accompanied by adequate research support at the beginning of their careers. Specific and deliberate efforts are needed to encourage and facilitate entry into research careers and foster their early phases of career development for pediatric physician–scientists, especially for those who are underrepresented in the extramural scientific workforce. However, more evidence is needed on funding trends, unmet research needs, quality of research mentorship, and outcomes from pediatric physician–scientist career development pathway programs to inform future efforts to support careers in research. Therefore, the committee makes the following recommendations:

RECOMMENDATION 6-1 The National Institutes of Health (NIH) Pediatric Research Consortium, with leadership from the National Institute of Child Health and Human Development and input from the NIH's Scientific Workforce Diversity Office, and with appropriate additional funding, should engage with other government and nongovernment pediatric research funders to create and maintain a publicly available central repository for qualitative and quantitative data on pediatric physician–scientists' funding and success throughout their careers (e.g., tracking research funding rates and attrition rates by pediatric subspecialty), including the development of new measures as needed to understand the initial success and retention of pediatric physician–scientists. The Association of Medical School Pediatric Department Chairs should provide supplemental data as needed.

Examples of data needed include the following:

- Quantitative data on the funding rates of career development and subsequent awards and the tracking of research careers by demographic factors, such as sex/gender, race, ethnicity, disability status, geography, type of science across the research continuum (e.g., basic, clinical, translational, implementation, health services research), topic/subspecialty, and professional background of the principal investigator; and
- Qualitative data on successful researchers and those who leave the research track, including the quality of relationship with mentors; types of support received from their institutions; availability of statistical, epidemiologic, academic and grant writing training and support; availability of funding to present and publish research; satisfaction with career progression; and reasons for attrition or retention.

RECOMMENDATION 6-2 The National Institutes of Health and the Agency for Healthcare Research and Quality should increase the number of career development grants in pediatrics, particularly institutional training awards (e.g., the Pediatric Scientist Development Program), the Pediatric Loan Repayment Program, and K awards, with attention to providing such grants to physician–scientists from backgrounds that are underrepresented in the scientific workforce and for high-priority subspecialties in pediatric research. Funding for individual K awards should be increased to reflect current salaries and research project expenses and should include additional explicit funding for mentorship.

CONCLUSION

The current health care system is expensive, not equitably accessible, and not fully satisfying to either the people who work in it or the patients and families it is intended to serve. This report outlines recommendations that, if fully implemented, can improve the quality of pediatric medical subspecialty care and the quality of the care experience for patients, families, and clinicians. Achieving a robust subspecialty workforce will require concerted efforts across federal and state governments, pediatric professional societies, major pediatric education and training organizations, medical schools and fellowship programs, and health systems, with input from patients and families. It will also require a willingness to adapt to the changing needs of children and clinicians and a changing health care delivery system, while investing in the necessary time and resources. Implementing all of these recommendations in combination with other necessary supports to primary care will result in a health care system that serves the needs of all children and improves the health of the nation.

1

Introduction

For many children, pediatric subspecialty care is essential to their survival, health, and well-being. When children require preventive care or experience illness, injury, or a limitation in their functioning, a wide variety of health professionals provide expert care to maintain and promote their health and well-being. In particular, pediatric subspecialists (physicians who typically complete a pediatric residency and then receive additional fellowship training in discrete areas) are critical to ensuring state-of-the-science care and pursuing research to improve prevention, diagnosis, and treatment for children. Tremendous advances in pediatric care have resulted in an increasing number of children living with chronic health conditions or surviving illnesses that previously would have meant death, a shortened lifespan, or a poor quality of life. Pediatric subspecialists focus their clinical practice on the ever-increasingly complicated subpopulation of acutely and chronically ill children. Primary care clinicians such as general pediatricians, advanced practice providers (e.g., advanced practice registered nurses, physician assistants), and family medicine physicians work closely with subspecialists in a way that complements the subspecialists' expertise. However, widespread inefficiencies are present in the interactions between primary care and subspecialty care.

Tremendous advances in research have resulted in a pediatric population with new and complex challenges. The resultant changing health care needs of children and the increasing complexity of their care—combined with perceived shortages of primary care clinicians, pediatric subspecialty physicians, and pediatric physician–scientists, as well as changing practice patterns—raised concerns about the current and future availability of pediatric subspecialty care and research (Mayer and Skinner, 2009; Stockman and Freed, 2009; Vinci, 2021) and adverse impacts on child health.

STUDY ORIGIN AND STATEMENT OF TASK

Several health care organizations with an interest in pediatric care approached the National Academies of Sciences, Engineering, and Medicine (National Academies) to examine clinical subspecialty workforce trends related to the health care needs of infants, children, and adolescents, and the impact of those trends on child health and well-being as well as trends in the pediatrician-scientist pipeline and the impact on the scope of child and adolescent health research. Those organizations included

- American Academy of Pediatrics,
- American Board of Pediatrics,
- Association of Medical School Pediatric Department Chairs,
- Children's Hospital Association,
- Council of Pediatric Subspecialties,
- Eunice Kennedy Shriver National Institute of Child Health and Human Development (NICHD),
- Robert Wood Johnson Foundation, and
- The Annie E. Casey Foundation.

In response, in 2022 the National Academies formed the Committee on the Pediatric Subspecialty Workforce and Its Impact on Child Health and Well-Being. The sponsors' charge to the committee is presented in Box 1-1.

DEFINITIONS AND TERMINOLOGY

The following sections provide a framework of definitions and distinctions in terminology used throughout this report.

Infants, Children, and Adolescents

A policy statement from the American Academy of Pediatrics (AAP) states that "pediatrics is a multifaceted specialty that encompasses children's physical, psychosocial, developmental, and mental health" (Hardin et al., 2017, pg. 1). The field of pediatrics covers a broad age range, and several groups have developed guidelines for defining the ages for the stages of infancy, childhood, and adolescence (FDA, 2022; Hardin et al., 2017; NIH, 2022a; Williams et al., 2012). However, these guidelines lack overall consensus. Furthermore, the upper limit of "pediatric" care has increased

BOX 1-1
Statement of Task

An ad hoc committee of the National Academies of Sciences, Engineering, and Medicine will examine pediatric subspecialty workforce trends related to the health care needs of infants, children, and adolescents, and the impact of those trends on child health and well-being. The committee will recommend strategies and actions to ensure an adequate pediatric subspecialty workforce to support broad access to high-quality care and a robust research portfolio to advance the care of all children and youth.

Topics to be considered by the committee will include, but will not be limited to, the following:

- How the pediatric workforce has evolved over time in general pediatrics and pediatric subspecialties, including a focus on diversity and geographic distribution
- Trends in the pediatrician-scientist pipeline and the impact on the scope of child and adolescent health research and improvements in child and adolescent health
- The changing demographics of the pediatric population in the United States (including race, ethnicity, rurality, immigration status, age, and prevalence of chronic conditions)
- Gaps in the pediatric workforce that may hinder optimal outcomes for pediatric patients, and strategies and technologies (such as telehealth) to ensure equitable patient access to pediatric expertise
- Trends in the selection of pediatric residency training and fellowships in pediatric subspecialties, and factors such as debt burden, cost of training, lifetime earning potential, and others that influence those trends
- The impact of reimbursement on the financial stability of pediatric health care, on pediatrician salaries, and on trainee selection of pediatrics and pediatric subspecialities
- Data on other clinicians who provide care for children, such as family medicine physicians, nurse practitioners, and physician assistants
- Strategies to better align clinician specialty selection with the existing and future medical and behavioral health needs of infants, children, and adolescents
- The role of state and federal policies and resources in developing and supporting a well-trained pediatric clinical and research subspecialty workforce with appropriate competencies to improve child health

over time, and more recent efforts have expanded the scope of adolescent medicine to define "adolescent and young adult medicine," which includes patients up to age 25 (Moreno and Thompson, 2020). However, in some cases, patients outside of these age ranges may continue to be cared for by pediatric providers. For the purposes of this report, the committee uses the terms "pediatric" and "child" to refer to individuals roughly under age 21; ages are included as appropriate in citation of specific studies.

Generalists, Specialists, and Subspecialists

Generalist physicians who are involved in the care of children include physicians such as general pediatricians and family physicians. Specialist physicians who care for children include professionals such as psychiatrists, surgeons (all types), and anesthesiologists, who complete a general residency and then receive training in the care of children and adolescents. The largest group of specialists who care for children complete a pediatric residency and then pursue additional training in discrete areas of medicine (e.g., rheumatology, endocrinology, adolescent medicine). In this report, the committee primarily uses the term "pediatric subspecialist" to refer to physicians with certification in specialty areas granted by the American Board of Pediatrics, the American Osteopathic Board of Pediatrics, or, in some cases, by another American Board of Medical Specialties (ABMS) board (see later in this chapter for a discussion of pathways for subspecialty certification). The committee's definition of the term excludes general pediatricians, family physicians, advanced practice providers (e.g., advanced practice registered nurses, physician assistants), adult-trained subspecialists, and others who provide specialized care for children. See later in this chapter for a discussion of the committee's focus, including primary attention to medical subspecialties (as opposed to surgical subspecialties).

Underrepresented Populations

The Association of American Medical Colleges (AAMC) defines underrepresented in medicine (URiM) as "those racial and ethnic populations that are underrepresented in the medical profession relative to their numbers in the population" (AAMC, 2023). The AAMC recognized the need to allow the term to be used flexibly in response to changing demographics, including variation at the regional or local level. In their workforce-related demographic data collections used widely in this report, the American Board of Pediatrics (ABP) includes the following categories: American Indian or Alaska Native; Black or African American; Hispanic, Latino, or Spanish Origin; and Native Hawaiian or Other Pacific Islander (ABP, 2023a). For the purposes of this report, the committee uses URiM broadly to allow for inclusion of a wide array of groups and not necessarily based on racial and ethnic demographics alone. For example, individuals from economically disadvantaged backgrounds may be considered to be URiM and would be included in this broad definition. However, the committee separately refers to this population in certain discussions (e.g., loan repayment).

The National Institutes of Health describes populations underrepresented in the extramural scientific workforce (including the biomedical, clinical, behavioral, and social sciences workforces) (NIH, 2022b). This includes certain racial and ethnic groups, individuals with disabilities, individuals from economically disadvantaged backgrounds, and others (depending upon the discipline). While the committee uses URiM throughout the report, they note that underrepresentation may be different for the clinical subspecialties than for subspecialists who focus on research.

High-Priority Subspecialties

In their evaluation of the available data, the committee concluded that the need for interventions to support and optimize the pediatric subspecialty workforce varies substantially and dynamically across subspecialties over time. Some subspecialties receive many fellowship applicants, while others have a dearth. The anticipated earnings vary by subspecialty, and individuals who train in critical care and other procedure-based subspecialties have incomes that are far above those for non-procedural pediatric subspecialties. The number and proportion of individuals who are extramurally funded physician–scientists vary substantially by pediatric subspecialty. Waiting times to access care also vary among pediatric subspecialties, from days for some to months for others, and by geographic location. While there are few URiM pediatric subspecialists, some fields have been more successful in advancing diversity. Given these variables, the groups referenced as "high-priority subspecialties" in the ensuing chapters and recommendations will differ within the specific context and may change over time. Thus, this report does not employ a single definition for "high-priority."

STUDY CONTEXT

The pediatric-specific pattern of disorders, infancy's anatomic challenges, children's rapid physical, cognitive, and socioemotional development, and the triadic clinician-parent-child relationship create unique challenges and provide strong justification for a pediatric health care system with its own workforce. To examine whether the current and future pediatric workforce is adequate to meet children's needs, it is important to understand the history of children's health, have a general overview of the health and demographics of today's children, and understand the development and evolution of pediatrics and pediatric subspecialties.

History of Children's Health

In the nineteenth and twentieth centuries, infant, child, and adolescent morbidity and mortality fell dramatically because of awareness of and improvements in public health (e.g., sanitation) as well as the impact of poverty and child labor (Bhatia et al., 2019; Connolly, 2023). The U.S. Children's Bureau was established in 1912 to improve the health of mothers and children, and the Sheppard-Towner Act, enacted in 1921, provided grants to states to develop health services for mothers and children (Brosco, 2012; Mahnke, 2000). However, due to opposition to the Act, it lapsed in 1929 (Mahnke, 2000).

The advent of antibiotics in the mid-twentieth century, combined with the development and routine immunization of the majority of children with effective vaccines, led to reduction of serious morbidity and mortality due to infectious diseases (Bhatia et al., 2019; Brosco, 2012; Thompson, 1984). This was followed by the development of effective drugs to treat childhood leukemias and other cancers, and advances in technology such as incubators and ventilators for the care of premature infants (Jessop, 2015; Thompson, 1984). As noted by Phoon (2018), "the establishment of the [NICHD] in 1962 underscored the importance of investigating human development throughout the entire life process, starting even before birth and with a critical role of health in childhood." With substantial improvement in child survival, there has been a conceptual shift to address the needs of children with chronic medical conditions and more recently, children with special health care needs. There has also been a growing understanding of the mental, behavioral, and developmental needs of children, as well as their comorbidity with physical health. (See Chapter 2 for more on children's changing health care needs.)

Overview of Children's Health and Demographics Today

The health of today's children sets the foundation for the future health of the nation (NRC and IOM, 2004). A child's health and well-being (or lack thereof) can have lifelong health effects (Barker, 2004; Boyce et al., 2021; Halfon and Hochstein, 2002; Halfon et al., 2014; Halfon et al., 2018; Lebrun-Harris et al., 2022; Shonkoff et al., 2021). Investing in children's health enhances the nation's future economic productivity, reduces rates of adult disorders and their associated disability, and improves the well-being of the children and their families. However, children face a host of threats linked to unhealthy lifestyles and diets, injury and violence, inequality, pollution, and climate change (WHO, 2020). Furthermore, many children live in families and communities that experience stress associated with poverty, language barriers, interpersonal and structural racism, and adverse social influences on health, which directly harm children and create challenges for parents and health care providers (Beech et al., 2021; NASEM, 2017; Trent et al., 2019). The COVID-19 pandemic exacerbated many of these problems for vulnerable children, and increased the burden of mental, emotional, and behavioral health as summarized in a recent National Academies report (NASEM, 2023).

In 2020, children (individuals younger than 18 years) in the United States numbered more than 73.1 million and accounted for 22.1 percent of the total population (U.S. Census Bureau, 2021). This represents a 1.4 percent decrease (more than 1.075 million children) since 2010, when children younger than 18 years represented 24 percent of the population. However, children today are increasingly diverse. In 2020, only 53 percent of the population under age 18 reported race as "White alone" (compared with 65.3 percent of children in 2010 and compared with 74.7 percent of adults 18 years and older) (Jones et al., 2021). Furthermore, 15.1 percent of children reported being "two or more races" in 2020 (compared with 5.6 percent in 2010). These changing demographics are particularly important because racial and ethnic disparities in children's health are persistent, widespread, and long lasting (Braveman and Barclay, 2009; Cheng et al., 2015; Flores and The Committee on Pediatric Research, 2010) and have great influence on the need for pediatric subspecialty care.

Organizations such as AAP have issued policy statements that emphasize the need for strategies to address health and development issues across the pediatric lifespan regarding ethnicity, culture, and circumstance, issues that are critical to reducing health disparities (Trent et al., 2019). In addition, children remain the poorest population subgroup in the United States. In 2021, the child poverty rate (for people under age 18) was 16.9 percent, 4.2 percentage points higher than the national rate (Benson, 2022). The large proportion of U.S. children who live in poverty, coupled with structural racism, has significant negative effects on children's health and well-being (Trent et al., 2019). Compared with other advanced nations, U.S. children experience more unfavorable outcomes across numerous health and social indicators such as mortality, family poverty, access to health care, and exposure to crime and violence (Anderson et al., 2022; Martorano et al., 2014; Thakrar et al., 2018).

Brief History of Pediatrics and the Development of Medical Subspecialties

The earliest pediatricians in the United States championed the importance of preventive medicine, the interrelationship between child and maternal health, and social determinants of health to reduce child and maternal mortality and morbidity (Faber and McIntosh, 1966; Mahnke, 2000). In 1860, Dr. Abraham Jacobi first lectured on the diseases of childhood (Connolly, 2023). At the time, specialists focused on a specific organ or technology, but Jacobi argued that the role of pediatricians should go beyond diseases and instead look holistically at child health. In 1880, a group of physicians founded the American Medical Association's section on the diseases of children, followed in 1888 by the American Pediatric Society (APS, 2022; Connolly, 2023). In the late 1800s, children's hospitals, originally designed for social welfare, began to focus more on the care of children with medical and surgical needs (Connolly, 2023).

In the early twentieth century, physicians could "self-declare" as a pediatrician without completing any specific training (ABP, 2023b). In response to such concerns, medical schools began offering training in certain specialties, and specialty boards were developed (ABP, 2023b). In 1931, the AAP was formed, followed by ABP in 1933 (ABP, 2023b,c). The ABP focused on "reviewing accreditation of training programs, developing criteria for those to be certified, and examining applicants" (ABP, 2023b). Originally, pediatricians were certified once, at the beginning of practice. In 1988, ABP began to require certification every 7 years; the time requirement changed in 2006 to align with the maintenance of certification requirements of the American Board on Medical Specialties, and as of 2019, pediatricians must recertify every 5 years (ABP, 2023b).

The development of pediatric medical subspecialties and the requirements and expectations for training and certification in those subspecialties have reflected the consensus of the pediatric community and specialty organizations on how best to address medical needs of children and advances in their diagnosis and care. Pediatric subspecialties grew out of clinics within medical schools in the 1930s and 1940s (ABP, 2023b). Before 1978, trainees were eligible for subspecialty certification after fellowship training following a minimum of 2 years of general pediatric training (Jones, Jr., et al., 2001; Stevenson et al., 2014). During these years, most fellowships would be best described as apprenticeships where trainees and mentors, usually partnered by reputation, areas of expertise, and personal connections would work together using broadly defined expectations of the field in the clinical and research activities of the mentor. Oversight by regulatory bodies was present, but less distinctly outlined, as the definition of program requirements did not develop until after the founding of the ACGME in 1981.

In 1978, the Task Force on the Future of Pediatric Education (FOPE) drove sweeping changes in pediatric residency training, including the need for a 3-year residency program; enhanced experiences in ambulatory settings; increased attention to developmental, behavioral, and adolescent health; and improved skill development in team-based care (Kempe et al., 1978). In 2000, *The Future of Pediatric Education II (FOPE II)* stated that subspecialty training should embrace providing experiences in clinical care, teaching, and research; the report also reconfirmed many of the recommendations and concepts provided in 1978 and continued to underscore the uneven geographic distribution of U.S. pediatricians (Chang and Halfon, 1997; DeAngelis et al., 2000; Gruskin et al., 2000).

Medical Subspecialty Certification Today

As shown in Table 1-1, the first subspecialty in pediatrics to be recognized by ABP for certification was cardiology (in 1961) followed by hematology/oncology, nephrology, and endocrinology (all in the 1970s) (Macy et al., 2021). The ABP currently grants certification for 15 medical subspecialties. For more on pediatric subspecialty education and training, see Chapters 4 and 5.

In addition to the 15 ABP-certified subspecialties, ABP recognizes 5 subspecialties administered by other co-sponsoring ABMS boards, and offers several combined training programs and non-standard pathways for subspecialization (see Table 1-2) (ABP, 2023d,e,f). The American Osteopathic Board of Pediatrics (AOBP) grants subspecialty certification in neonatology and adult and pediatric allergy and immunology (AOBP, 2023a,b). Other ABMS boards offer medical subspecialty certification in the care of children without collaboration with ABP (e.g., pediatric dermatology). Some subspecialties do not have formal certifications but are widely recognized by the pediatric community (e.g., obesity medicine). A variety of surgical subspecialties are also involved in the care of infants, children, and adolescents.

STUDY FOCUS

The committee recognizes the important contribution of many different types of clinicians towards the care of children; however, based on the statement of task and discussions with study sponsors, this report focuses on the medical subspecialty physician workforce. The committee particularly focused on the 15 medical subspecialties certified by the American Board of Pediatrics (ABP) (see Table 1-3). These represent the bulk of pediatric subspecialty physicians and share common pathways for education and training; furthermore, many of these subspecialties experience significant challenges in recruitment and retention. When appropriate and relevant, the

TABLE 1-1 Pediatric Medical Subspecialties by First Year of Certification

Subspecialty	Year of First Board Examination	Description
Pediatric Cardiology	1961	Care for pediatric patients with congenital or acquired cardiac and cardiovascular abnormalities.
Pediatric Hematology/Oncology	1974	Diagnose and treat children with cancer and blood disorders that range from severe conditions such as genetic disorders of coagulation or more benign conditions such as nutritional anemia.
Pediatric Nephrology	1974	Care for pediatric patients with various acuities of kidney-related disorders. This can include dialysis, management of chronic conditions such as kidney disease, or transplants.
Neonatal-Perinatal Medicine	1975	Care for critically ill newborn and premature infants typically just before and after birth.
Pediatric Endocrinology	1978	Care for pediatric patients who have metabolic or other hormonal disorders, such as diabetes, hormone and gland disorders, and differences in sex development.
Pediatric Pulmonology	1986	Care for pediatric patients with various acuities of respiratory and lung-related disorders. Conditions can range from asthma to lung transplants, cystic fibrosis, or even sleep medicine.
Pediatric Critical Care Medicine	1987	Care for pediatric patients who require high levels of inpatient care and monitoring, such as those who have seizures, cardiac failure, or traumatic injuries.
Pediatric Gastroenterology	1990	Care for pediatric patients to manage their digestive health. This can include acute disorders such as gastrointestinal bleeding or chronic issues such as Crohn's disease and irritable bowel syndrome.
Pediatric Emergency Medicine	1992	Care for pediatric patients who come into the emergency department for a wide range of conditions of varying degrees of complexity.
Pediatric Rheumatology	1992	Care for children with illnesses affecting their muscles, bones, joints, ligaments, and tendons such as lupus, autoinflammatory diseases, or arthritis.
Adolescent Medicine	1994	Combine clinical and non-clinical work to address various aspects of adolescent health, including disorders of puberty, eating disorders, chronic illnesses, and reproductive and sexual health.
Pediatric Infectious Diseases	1994	Prevent and treat infectious diseases among pediatric patients.

TABLE 1-1 Continued

Subspecialty	Year of First Board Examination	Description
Developmental-Behavioral Pediatrics	2002	Evaluate and treat developmental and behavioral disorders in pediatric patients based on an understanding of social, educational, and cultural influences on the biological and social factors of children.
Child Abuse Pediatrics	2009	Care for infants, children, and adolescents who are suspected victims of any form of child maltreatment, including physical, sexual, medical, or emotional child abuse.
Pediatric Hospital Medicine	2020	Care for pediatric patients in a hospital in various pediatric units, including labor and delivery, the intensive care unit, or acute care areas.

SOURCES: ABP, 2023d; CoPS, 2022a,b,c,d,e,f,g,h,i,j,k,l,m,n,o; Macy et al., 2021.

committee also considered other pediatric medical subspecialties, including those certified by the American Osteopathic Board of Pediatrics (AOBP), subspecialties that are cosponsored by ABP but certified by other boards within the American Board of Medical Specialties (ABMS), subspecialties that are pursued through ABP non-standard pathways and combined training programs, subspecialties that are certified by other ABMS boards (without collaboration of ABP), and emerging medical subspecialties.

As a secondary focus, the committee discussed the interaction and collaboration between pediatric medical subspecialty physicians and primary care clinicians because these types of physicians commonly collaborate with each other on patient management. Other members of the health care workforce—including pediatric surgical subspecialists, adult-trained subspecialists who provide some care for children, and child and adolescent psychiatrists, among others—are also involved in the care of infants, children, and adolescents but not a primary focus for this report.

The committee recognized that advanced practice providers are increasingly used to provide both inpatient and outpatient pediatric subspecialty care and an important part of the pediatric workforce, especially in children's hospitals. However, their training and certification is separate from that of pediatric physicians and therefore not a primary focus in this report. The committee is also aware that scientists conducting research on conditions that occur in the pediatric age group represent a diverse group of individuals. Following the charge, the committee's focus for research was on the recruitment, training, funding, and retention of pediatric physician–scientists.

TABLE 1-2 Pediatric Medical Subspecialties Engaged with ABP and AOBP

ABP Certified Subspecialties	
• Adolescent Medicine*	• Pediatric Gastroenterology*
• Child Abuse Pediatrics*	• Pediatric Hematology/Oncology*
• Developmental-Behavioral Pediatrics*	• Pediatric Hospital Medicine*
• Neonatal-Perinatal Medicine*	• Pediatric Infectious Diseases*
• Pediatric Cardiology*	• Pediatric Nephrology*
• Pediatric Critical Care Medicine*	• Pediatric Pulmonology*
• Pediatric Emergency Medicine*	• Pediatric Rheumatology*
• Pediatric Endocrinology*	
AOBP-Certified Subspecialties	
Adult and Pediatric Allergy and Immunology*	Neonatology*
ABP Co-Sponsored Subspecialties (Certified by Another ABMS Specialty Board)	
• Hospice and Palliative Medicine	• Sleep Medicine
• Medical Toxicology	• Sports Medicine
• Pediatric Transplant Hepatology	
ABP Non-Standard Pathways and Combined Training Programs	
• Allergy and Immunology*	• Pediatrics-Neurodevelopmental Disabilities
• Medicine-Pediatrics	• Pediatrics-Neurology*
• Pediatrics-Anesthesiology	• Pediatrics-Physical Medicine and Rehabilitation
• Pediatrics-Emergency Medicine*	
• Pediatrics-Medical Genetics	• Pediatrics-Psychiatry/Child and Adolescent Psychiatry

NOTE: *indicates subspecialties (in addition to "academic generalist") represented in the Council of Pediatric Subspecialties (CoPS, 2023).
SOURCE: Committee generated.

The committee's task was not to redesign the overall health system of pediatric care delivery, including transitions to adult care, but rather to focus on equitable access to pediatric subspecialty care. Furthermore, the committee recognizes the importance of high-quality primary care as a foundation for high-quality subspecialty care. Although the committee did examine some new models of subspecialist–primary care clinician interaction for patient care, the 2021 National Academies report *Implementing High-Quality Primary Care: Rebuilding the Foundation of Health Care* addresses strategies to improve primary care broadly, including the use of interprofessional teams, and the committee considered its work to build upon that study. The committee also recognizes a study in progress at the

TABLE 1-3 Primary and Secondary Focus of Report

Focus	Grouping	Examples
Primary Focus	American Board of Pediatrics (ABP)–Certified Pediatric Medical Subspecialty Physicians (Clinicians and Researchers)	• Adolescent Medicine • Child Abuse Pediatrics • Developmental-Behavioral Pediatrics • Neonatal-Perinatal Medicine • Pediatric Cardiology • Pediatric Critical Care Medicine • Pediatric Emergency Medicine • Pediatric Endocrinology • Pediatric Gastroenterology • Pediatric Hematology/Oncology • Pediatric Hospital Medicine • Pediatric Infectious Diseases • Pediatric Nephrology • Pediatric Pulmonology • Pediatric Rheumatology
	Other Pediatric Medical Subspecialty Physicians (Clinicians and Researchers)	• American Osteopathic Board of Pediatrics–certified subspecialties • ABP co-sponsored subspecialties (certified by another board of the American Board of Medical Specialties [ABMS]) • ABP nonstandard pathways and combined training programs* • Subspecialties certified by other ABMS boards without collaboration of ABP (e.g., pediatric dermatology) • Emerging medical subspecialties (e.g., obesity)
Secondary Focus	Primary – Subspecialty Care Interface	Interaction of subspecialists with primary care clinicians, including the following: • General Pediatricians • Advanced Practice Providers (e.g., Advanced Practice Registered Nurses, Physician Assistants) • Family Medicine Physicians

NOTE: *Although the ABP recognizes a combined training program for child and adolescent psychiatry, very few physicians choose this pathway, so it is not included as part of the committee's primary focus.
SOURCE: Committee generated.

National Academies that is charged to address "innovations that can be implemented in the health care system to improve the health and wellbeing of children and youth," including workforce development and team-based care.[1]

PREVIOUS WORK OF THE NATIONAL ACADEMIES

Many previous National Academies reports are relevant to this current study. For example:

- *Children's Health, the Nation's Wealth* (2004) reflects on inadequacies in the ways in which the nation monitors and optimizes the health of children. Specifically, the report notes the need to measure and monitor trends in health, in part to anticipate the need for specific services (NRC and IOM, 2004).
- *Graduate Medical Education That Meets the Nation's Health Needs* (2014) highlights concerns about a mismatch between population health needs and the specialty makeup of the physician workforce, physicians' geographic maldistribution, insufficient diversity, gaps between new physicians' knowledge and currently required competencies, and a lack of fiscal transparency (IOM, 2014).
- *The Promise of Adolescence: Realizing Opportunity for All Youth* (2019) emphasizes that adolescents undergo complex neurobiological and sociobehavioral transformations as they develop. Equity is brought to the forefront in ensuring the "promise of adolescence" for all adolescents and bridging the disparities in resources and supports that disadvantaged youth face (NASEM, 2019).
- *Implementing High-Quality Primary Care* (2021) aims to make high-quality primary care available to everyone by modifying payment approaches, expanding accessibility, strengthening community-based training of the workforce, improving the use of health information technology, and monitoring implementation of recommended approaches (NASEM, 2021).
- *Addressing the Long-Term Effects of the COVID-19 Pandemic on Children and Families* (2023) recommends improved data collection to monitor ongoing effects of COVID-19 on children and families and strengthening and expanding Medicaid at the federal level to ensure access to high-quality care (NASEM, 2023).

---

[1] For more information, see https://www.nationalacademies.org/our-work/improving-the-health-and-wellbeing-of-children-and-youth-through-health-care-system-transformation (accessed July 7, 2023).

STUDY APPROACH

The Committee on the Pediatric Subspecialty Workforce and Its Impact on Child Health and Well-Being consisted of 17 members with a broad range of expertise, including general and subspecialty pediatrics, primary care, family medicine, nursing, clinician training and education, health services research, clinical research, bench research, health policy, health disparities, and health economics. Appendix A provides brief biographies of the committee members and staff.

The committee deliberated during seven hybrid meetings, many working group calls, and multiple ad hoc meetings between May 2022 and June 2023. Additionally, the committee held six virtual public webinars and invited speakers to offer comments or make presentations to inform the committee's deliberations. The speakers provided valuable input on a broad range of topics, including patient and family perspectives, emerging issues in child health, innovative approaches in education and training, early career perspectives on the subspecialty pipeline, meeting community needs, modeling the future subspecialty workforce, the pediatric physician–scientist and research pathway, and innovative clinical practices to improve access.

The committee also completed an extensive search of the peer-reviewed literature and the gray literature, including publications by private organizations, advocacy groups, and government entities. In addition, the committee established an online system for collecting narratives on patient and family experiences with pediatric subspecialty care as well as perspectives from clinicians on why they selected their subspecialty and what barriers they faced. This "call for perspectives" was posted on the project website, announced at all public meetings, and shared with project sponsors; it included two open-ended questions. Patients and families were asked to comment on "what has been your experience with seeking pediatric subspecialty care?" Trainees and clinicians were asked "why do you want or why did you decide to go into your chosen pediatric subspecialty? What barriers, if any, do you or did you face?" There was also an opportunity to submit any additional thoughts on pediatric subspecialty care. A total of 166 sets of comments were submitted, and most came from the pediatric subspecialty trainees and clinicians themselves. Selected quotes from these narratives are included in boxes throughout this report.[2] Finally, the committee commissioned a data analysis to better understand the patterns of children's uses of medical subspecialty care. The commissioned analysis examined health plan administrative files for commercially insured individuals. Two other data analyses were submitted to the committee: one examined patterns for children who received subspecialty care in academic medical centers while

---

[2] The full list of submissions can be found in the project's public access file.

Vision of High Quality of Care

To achieve the goal of a high-quality pediatric subspecialty workforce for clinical care and research, the committee envisions an accessible and efficient health system that enables all children to receive the appropriate type and amount of primary and specialty care whenever they need it. Such a system would value high-quality care for all children, with care that embodies the six elements for quality defined by the Institute of Medicine[3]: safety, timeliness, effectiveness, efficiency, equity, and patient-centeredness. High-quality pediatric subspecialty care is *safe* when the referral, or lack of referral, does not result in harm. It is *timely* when diagnosis and treatment alleviate anxiety and symptoms as quickly as feasible and avoid delays that exacerbate symptoms or functional limitations attributable to the disease or its course. It is *effective* when patient and family questions and concerns are fully addressed and it produces the best possible health outcomes. It is *efficient* when the diagnostic and treatment journey does not create unneeded testing or treatments or delays in delivery of appropriate services. It is *equitable* when the access to necessary knowledge and the use of appropriate treatment is provided according to patient need, rather than social determinants of health. It is *patient- and family-centered* when patients, families, and clinicians are considered partners in determining goals of care and shared decision making is incorporated when appropriate.

High-quality pediatric subspecialty care requires a well-supported, superbly trained, and appropriately used primary care, subspecialty, and physician–scientist workforce achieved through effective education and training, well-designed care models, and continued attention to the changing health care and economic landscapes. In addition, all clinicians need to be able to practice at the top of their scope with appropriate reimbursement for their administrative and clinical work. Increased opportunities are needed for implementation of innovative delivery system models and health care technologies, and flexible training pathways are needed to train the workforce in response to the changing medical and behavioral health needs of infants, children, and adolescents.

---

[3] As of March 2016, the Health and Medicine Division of the National Academies of Sciences, Engineering, and Medicine (National Academies) continues the consensus studies and convening activities previously carried out by the Institute of Medicine (IOM). The IOM name is used to refer to reports issued prior to July 2015.

Data Limitations

Concerns about significant shortages in the availability of the entire pediatric workforce, which may affect access to care, are prevalent in the literature. However, research and data on the pediatric subspecialty workforce remain limited in many key areas (which are noted throughout the report). Previous studies on the pediatric subspecialty physician workforce are often outdated (i.e., more than 10 years old), use limited sampling methods, have low response rates to surveys (leading to concerns about response bias), and do not distinguish between subspecialists and general pediatricians.

The committee also noted several other challenges of the literature. First, there is mixed use of the terms "specialist" and "subspecialist," and many reports and datasets do not use a standard set of subspecialties when speaking to subspecialties broadly in their research. In some cases, only a subset of ABP-certified subspecialties are included, or they are included in combination with other pediatric subspecialties, or even in combination with specialties and subspecialties outside of pediatrics. As noted by Laurel Leslie, vice president of research for ABP, in her presentation to this committee in a public webinar:

> Most national models clump all pediatric subspecialists together as if they were one group, and we were very aware from our data that each of the [subspecialties] functions independently and has very different profiles with respect to the workforce.[4]

Additionally, for some surveys, the definition of a specialist might be subject to interpretation by patients and families. For example, the National Survey of Children's Health defined specialists as "doctors like surgeons, heart doctors, allergy doctors, skin doctors, and others who specialize in one area of health care" (CAHMI, 2023). Finally, the committee noted a lack of robust data on patient outcomes associated with subspecialist care and lack of standard definitions for measures within those studies.

Organization of the Report

The committee structured its report around the main issues challenging the pediatric medical subspecialty workforce. This introductory chapter has described the study context, charge to the committee, and the scope and methods of the study. Chapter 2 provides an overview of access to pediatric subspecialty care and its connection to child health while Chapter

---

[4] The webinar recording can be accessed at https://www.nationalacademies.org/event/11-02-2022/the-pediatric-subspecialty-workforce-and-its-impact-on-child-health-and-well-being-webinar-3.

3 presents the three data analyses considered by the committee to better understand the usage of pediatric subspecialty services. Chapter 4 focuses on the pediatric subspecialty workforce itself, including basic demographics and how subspecialists are trained, and offers a high-level summary of the overall health care workforce for children. Chapter 5 considers the factors that influence the choices of physicians to pursue a career in a pediatric subspecialty, and Chapter 6 specifically explores the pediatric subspecialty research workforce. Chapter 7 explores the interface between pediatric subspecialists and the broader child health care workforce, particularly the interface between primary care clinicians and pediatric subspecialists. Finally, Chapter 8 examines financing of child health. In addition to the main report, Appendix A contains committee, fellow, and staff biographies.

REFERENCES

AAMC (Association of American Medical Colleges). 2023. *Underrepresented in medicine definition*. https://www.aamc.org/what-we-do/equity-diversity-inclusion/underrepresented-in-medicine (accessed April 27, 2023).

ABP (American Board of Pediatrics). 2023a. *Latest race and ethnicity data for pediatricians and pediatric trainees: Estimates by subpopulations as distinct groups*. https://www.abp.org/dashboards/latest-race-and-ethnicity-data-pediatricians-and-pediatric-trainees (accessed April 23, 2023).

ABP. 2023b. *History of the ABP*. https://www.abp.org/content/history-abp (accessed May 5, 2023).

ABP. 2023c. *About us*. https://www.abp.org/content/about-us (accessed May 5, 2023).

ABP. 2023d. *Subspecialty certifications and admission requirements*. https://www.abp.org/content/subspecialty-certifications-and-admission-requirements (accessed April 22, 2023).

ABP. 2023e. *Combined programs*. https://www.abp.org/content/combined-programs (accessed April 22, 2023).

ABP. 2023f. *Non-standard pathways and combined programs*. https://www.abp.org/content/non-standard-pathways-and-combined-programs (accessed May 5, 2023).

Anderson, N. W., D. Eisenberg, N. Halfon, A. Markowitz, K. A. Moore, and F. J. Zimmerman. 2022. Trends in measures of child and adolescent well-being in the U.S. from 2000 to 2019. *JAMA Network Open* 5(10):e2238582.

AOBP (American Osteopathic Board of Pediatrics). 2023a. *Welcome to the American Osteopathic Conjoint Examination Committee on pediatric and adult allergy and immunology*. https://certification.osteopathic.org/allergy-immunology (accessed May 5, 2023).

AOBP. 2023b. *Subspecialty certification: Neonatology*. https://certification.osteopathic.org/pediatrics/certification-process/neonatology (accessed May 5, 2023).

APS (American Pediatric Society). 2022. *American Pediatric Society*. https://www.aps1888.org (accessed April 22, 2023).

Barker, D. J. 2004. The developmental origins of well-being. *Philosophical Transactions of the Royal Society B* 359(1449):1359-1366.

Beech, B. M., C. Ford, R. J. Thorpe, M. A. Bruce, and K. C. Norris. 2021. Poverty, racism, and the public health crisis in America. *Frontiers in Public Health* 9: 699049.

Benson, C. 2022. *Poverty rate of children higher than national rate, lower for older populations*. https://www.census.gov/library/stories/2022/10/poverty-rate-varies-by-age-groups.html (accessed January 31, 2023).

Bhatia, A., N. Krieger, and S. V. Subramanian. 2019. Learning from history about reducing infant mortality: Contrasting the centrality of structural interventions to early 20th-century successes in the United States to their neglect in current global initiatives. *Milbank Quarterly* 97(1):285-345.

Boyce, W. T., P. Levitt, F. D. Martinez, B. S. McEwen, and J. P. Shonkoff. 2021. Genes, environments, and time: The biology of adversity and resilience. *Pediatrics* 147(2):e20201651.

Braveman, P., and C. Barclay. 2009. Health disparities beginning in childhood: A life course perspective. *Pediatrics* 124(Suppl 3):S163-S175.

Brosco, J. P. 2012. Navigating the future through the past: The enduring historical legacy of federal children's health programs in the United States. *American Journal of Public Health* 102(10):1848-1857.

CAHMI (Child and Adolescent Health Measurement Initiative). 2023. *2020 National Survey of Children's Health (NSCH) data query: Indicator 4.5: During the past 12 months, did this child see a specialist other than a mental health professional?* https://www.childhealthdata.org/browse/survey/results?q=9391&r=1&g=1000 (accessed April 21, 2023).

Chang, R. K., and N. Halfon. 1997. Geographic distribution of pediatricians in the United States: An analysis of the fifty states and Washington, DC. *Pediatrics* 100(2 Pt 1):172-179.

Cheng, T. L., M. A. Emmanuel, D. J. Levy, and R. R. Jenkins. 2015. Child health disparities: What can a clinician do? *Pediatrics* 136(5):961-968.

Connolly, C. A. 2023. *Late-nineteenth and early-twentieth century pediatrics.* https://www.nursing.upenn.edu/nhhc/home-care/late-nineteenth-and-early-century-pediatrics (accessed April 22, 2023).

CoPS (Council of Pediatric Subspecialties). 2022a. *Child abuse pediatrics.* https://www.pedsubs.org/about-cops/subspecialty-descriptions/child-abuse (accessed April 14, 2022).

CoPS. 2022b. *Developmental and behavioral pediatrics.* https://www.pedsubs.org/about-cops/subspecialty-descriptions/developmental-and-behavioral (accessed April 14, 2022).

CoPS. 2022c. *Pediatric adolescent medicine.* https://www.pedsubs.org/about-cops/subspecialty-descriptions/adolescent-medicine/#Ques1 (accessed April 14, 2022).

CoPS. 2022d. *Pediatric cardiology.* https://www.pedsubs.org/about-cops/subspecialty-descriptions/cardiology (accessed April 14, 2022).

CoPS. 2022e. *Pediatric critical care.* https://www.pedsubs.org/about-cops/subspecialty-descriptions/critical-care (accessed April 14, 2022).

CoPS. 2022f. *Pediatric emergency medicine.* https://www.pedsubs.org/about-cops/subspecialty-descriptions/emergency-medicine (accessed April 14, 2022).

CoPS. 2022g. *Pediatric endocrinology.* https://www.pedsubs.org/about-cops/subspecialty-descriptions/endocrinology (accessed April 14, 2022).

CoPS. 2022h. *Pediatric gastroenterology.* https://www.pedsubs.org/about-cops/subspecialty-descriptions/gastroenterology (accessed April 14, 2022).

CoPS. 2022i. *Pediatric hematology/oncology.* https://www.pedsubs.org/about-cops/subspecialty-descriptions/hematology-oncology (accessed April 14, 2022).

CoPS. 2022j. *Pediatric hospitalist.* https://www.pedsubs.org/about-cops/subspecialty-descriptions/hospitalist (accessed April 14, 2022).

CoPS. 2022k. *Pediatric infectious diseases.* https://www.pedsubs.org/about-cops/subspecialty-descriptions/infectious-diseases (accessed April 14, 2022).

CoPS. 2022l. *Pediatric neonatology.* https://www.pedsubs.org/about-cops/subspecialty-descriptions/neonatology (accessed November 22, 2022).

CoPS. 2022m. *Pediatric nephrology.* https://www.pedsubs.org/about-cops/subspecialty-descriptions/nephrology (accessed April 14, 2022).

CoPS. 2022n. *Pediatric pulmonary medicine.* https://www.pedsubs.org/about-cops/subspecialty-descriptions/pulmonary-medicine (accessed April 14, 2022).

CoPS. 2022o. *Pediatric rheumatology.* https://www.pedsubs.org/about-cops/subspecialty-descriptions/rheumatology (accessed April 14, 2022).

CoPS. 2023. *Subspecialty descriptions.* https://www.pedsubs.org/about-cops/subspecialty-descriptions (accessed May 5, 2023).

DeAngelis, C., R. Feigin, T. DeWitt, L. R. First, E. A. Jewett, R. Kelch, R. W. Chesney, H. J. Mulvey, J. L. Simon, and E. R. Alden. 2000. Final report of the FOPE II pediatric workforce workgroup. *Pediatrics* 106(5):1245-1255.

Faber, H., and A. R. McIntosh. 1966. *History of the American Pediatric Society.* New York: McGraw-Hill.

FDA (U.S. Food and Drug Administration). 2022. *Pediatric medical devices.* https://www.fda.gov/medical-devices/products-and-medical-procedures/pediatric-medical-devices#:~:text=Neonates%20%2D%20from%20birth%20through%20the,not%20including%20the%2022nd%20birthday) (accessed April 21, 2023).

Flores, G., and The Committee on Pediatric Research. 2010. Racial and ethnic disparities in the health and health care of children. *Pediatrics* 125(4):e979-e1020.

Gruskin, A., R. G. Williams, E. R. McCabe, F. Stein, J. Strickler, R. W. Chesney, H. J. Mulvey, J. L. Simon, and E. R. Alden. 2000. Final report of the FOPE II pediatric subspecialists of the future workgroup. *Pediatrics* 106(5):1224-1244.

Halfon, N., C. B. Forrest, R. M. Lerner, and E. M. Faustman. 2018. *Handbook of life course health development.* Edited by N. Halfon, C. B. Forrest, R. M. Lerner and E. M. Faustman, Cham (CH): Springer.

Halfon, N., and M. Hochstein. 2002. Life course health development: An integrated framework for developing health, policy, and research. *Milbank Quarterly* 80(3):433-479, iii.

Halfon, N., K. Larson, M. Lu, E. Tullis, and S. Russ. 2014. Life course health development: Past, present and future. *Maternal and Child Health Journal* 18(2):344-365.

Hardin, A. P., J. M. Hackell, Committee on Practice and Ambulatory Medicine, G. R. Simon, A. D. Arauz Boudreau, C. N. Baker, G. A. Barden, III, K. E. Meade, S. B. Moore, and J. Richerson. 2017. Age limit of pediatrics. *Pediatrics* 140(3):e20172151.

IOM (Institute of Medicine). 2014. *Graduate medical education that meets the nation's health needs.* Edited by J. Eden, D. Berwick, and G. Wilensky. Washington, DC: The National Academies Press.

Jessop, E. 2015. The *history of childhood cancer research.* https://www.stbaldricks.org/blog/post/the-history-of-childhood-cancer-research (accessed April 22, 2023).

Jones, M. D., Jr., T. F. Boat, J. A. Stockman, E. B. Clark, K. Minaga-Miya, G. S. Gilchrist, R. Colletti, and H. S. Winter. 2001. Federation of Pediatric Organizations Subspecialty Forum. *The Journal of Pediatrics* 139(4):487-493.

Jones, N., R. Marks, R. Ramirez, and M. Rios-Vargas. 2021. *2020 Census illuminates racial and ethnic composition of the country.* https://www.census.gov/library/stories/2021/08/improved-race-ethnicity-measures-reveal-United-States-population-much-more-multiracial.html (accessed January 3, 2023).

Kempe, C. H. 1978. The 1978 presidential address of the American Pediatric Society: The future of pediatric education. *Pediatric Research* 12(12):1149-1151.

Lebrun-Harris, L. A., R. M. Ghandour, M. D. Kogan, and M. D. Warren. 2022. Five-year trends in U.S. children's health and well-being, 2016-2020. *JAMA Pediatrics* 176(7):e220056.

Macy, M. L., L. K. Leslie, A. Turner, and G. L. Freed. 2021. Growth and changes in the pediatric medical subspecialty workforce pipeline. *Pediatric Research* 89(5):1297-1303.

Mahnke, C. B. 2000. The growth and development of a specialty: The history of pediatrics. *Clinical Pediatrics* 39(12):705-714.

Martorano, B., L. Natali, C. de Neubourg, and J. Bradshaw. 2014. Child well-being in advanced economies in the late 2000s. *Social Indicators Research* 118(1):247-283.

Mayer, M. L., and A. C. Skinner. 2009. Influence of changes in supply on the distribution of pediatric subspecialty care. *Archives of Pediatrics & Adolescent Medicine* 163(12):1087-1091.

Moreno, M., and L. Thompson. 2020. What is adolescent and young adult medicine? *JAMA Pediatrics* 174(5):512.

NASEM (National Academies of Sciences, Engineering, and Medicine). 2017. *Communities in action: Pathways to health equity*. Edited by J. N. Weinstein, A. Geller, Y. Negussie, and A. Baciu. Washington, DC: The National Academies Press.

NASEM. 2019. *The promise of adolescence: Realizing opportunity for all youth*. Edited by R. J. Bonnie and E. P. Backes. Washington, DC: The National Academies Press.

NASEM. 2021. *Implementing high-quality primary care: Rebuilding the foundation of health care*. Edited by L. McCauley, R. L. Phillips, Jr., M. Meisnere, and S. K. Robinson. Washington, DC: The National Academies Press.

NASEM. 2023. *Addressing the long-term effects of the COVID-19 pandemic on children and families*. Edited by T. R. Coker, J. A. Gootman, and E. P. Backes. Washington, DC: The National Academies Press.

NIH (National Institutes of Health). 2022a. *NIH style guide: Age*. https://www.nih.gov/nih-style-guide/age (accessed April 21, 2023).

NIH. 2022b. *Populations underrepresented in the extramural scientific workforce*. https://diversity.nih.gov/about-us/population-underrepresented (accessed July 10, 2023).

NRC and IOM (National Research Council and Institute of Medicine). 2004. *Children's health, the nation's wealth: Assessing and improving child health*. Washington, DC: The National Academies Press.

Phoon, C. 2018. The origins of pediatrics as a clinical and academic specialty in the United States. https://hekint.org/2018/03/15/origins-pediatrics-clinical-academic-specialty-United-States (accessed April 22, 2023).

Shonkoff, J. P., N. Slopen, and D. R. Williams. 2021. Early childhood adversity, toxic stress, and the impacts of racism on the foundations of health. *Annual Review of Public Health* 42:115-134.

Stevenson, D. K., G. A. McGuinness, J. D. Bancroft, D. M. Boyer, A. R. Cohen, J. T. Gilhooly, M. F. Hazinski, E. S. Holmboe, M. D. Jones, Jr, M. L. Land, Jr, S. S. Long, V. F. Norwood, D. J. Schumacher, T. C. Sectish, J. W. St. Geme, III, and D. C. West. 2014. The initiative on subspecialty clinical training and certification (SCTC): Background and recommendations. *Pediatrics* 133(Supplement_2):S53-S57.

Stockman, J. A., III, and G. L. Freed. 2009. Adequacy of the supply of pediatric subspecialists: So near, yet so far. *Archives of Pediatrics & Adolescent Medicine* 163(12):1160-1161.

Thakrar, A. P., A. D. Forrest, M. G. Maltenfort, and C. B. Forrest. 2018. Child mortality in the U.S. and 19 OECD comparator nations: A 50-year time-trend analysis. *Health Affairs* 37(1):140-149.

Thompson, H. C. 1984. 20th century U.S. child health care: Past, present, future. *American Journal of Diseases of Children* 138(9):804-809.

Trent, M., D. G. Dooley, J. Dougé, Section on Adolescent Health, Council on Community Pediatrics, Committee on Adolescence, R. M. Cavanaugh, Jr., A. E. Lacroix, J. Fanburg, M. H. Rahmandar, L. L. Hornberger, M. B. Schneider, S. Yen, L. A. Chilton, A. E. Green, K. J. Dilley, J. R. Gutierrez, J. H. Duffee, V. A. Keane, S. D. Krugman, C. D. McKelvey, J. M. Linton, J. L. Nelson, G. Mattson, C. C. Breuner, E. M. Alderman, L. K. Grubb, J. Lee, M. E. Powers, M. H. Rahmandar, K. K. Upadhya, and S. B. Wallace. 2019. The impact of racism on child and adolescent health. *Pediatrics* 144(2):e20191765.

U.S. Census Bureau. 2021. *The U.S. adult and under-age-18 populations: 2020 Census.* https://www.census.gov/library/visualizations/interactive/adult-and-under-the-age-of-18-populations-2020-census.html (accessed December 22, 2022).

Vinci, R. J. 2021. The pediatric workforce: Recent data trends, questions, and challenges for the future. *Pediatrics* 147(6):e2020013292.

WHO (World Health Organization). 2020. *Children: New threats to health.* https://www.who.int/news-room/fact-sheets/detail/children-new-threats-to-health (accessed December 21, 2022).

Williams, K., D. Thomson, I. Seto, D. Contopoulos-Ionnidis, J. Ionnidis, S. Curtis, E. Constantin, G. Batmanabane, L. Hartling, and T. Klassen. 2012. Standard 6: Age groups for pediatric trials. *Pediatrics* 129(Suppl 3):153-160.

2

Children's Health Care Needs and Access to Subspecialty Care

Pediatric subspecialty physicians fill a major role for children with health conditions that occur too infrequently for primary care clinicians to gain and maintain sufficient, up-to-date clinical knowledge; for common conditions with high disease severity; or for conditions that require technical procedures and use specialized equipment and procedures. Children's rapid development renders them particularly vulnerable as delays in addressing health needs or deferring care altogether may lead to harmful effects both during childhood and much later as adults, particularly if they occur during critical periods of development. For example, high blood pressure in childhood and adolescence has been associated with morbidity at older ages (due to heart and kidney disease) and premature death (Leiba et al., 2019; Franks et al., 2010; Yang et al., 2020). Given the low prevalence of individual conditions, pediatric subspecialists see enough cases concentrated from a very large population to give them the experience needed to diagnose and treat these conditions effectively. However, while children have relatively high rates of access for common preventive care such as well-child visits (CDC, 2020), their access to care for rarer conditions may be more complicated. A well-functioning health system needs to be organized to ensure good access to care for both common and uncommon acute and chronic health problems. While this chapter discusses some issues of access to health care in general, a framework is presented for understanding access to pediatric subspecialty physician care specifically in the context of the changing health care needs of infants, children, and adolescents.

FRAMEWORK

Ensuring access to high-quality pediatric subspecialty care benefits the health and well-being of millions of children both for children themselves and the adults they will become. As seen in Figure 2-1, the committee developed a framework to help understand the connection between pediatric subspecialty care and children's health, including demand and need for

Demand and Need	• Changing health care needs
	• Sources of demand
	  ○ Patients and families
	  ○ Primary care clinicians
	  ○ Subspecialists
	  ○ Inpatient care

Access	• Workforce supply
	• Financial accessibility
	  ○ Insurance type
	  ○ Out-of-pocket costs
	  ○ Other financial factors
	• Geospatial accessibility
	  ○ Geographic distribution
	  ○ Regionalization of care
	  ○ Inpatient vs. outpatient settings
	• Organizational accessibility
	  ○ Wait times
	• Demographic and Cultural Factors
	  ○ Racial/ethnic concordance
	  ○ Language barriers
	• Transitions from pediatric to adult care

Use	• Short-term non-procedural consultation • Short-term procedural consultation • Long-term co-management • Principal care

Outcomes	• Patient outcomes
	  ○ Clinical outcomes
	  ○ Survival
	  ○ Well-being
	• Family well-being
	• Clinician well-being*

FIGURE 2-1 Framework for understanding overall access to pediatric subspecialty care.
NOTES: *Clinician outcomes of job satisfaction and well-being are discussed in Chapter 5. While *consultation* typically refers to a short-term situation and *referral* may imply a long-term scenario for co-management or shifting of care management, the committee generally uses the term *referral* to apply to both situations.
SOURCE: Committee generated.

services; access to care; use of subspecialty services; and patient, family, and provider outcomes.

DEMAND AND NEED

Understanding the need for health care is an important step toward quantifying demand for health care and its future trends. The process of obtaining subspecialty care begins with a perceived need—that is, demand for these services. An individual who thinks they need a service has a demand for it. However, demand is not the same as need. Demand relates to the desire to receive health care while need refers to the capacity to benefit from health care, meaning that the care is effective in "improving, maintaining, or slowing the deterioration of health" (Rodriguez Santana et al., 2023). Need may be recognized by an individual, their health care team, or both. One of the core functions of primary care is recognition of new health problems and selection of the most appropriate treatment setting for the care of that problem or the ruling out of health problems that may require subspecialty care.

For example, consider this hypothetical example drawn from the collective experience of the authoring committee: a primary care physician evaluates a patient with a history of chronic diarrhea, weight loss, and intermittent abdominal pain. The physician is concerned about possible celiac disease, and initial testing supports this presumptive diagnosis; the patient has a *need* for subspecialty care to definitively make this diagnosis and provide consultation on nutritional management and best available treatments. The patient will benefit from long-term co-management between the primary care clinician and pediatric gastroenterologist, who provides episodic consultation over time related to progression and optimal treatments. In an alternative hypothetical example of a healthy child who is growing and developing well but has infrequent hard stools, a primary care physician makes a diagnosis of constipation and counsels the family that the constipation will likely resolve with hydration, dietary changes, and over-the-counter medication. However, the family remains concerned and self-refers to a pediatric gastroenterologist. This patient has demand, but likely no need for subspecialty care. Thus, demand is a belief that care is required, while need refers to a capacity to benefit from a particular type of health care service.

Patients can have needs, but no demand (i.e., unmet need). The patient with likely celiac disease described above had a need for subspecialty care, but may have deferred treatment if they experienced disincentives to seeking such care, such as high deductibles or long wait times. Patients can also have demand, but no need, which leads to overuse of services. In both cases, patients may experience harm. A high-functioning health system will align demand with need as much as possible.

The Changing Health Care Needs of Infants, Children, and Adolescents

Over the past two decades, there have been significant changes in the physical, mental, and behavioral health needs of the pediatric population. For example, among American infants, children, and adolescents:

- In 2017–2020, obesity affected 19.7 percent of children aged 2–19 (Stierman et al., 2021), up from 13.9 percent of children in 1999–2000 (Sanyaolu et al., 2019). Early studies show significant increases in weight and body mass index among children during the COVID-19 pandemic (Lange et al., 2021; Woolford et al., 2021).
- In 2015–2017, 17.8 percent of children aged 3–17 had a developmental disability (up from 16.2 percent in 2009 to 2011) (Zablotsky et al., 2019).
- In 2001–2017, the prevalence of type 2 diabetes among children aged 10–19 years doubled (from 0.34 to 0.67 per 1,000) (Lawrence et al., 2021).
- Between 2016 and 2020, there were significant increases in anxiety (27 percent increase) and depression (24 percent increase) in children (Lebrun-Harris et al., 2022).
- From 2009 to 2019, the percentage of pediatric mental health hospitalizations with attempted suicide, suicidal ideation, or self-injury diagnoses increased from 30.7 percent to 64.2 percent (Arakelyan et al., 2023).

Overall, serious congenital conditions that were previously lethal or disabling are now treatable and even curable, thanks to scientific innovations. For example, immunizations have eradicated or significantly reduced a number of deadly infections, such as diphtheria, smallpox, measles, bacterial meningitis, pertussis, and many other diseases (CDC, 2022). On the other hand, today's children experience a wide variety of chronic, often lifelong, illnesses (Anderson and Horvath, 2002; Gerteis et al., 2014; Van Cleave et al., 2010; Wise, 2007). Although the most common health conditions that affect children today are acute and recurrent illnesses (e.g., otitis media, respiratory viral illnesses, gastroenteritis), a growing proportion of children are affected by long-term (i.e., expected to last more than one year) medical and behavioral health conditions. Additionally, there are a sizable number of children afflicted with less common diseases, such as nephrotic syndrome, congenital heart disease, sickle cell disease, cystic fibrosis, muscular dystrophy, and complications associated with premature birth. Rare diseases comprise a clinically heterogeneous group of disorders, each one occurring in fewer than 200,000 persons in the United States. They are commonly diagnosed during childhood (70 percent have an exclusive pediatric onset), are frequently genetic in origin, and can have deleterious effects on both immediate and long-term health (Nguengang Wakap et al., 2020). Children also have a variety of mental, behavioral, and social care needs.

A variety of terms have been used to describe the complex care needs of some children, including chronic illness, special health care needs, and medical complexity. Although all have somewhat different definitions, of these types of health care, needs are rising and create challenges for care coordination, referral, and the time needed for subspecialists to assess and treat these patients.

Chronic Conditions

More than one-third (38 percent) of children in middle childhood and adolescence have at least one chronic health condition (CAHMI, 2023a). Many of these individuals are affected by mental health and neurodevelopmental conditions such as anxiety, depression, attention deficit hyperactivity disorder (ADHD), and developmental delay. Others are affected by common chronic medical conditions such as asthma, headaches, and allergies.

Chronic pediatric conditions traditionally have been conceptualized as stratified by physical or mental health conditions, but over the past decades there has been greater awareness of the comorbidity of physical and mental health conditions (Berg et al., 2017; Bright et al., 2016; Butwicka et al., 2016; Muskens et al., 2017; Rankin et al., 2016; Rubinstein et al., 2018). In children with physical and mental health comorbidities, mental health issues may make care and control of the medical condition like diabetes difficult unless both are treated together. An important note, however, is that while children with chronic conditions have worse general health (including function and symptom burden) than those without chronic conditions, life satisfaction appears the same for both groups (Blackwell et al., 2019; Forrest et al., 2022). Therefore, pediatric subspecialty care can help children with chronic conditions to maintain and optimize their quality of life by maximizing their function and minimizing symptom burden.

Children and Youth with Special Health Care Needs

Children [and youth][1] with special health care needs (CYSHCN) is purposively broadly defined as "those who have or are at risk for a chronic physical, developmental, behavioral, or emotional condition and who also require health and related services of a type or amount beyond that required by children generally" (McPherson et al., 1998). While the "at

---

[1] Originally defined as children with special health care needs.

risk" component of this definition has not been adequately quantified or measured, it is important to acknowledge that CYSHCN status can change over time and patients may require services to prevent a chronic condition among those at risk. Special health care needs can include "physical, intellectual, and developmental disabilities, as well as long-standing medical conditions such as asthma, diabetes, a blood disorder, or muscular dystrophy" (CDC, 2021). In 2019-2020, about 20 percent of U.S. children had a special health care need, with needs being more prevalent in non-Hispanic Black children and children with multiple adverse childhood experiences (HRSA, 2022). In 2019–2020, 32.2 percent of CYSHCN received care from a specialist[2] doctor compared with 7.4 percent of non-CYSHCN (CAHMI, 2023b). CYSHCN were nearly four times more likely to have unmet health care needs in the past year compared with non-CYSHCN and more likely to have unmet needs across every type of need, the largest gap being observed in mental health care. The most commonly reported reasons for unmet need included cost (49 percent) and appointment availability (54 percent). Fewer than two-thirds of CYSHCN and their families had adequate insurance to cover the needed services and less than a quarter received health care transition planning to adult care (HRSA, 2022).

Mental Health

Mental and behavioral health conditions are prevalent among the children cared for by pediatric subspecialists, particularly children with chronic medical conditions (Reardon et al., 2020). The severity of mental health conditions occurs on a continuum, from mild conditions that do not necessarily require any treatment, to more severe conditions that can cause impairment. Many disorders typically start in early childhood, although symptoms may not be recognized until later (Amminger et al., 2011; Kessler et al., 2005; Schimmelmann et al., 2007; Shear et al., 2006).

Globally, mental health disorders among children and adolescents contribute to disability and self harm (Kyu et al., 2016). Approximately one in six U.S. children have a diagnosable mental, behavioral, or developmental disorder (Cree et al., 2018; Whitney and Peterson, 2019). The most common disorders among children and adolescents (aged 3–17) are ADHD, anxiety, disruptive behavior problems, and depression (Bitsko et al., 2022; Ghandour et al., 2019). In 2016, nearly 10 percent of U.S. children had a diagnosis of ADHD (Danielson et al., 2018). In 2020, one in 36 children met the case definition for autism (up from one in 59 in 2014) (Baio et al.,

---

[2] In the National Survey of Children's Health, specialist doctors were defined as "doctors like surgeons, heart doctors, allergy doctors, skin doctors, and others who specialize in one area of health care."

2018; Maenner et al., 2023). One-fifth (20 percent) of adolescents (aged 12–17) experienced a major depressive episode between 2013 and 2019, and more than one-third (37 percent) reported "persistently feeling sad or hopeless in the past year" (Bitsko et al., 2022). Some conditions commonly occur together. For example, about 74 percent of children with depression also have anxiety (CDC, 2023). Suicide rates among children and adolescents aged 10–24 years have increased dramatically since 2007—reaching nearly 0.11 percent in 2018 (Curtin, 2020). Physical and mental health comorbidities are also common in children (Chavira et al., 2008; Merikangas et al., 2015; Romano et al., 2021). Transgender and non-binary youth are at increased risk for depression, suicidality, and self-harm (Connolly et al., 2016; Price-Feeney et al., 2020; Rimes et al., 2019).

The COVID-19 pandemic increased mental health risks in children and adolescents, particularly those from disadvantaged backgrounds (Fegert et al., 2020; NASEM, 2023). Children in the United States were more likely to experience anxiety or depression during the first year of the pandemic (as compared with previous years), with 5.6 million children diagnosed with anxiety and 2.4 million children diagnosed with depression in 2020 (AECD, 2022; Lebrun-Harris et al., 2022). From 2019 to 2020, there was a 21 percent year-over-year increase in diagnoses of behavior or conduct problems (Lebrun-Harris et al., 2022). In addition, the disruption of schooling for most children in 2020–2021 due to the states' and communities' response to the pandemic has had and will likely continue to have serious consequences for children for a number of years (NASEM, 2023). For example, the rate of teen suicide and the burden of pediatric mental health problems increased during the COVID-19 pandemic (Charpignon et al., 2022; Yard et al., 2021).

Even before the COVID-19 pandemic, improving access to and quality of child mental health care has been a national priority area (Hoagwood and Olin, 2002; Hogan, 2003; NRC and IOM, 2004; Stroul and Friedman, 1986) supported by evidence that the child mental health care system is often inaccessible, ineffective, and inequitable (Coker et al., 2016; Danielson et al., 2018; Epstein et al., 2014; Kalb et al., 2019; Whitney and Peterson, 2019; Zima et al., 2010). Among children and adolescents aged 3–17 years, about 10 percent had received mental health services, and nearly 8 percent had taken medication for their disorder (Bitsko et al., 2022). However, while evidence based-treatments (e.g., psychotherapy, parent training, applied behavior analysis, psychotropic medications) are effective for common child mental health disorders (AHRQ, 2017, 2022; Cheung et al., 2013; Fristad and MacPherson, 2014; Müller et al., 2014; Slocum et al., 2014), nearly half (49.4 percent) of children with a mental health disorder do not receive needed treatment or counseling (Whitney and Peterson, 2019). Treatment status can also vary by disorder. For example, nearly 80 percent of children with depression report receiving treatment within the past year, but only 59 percent of children with anxiety reported receiving treatment (Ghandour et al., 2019). The adverse consequences of untreated or inadequately treated mental health disorders include increased child risk for suicide (Siffel et al., 2020), school failure (Finning et al., 2019; Kuriyan et al., 2013; Loe and Feldman, 2007), and traumatic injury (Brunkhorst-Kanaan et al., 2021; Chang et al., 2018a). Furthermore, nearly 10 percent of U.S. pediatric hospitalizations are for a primary mental health diagnosis, and rates continue to rise (Bardach et al., 2014). Among hospitalizations, the most frequent and costly diagnoses are depression (44 percent; $1.33 billion), bipolar disorder (18 percent; $702 million), and psychosis (12 percent; $540 million) (Bardach et al., 2014). The 10-year rise in U.S. children's hospitalizations was five times greater for mental health diagnoses compared with other conditions, costing $1.6 billion (Zima et al., 2016). Following COVID-19 school closure orders, among 44 U.S. children's hospitals, hospitalizations for suicide attempt or self-injury rose by 42 percent (Zima et al., 2022).

Source of Demand for Subspecialty Care

Subspecialty consultation and referral demand can be driven by patients, families, or primary care clinicians who perceive a need for consult with a subspecialist. Demand for subspecialty services also results from patient visits to emergency departments, between subspecialists themselves (cross-referral), or from subspecialty-generated return appointments.

Patients and Families

Patients and families may induce demand by directly seeking subspecialty care (self-referral) or consult with their primary care clinician about the need for referral to a subspecialist. Primary care clinicians report that patient/parent pressure is a common reason for a referral (Kaul et al., 2015; Kunin et al., 2018; Little et al., 2004), and as a result, they may refer in order to maintain patient satisfaction, which is often incentivized by health systems. For example, "readiness to refer your child to another physician in a timely manner?" is included as a question to rate professional competence on a validated standardized questionnaire for patient satisfaction in the pediatric outpatient setting (Bitzer et al., 2012). In a survey of pediatricians, 4 in 10 reported that they sometimes or often made unnecessary referrals to specialists based on patient request (Kaul et al., 2015). Patient demand for subspecialty care may also increase via self-referral if there is constrained access to primary care or if they feel that referral for care of a particular problem is inevitable. Ray et al. (2016) identified five desired outcomes for subspecialty referrals: improved current health status, improved long-term health outcomes, increased knowledge and understanding of their disease and/or treatment, informed family expectations for care goals, and reduced anxiety regarding changes in their child's health status. During one of the committee's public webinars, LaToshia Rouse, birth and postpartum doula (Birth Sisters Doula Services), patient and family engagement consultant, and parent to children who have needed subspecialty care, stated:

> I would love to have a system that would allow me to go when I needed to go, but also have those telehealth system[s] when it was necessary. Some appointments could have been an e-mail. Some appointments could have been a test or a chart message. But some of them, I need you to see this, I need to see you.[3]

Primary Care Clinicians

Primary care clinicians may believe a subspecialty referral is needed if the health condition is rare and they lack the necessary expertise, they need advice on diagnosis or treatment for a complex problem, the patient needs a technical procedure, the patient needs ancillary services provided by a subspecialty team, or the patient has not responded to conventional therapy in primary care settings. An important determinant of primary care physicians' subspecialty referral behavior, which drives demand, is the breadth of their service provision. As the number of pediatric subspecialties has grown, many pediatricians may refer for conditions they might have treated themselves in the past. Pediatricians may also refer to subspecialists in response to disincentives to initiate care for certain patients such as lack of time to invest in patients with complex care needs and fear of malpractice for "failure to refer" (Pho, 2012).

Subspecialists

Subspecialists induce demand largely due to follow-up or return visits. One older study found that 75 percent of visits to medical subspecialists for children were for continuing care, with just 25 percent reported to be for new patients, and 73 percent of all visits resulted in a specialist request for a follow-up visit (Valderas et al., 2009). There is limited evidence to guide decision making on the frequency and timing of return subspecialty visits, resulting in wide practice variation. Administrative quotas for visit and

---

[3] The webinar recording can be accessed at https://www.nationalacademies.org/event/07-19-2022/the-pediatric-subspecialty-workforce-and-its-impact-on-child-health-and-well-being-webinar-1.

procedure volume may incentivize specialists to induce demand, although the extent to which this occurs is unknown and merits examination.

Subspecialists can create additional demand by cross-referring to other specialists and converting primary care clinician-requested, short-term consults into longer term co-managed care, which often makes primary care clinicians' coordination of the referral more challenging. Some specialist-induced demand is necessary, such as during diagnostic evaluations and to ascertain treatment responsiveness. On the other hand, some follow-up visits may be unnecessary, or may be more appropriately performed in primary care settings. (For more on primary care–subspecialty collaboration and referrals, see Chapter 7.)

Hospitalization and Inpatient Consultations

Inpatient pediatric subspecialty consultation is not well described in the literature, but existing studies indicate there is likely wide variation in consultative practice related to patient, provider, and system factors (Darby et al., 2019; Kern-Goldberger et al., 2023; Sump et al., 2020). In children with medical complexity, inpatient consultations may decrease length of stay, cost of care, and subsequent hospitalizations (Mosquera et al., 2021). However, there are likely opportunities to be more judicious with inpatient consultation (Kern-Goldberger et al., 2021). Parallels exist to primary care consultation, including challenges ensuring clear communication between a primary inpatient clinician and the pediatric subspecialty consultant, consultations at the request of families, and because of medicolegal concerns (Kern-Goldberger et al., 2021).

ACCESS TO SUBSPECIALTY CARE

Access can be evaluated from the vantage of patients/families (how easy or difficult it is to obtain care), providers (organization of subspecialty care to make it available for patients), or the health system (how its financing and organization influence the equitable distribution of subspecialty services). Access can also be evaluated across multiple dimensions of experience: geospatial accessibility (e.g., location of providers), financial accessibility (e.g., out-of-pocket costs, insurance design), organizational accessibility (e.g., wait times), and equity (e.g., whether patients' opportunities to access subspecialty services are based on need, rather than socially determined characteristics). Chapter 7 provides more insights on access to care due to challenges at the primary care–subspecialty interface (i.e., consultation and referral between primary care clinicians and pediatric subspecialists). See Box 2-1 for family and clinician perspectives on access to subspecialty care.

> **BOX 2-1**
> **Family and Clinician Perspectives—**
> **Access to Subspecialty Care**
>
> "Patients in rural areas have no access within a several hour drive for certain subspecialties. Telehealth options should be offered/expanded to rural areas to meet the need for patients who live far from pediatric subspecialists."
> **– Pediatric Emergency Medicine Faculty, Houston, TX**
>
> "Pediatricians can be great gatekeepers for referrals, but whether that referral is accessible geographically or covered by insurance is another puzzle. They can also be difficult to get appointments with, especially as a new patient for a month or two. Even once you get those appointments, each specialist only looks at their particular system, so there's never a complete picture of what's happening in the body. Everything is always fragmented."
> **– Mother of a Patient**
>
> "Currently as a DBP I have a waitlist of over 700 patients for my next available new patient visit. If you are referred today, it is likely you would receive your final diagnosis in 18 months. This is a national tragedy in a time of a mental health crisis for youth."
> **– Developmental-Behavioral Pediatrician, Boston, MA**
>
> "In southern California, there is a backlog of many [pediatric subspecialists], which results in long, worrisome at times, waits for families, especially in the realms of neurology, endocrinology, dermatology, rheumatology, and autism care."
> **– Pediatric Nurse Practitioner, Orange County, CA**
>
> *These quotes were collected from the committee's online call for trainee, clinician, and family perspectives.*

Geospatial Accessibility

Patients and families are responsible for getting to the subspecialist and they may experience difficulty in traveling there because of the geographic distribution of subspecialists.[4] At the health-system level, the geospatial

---

[4] Technological innovations like telehealth may help reduce this access barrier for some patients, but not all. See Chapter 7 for more information on strategies and technologies to ensure equitable patient access to pediatric expertise.

distribution per population is a key factor. Turner et al. (2020) found that the number of pediatric subspecialists in the United States increased by 77 percent between 2003 and 2019, with increases varying across subspecialties. During the same period, the number of children in the United States remained the same, but the changing population density of children varied across the country (see Figure 2-2).

Driving Distance and Regionalization of Care

Driving distance is typically presented as a measure of geographic accessibility. Between 2003 and 2019, the mean driving distance for children decreased among all pediatric subspecialties, but the benefits of increased numbers of subspecialists on travel distance were not uniformly distributed across the United States or by subspecialty (Turner et al., 2020). Depending on the subspecialty, an estimated 1 million to 39 million children (2 to 53 percent) resided 80 miles or more from a subspecialist (Turner et al., 2020). Analyses by the American Board of Pediatrics also show variation in mean driving distance to care by subspecialty (ABP, 2023). However,

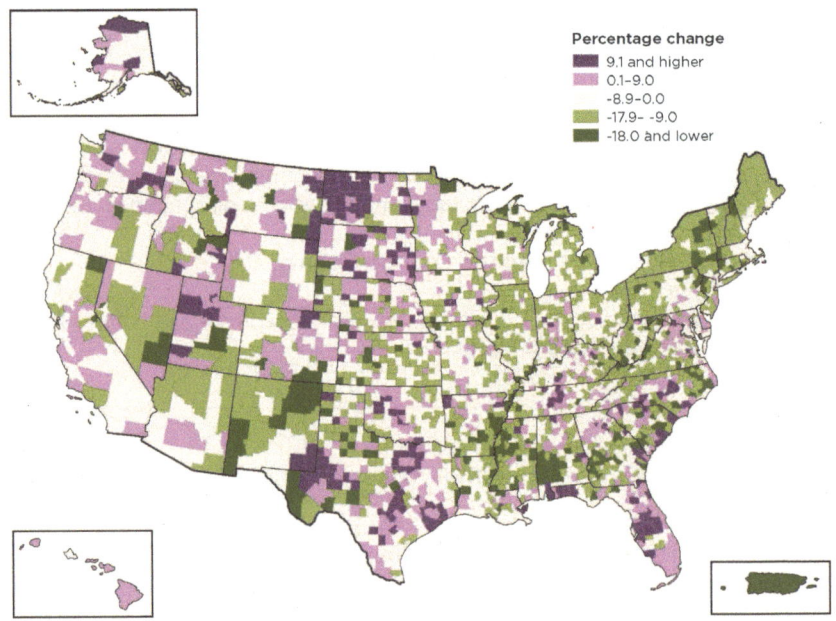

FIGURE 2-2 Percentage change among the population under age 18: 2010 to 2019.
SOURCE: U.S. Census Bureau, 2020. Modified and reprinted with permission from U.S. Census Bureau.

driving distance may not be an accurate representation of the challenges patients and families face in receiving subspecialty care. For example, these measurements may not take certain sites of care into account such as outreach clinics from larger academic medical centers; in part, these locations may not be accounted for because there is limited data on their locations and use (Freed, 2021; Turner et al., 2022). During one of the committee's public webinars, Joanna Lewis, pediatric residency program director and director for mobile health services at Advocate Children's Hospital in Park Ridge, IL, described her program, which uses partnerships with hospitals and health systems to create multi-specialty pediatric ambulatory hubs (e.g., school-based health center, mobile unit) that provide local access to care.[5]

It is likely not a fair expectation for all children to live within a short distance of every type of subspecialist. As noted by Mayer (2006), "the practice locations of pediatric subspecialists parallel the geographic distribution of children in the United States." The committee recognizes that more rural communities, for example, will not likely support full subspecialty practices, and so traveling for subspecialty care will likely always be necessary for various populations. Factors contributing to the regionalization of subspecialists include "that highly specialized physicians would be unlikely to have enough patients to attend to in any single community" and that access to technologies and other resources for care would be more available in centralized care centers (Gans et al., 2013). Furthermore, concentration of subspecialty care into centralized pediatric care centers leads to a higher volume of experience with rarer conditions and is associated with better outcomes (as compared to centers that see fewer cases per condition) (Howell et al., 2007; Khan et al., 2015; Lasswell et al., 2010; Michelson et al., 2018; Myers et al., 2019). Associated with regionalization, partnerships between larger hospital and community-based settings can help improve access to care for some subspecialties. For example, neonatal intensive care units are typically tiered according to the intensity of care they provide; as a result, some less complicated services may be provided in community-based settings, allowing for partnerships between facilities to provide comprehensive care (Stark et al., 2023). Outreach clinics, as described above, may also help extend the reach of centralized subspecialty care. Finally, when it comes to geographic distribution, accessibility to pediatric subspecialists, especially for rural and frontier communities, may be more directly impacted by lack of transportation or the unavailability of telehealth options, including reliable broadband access (Cortelyou-Ward et

---

[5] The webinar recording can be accessed at https://www.nationalacademies.org/event/09-06-2022/the-pediatric-subspecialty-workforce-and-its-impact-on-child-health-and-well-being-webinar-2.

al., 2020; Marcin et al., 2016; Wolfe et al., 2020). (See Chapter 7 for more on the use of telehealth.)

Hospital Settings

Although most children receive pediatric subspecialty care in outpatient settings, inpatient care is another important access point for children who require pediatric subspecialty care. Overall, pediatric hospitalizations are decreasing, but children are admitted with increasing acuity and complexity of illness (Berry et al., 2013; Elixhauser, 2008; Horak et al., 2019; Witt et al., 2014). In addition, children are less likely to be cared for in non-academic, community hospitals, but instead are admitted to academic medical centers that offer tertiary care (i.e. comprehensive care across a wide range of conditions) (França and McManus, 2017). This change in care setting, driven in part by chronicity and complexity of illness as well as other health policies, resulted in an emerging trend in community hospitals closing their inpatient pediatric units, necessitating a shift in inpatient pediatric care to regional, tertiary-care children's hospitals (Krugman and Rauch, 2022). Closure of inpatient pediatric units impacts access to pediatric subspecialty inpatient care, but also limits outpatient pediatric subspecialty care in those communities as well (Chang, 2018; França and McManus, 2018; Krugman and Rauch, 2022; VonAchen et al., 2022). Wider implications including patient outcomes and cost of care are not yet clear.

Financial Accessibility

Cost of care, insurance status, and insurance design can impact whether and how quickly patients can obtain subspecialty care due to limited networks, high out-of-pocket payments, and broader financing issues that affect access. See Chapter 8 for more information on the financing of children's health care.

Barriers due to Insurance Type and Status

While all children may experience challenges in access to subspecialty care, these challenges may be magnified based on the specific type of insurance (i.e., Medicaid, Children's Health Insurance Program [CHIP], private) and insurance status (i.e., insured versus uninsured). In general, being insured improves access to subspecialty care (Davidoff et al., 2005; Skinner and Mayer, 2007). Indeed, expansions in insurance coverage over the past decades, including expanded Medicaid eligibility for children, CHIP, the Affordable Care Act, and other changes have been successful in removing the barrier of uninsurance for 95 percent of U.S. children (Tolbert et al., 2022).

In an older study by Bisgaier and Rhodes (2011), 66 percent of callers to specialty clinics were denied appointments when they reported Medicaid/CHIP insurance compared with 11 percent of callers who reported having commercial insurance. Among 89 clinics that accepted Medicaid/CHIP and private insurance, callers indicating Medicaid/CHIP enrollment were given on average a 22-day longer wait time. In a similar study, Bisgaier and colleagues (2012) found that callers with Medicaid/CHIP experienced lower rates of denial for appointments if the specialty clinic was affiliated with an academic medical center. However, callers with Medicaid/CHIP were given a 40-day longer wait time on average by these academic specialty clinics than callers with private insurance. Additionally, a meta-analysis of appointment availability audit studies that examined both pediatric and adult patients found that patients with Medicaid insurance experienced more difficulty securing an appointment for specialty care compared with primary care (Hsiang et al., 2019).

For both adults and children, Timbie et al. (2019) found that difficulty obtaining new patient specialty visits reported by community health centers varied by insurance type, with most respondents reporting difficulty for patients with no insurance (84 percent) or Medicaid (57 percent). The community health centers that reported difficulty obtaining specialty care for their patients insured by Medicaid rated several barriers as often or always contributing to poor access, including barriers related to "payment, coverage, and availability of appointments, including low Medicaid payment rates for specialists (78 percent), few specialists in Medicaid managed care organization (MCO) networks accepting new patients (69 percent), lack of Medicaid coverage for telemedicine (49 percent), and Medicaid MCOs' administrative requirements for obtaining specialist consults (49 percent)" (Timbie et al., 2019). More research is needed to determine whether these denial trends have improved, worsened, or stayed the same over the past decade, and whether there are different rates for children and adults.

Difficulties in Cross State Access due to Insurance Policies

For some patients, the distance to the closest pediatric subspecialist or academic medical center is much shorter in a neighboring state compared to one within their own state, particularly in certain rural areas. For these patients and families, an out-of-state hospital is often the closest and most convenient option, ensuring they can receive cutting-edge care while lessening their transportation burdens (Meyer, 2021). While the issue of out-of-state care affects all populations, it is particularly relevant in the field of pediatrics. A review examining Medicaid payment for out-of-state hospital services found that children's hospitals serve a higher share of patients from out of state than any other type of hospital, with nearly 90 percent of children's hospitals treating Medicaid patients that reside outside of their state compared to just under 60% of short-term acute care hospitals (MACPAC, 2020).

Health insurance may pose a barrier to accessing care out of state. Some health insurance plans may not cover out-of-state care or may have greater out-of-pocket costs if the out-of-state care is not considered in-network; this varies by type of insurance (e.g., commercial, or public) and by type of plan (e.g., Health Management Organizations, Preferred Provider Organizations, Exclusive Provider Organizations, Point of Service Plans) (Aetna, 2023).[6] (See Chapter 8 for more information on network adequacy and narrow networks.) In Medicaid, federal law requires states to cover out-of-state services under certain circumstances, including a medical emergency; cases in which the beneficiary's health would be at risk if they were required to travel to the state of residence; situations where services or resources are more readily available in another state; or instances where it is common practice for Medicaid recipients in a particular locality to use medical resources in another state (42 CFR § 431.52; MACPAC, 2020). However, administrative challenges may hinder provider availability to provide out-of-state care. Both clinicians and out-of-state hospitals must enroll with the patient's home state Medicaid program and fulfill screening requirements. The specific requirements, as well as the time needed for screening and enrolling out-of-state providers, vary widely from state to state in terms of their approach, operational processes, application procedures, and verification timelines (GAO 2019; MACPAC, 2020; Manetto et al., 2020).[7] Providers are routinely asked to enroll and re-enroll in multiple out-of-state Medicaid programs, and these administrative measures may result in delays in care (Manetto et al., 2020).

In addition, pediatric patients with Medicaid insurance may face additional obstacles in accessing out-of-state services due to state Medicaid regulations that restrict or limit out-of-state payments. States have some flexibility in determining reimbursement rates for out-of-state hospitals that may affect providers' willingness to serve out-of-state Medicaid beneficiaries. For physician services covered under fee-for-service Medicaid, 26 of 36 states for which information could be found pay the in-state rate to out-of-state providers; of the remaining ten states, three use the in-state rate

---

[6] Both health maintenance organizations and exclusive provider organizations have closed networks, meaning nonemergency care from out-of-network providers generally is not covered (Pollitz, 2022).

[7] All states implemented Section 1135 waivers to allow out-of-state providers with equivalent licensing in another state to provide care to Medicaid enrollees during the pandemic, though many states have let those waivers lapse. For more information, see Chapter 7.

as a floor for out-of-state payment (MACPAC, 2017). For payment under Medicaid managed care, plans set reimbursement rates (Meyer, 2021). Some states have established different payment rates for out-of-state hospitals located in specific geographical areas. For example, Vermont's Medicaid state plan designates some hospitals in neighboring states as "out-of-state in-network hospitals" (border hospitals) and pays them the same rate as in-state hospitals due to their close proximity and the general practice of Vermont residents to receive care at these hospitals (DVHA 2023), while making lower payments to other out-of-state hospitals that are not designated as border hospitals (MACPAC, 2020). Similar policies are being considered by other states, particularly for children's hospitals in neighboring states, with the aim of achieving near-parity with in-state facilities (Meyer, 2021).

In 2021, CMS issued guidance outlining best practices to ensure that children with complex medical conditions receive prompt care out of state when medically necessary, including (1) states should pursue an abbreviated timeline for provider screening and enrollment, (2) states should promote access to telehealth services from out-of-state providers, and (3) states should establish economic and efficient provider payment rates to "ensure access to care and services available under the state plan and, under certain circumstances, provide coverage and payment when services are provided by out-of-state providers who serve children with medically complex conditions, consistent with section 1902(a)(30)(A) of the Act and 42 CFR § 431.52. States use a variety of payment methods to set rates paid to out-of-state providers and these methods should be clearly described in the Medicaid state plan" (CMS, 2021). CMS also released guidance in 2022 on a new Medicaid health home benefit for children with medically complex conditions that includes providing access to the full range of pediatric specialty and subspecialty medical services, including services from out-of-state providers (CMS, 2022). (See Chapter 7 for more information.)

Out-of-Pocket Costs

Children forgo or reduce service use in response to various cost-sharing mechanisms such as health plan deductibles and co-payments, a finding first reported by the classic RAND Health Insurance Experiment (Leibowitz et al., 1985). Over the past 15 years, while the proportion of children insured has expanded, there has been a steady growth in the number of children enrolled in high-deductible health plans. A data analysis commissioned by this committee from HealthCore found that use of high-deductible plans increased from 0.5 percent of the study population with commercial insurance in 2006 to 26 percent in 2021.[8] (See Chapter 3 for more on this data

---

[8] Commissioned HealthCore data analysis can be accessed in the Public Access File.

analysis.) This increase was also reported by Larson et al. (2021); using data from the National Health Interview Survey, Larson and colleagues found that the proportion of children with private insurance who were enrolled in these plans increased from 18 percent in 2007 to 49 percent in 2018 (Larson et al., 2021). That study defined these plans as those with a minimum deductible of $2,700 per family per year. They also found that compared with children with conventional private insurance, those with high-deductible health plans were more likely to forgo needed medical care and reported problems paying medical bills. More work is needed to understand how these plans are shaping children's use of needed subspecialty care.

Another attribute of health plans that can increase costs of care for children is the composition of the provider network. Many plans include tiers of cost sharing, with reduced costs for using providers within a defined network and higher out-of-pocket costs for those providers who are out of network. Children with rare or complex diseases are more likely to need specialized providers who are not within a plan's network. A recent study of children enrolled in commercial insurance found that those with complex chronic diseases were most likely to obtain out-of-network care, incurring markedly higher costs (Xu et al., 2022).

Other Financial Factors

Other patient and family financial factors may influence accessibility to care. For example, the ability to receive care may be influenced by the ability to take time off work to attend a medical visit (and the associated lost wages), the cost for child care for other children in the family, and transportation costs (Chang et al., 2018b). Additionally, little is known about how financial incentives inherent in alternative physician payment systems influence subspecialists' decisions about use of specialized technology, frequency of follow-up visits, and availability of visits.

Organizational Accessibility

How subspecialty care is organized within a health care system contributes to the accessibility of that care, a dimension that can be monitored to some degree by appointment wait times. Most clinics monitor appointment wait time, often operationalized as the *time to first visit for new patients*. The number of subspecialists, the proportion of their time spent in clinical care, the balance of new versus follow-up visits, model of care (e.g., use of advanced practice registered nurses and generalists within the clinic), subspecialist-induced demand for follow-up, and the appointment system itself all influence appointment wait times. However, the relative contribution of each of these factors to overall pediatric subspecialty access is currently unknown.

In a survey of 8,583 pediatric medical subspecialists conducted from 2012 to 2015, 10 percent of respondents reported typical wait times of longer than 8 weeks, with highest levels reported for developmental-behavioral pediatrics (50 percent), neurology (30 percent), endocrinology (23 percent), and rheumatology (16 percent) (Rimsza et al., 2018). Long wait times to see a specialist are associated with increased chances of not attending the first visit with a specialist for a new health problem and forgoing needed care (Stephens et al., 2019).

One possible reason for the longer wait times in some subspecialties may be the changing epidemiology of pediatric disorders, noted earlier in this chapter. For example, it is possible that a contributing factor to the long wait times for subspecialties such as developmental-behavioral pediatrics and child neurology is the increasing number of children with diagnosed neurodevelopmental disorders (Visser et al., 2014), some of whom may be children who were born and survive at a greater severity of prematurity.

In 2017, the Children's Hospital Association surveyed 40 children's teaching hospitals to highlight the specialties with the longest appointment wait times and vacancies (i.e., staffing shortages) at their institutions (CHA, 2017). Developmental pediatrics, child and adolescent psychiatry, and pediatric neurology were ranked as the specialties with the largest shortages affecting ability to deliver care. The specialties with the longest appointment wait times included genetics (21 weeks), developmental pediatrics (19 weeks), pain management and palliative care (12 weeks), and child and adolescent psychiatry (10 weeks). See Chapter 7 for more on referral innovations to reduce wait times.

Accessibility Related to Demographic and Cultural Factors

A variety of demographic and cultural factors (e.g., race/ethnicity, language, gender identity, educational level) can influence a person's ability to access needed health care. Studies of implicit bias in health care (in general) show that "biases are likely to influence diagnosis and treatment decisions and levels of care in some circumstances" (FitzGerald and Hurst, 2017, p.1). While the literature base on these influences specific to pediatric medical subspecialty care is limited, the following sections provide an overview of several demographic and cultural factors that can influence access to care.

Racial and Ethnic Disparities in Access

As noted by Flores and Lin (2013), "minority children continue to experience multiple disparities in medical and oral health and healthcare."

In particular, they noted that all minoritized groups (except for Asian/Pacific Islander) had difficulty accessing specialty care (as compared with White children). Disparities by race and ethnicity persist for children's access to general and subspecialty physical and mental health care (Alberto et al., 2019; Burdick et al., 2023; Rodgers et al., 2022). For example, in one study of children with medical complexity insured by Medicaid, Black non-Hispanic and Hispanic children had lower outpatient visit rates as compared with White non-Hispanic children (Ming et al., 2022). Another study of children with ADHD concluded that "disparities in ADHD treatment among children from racial–ethnic minority populations may be driven primarily by disparities in access rather than in utilization." (Yang et al., 2022). (See Chapter 6 for more on diversity in research.)

Racial and ethnic disparities in access to care may be related to the fact that some patients have indicated a preference for racial/ethnic concordance in their health care practitioners (i.e., someone of their own rate or ethnicity), and racial/ethnic concordance has been associated with reduction in health care disparities and increased patient satisfaction (Alberto et al., 2021; Greenwood et al., 2020; Takeshita et al., 2020). However, the diversity of the pediatric health care workforce in general, and the pediatric subspecialty workforce specifically, does not reflect the diversity of the population it serves. (See Chapter 4 for more on workforce diversity.)

Immigration Status

Some limited evidence shows that immigration status may be associated with barriers to needed health care in general, such as policies that limit access to insurance (Perreira and Pedroza, 2019). This may be particularly important for pregnant women who are ineligible for Medicaid (because of their immigration status) and as a result receive inadequate prenatal care. Insurance eligibility expansions have been associated with increased use of prenatal care (Drewry et al., 2015; Fuentes-Afflick et al., 2006).

Language Barriers

Language-specific barriers can affect the ability of children to access needed subspecialty care (Cohen and Christakis, 2006; Flower et al., 2021; St. Amant et al., 2018; Wojcik et al., 2023; Yu et al., 2004). Particular challenges include lack of bilingual interpreters and difficulty for the child's parents in communicating over the phone. Language concordance care has been defined as "the provision of health care in a shared non-dominant minority language" (Lor and Martinez, 2020). In general, language concordance has been associated with levels of trust and patient satisfaction, but has mixed evidence for its impact on health outcomes (Hsueh et al., 2021; Lor and Martinez, 2020). In pediatrics specifically, language concordance, including the use of interpreters, has been associated with greater satisfaction, improved communication, and enhanced understanding (Dunlap et al., 2015; Gutman et al., 2018; Jaramillo et al., 2016). In addition, studies show underrepresentation of non-English-speaking children or children of non-English-speaking parents in pediatric research (Aristizabal et al., 2015; Chen et al., 2023).

Transitioning from Pediatric to Adult Care

Many adolescents with chronic conditions experience fragmented care as they transition from pediatric to adult subspecialty care and may receive care from pediatric clinicians into adulthood (Lebrun-Harris et al., 2018; McManus et al., 2020). The transition from child to adult medical and behavioral health care often is associated with poor outcomes among young adults, with challenges including discontinuities in care, differences between the child/adolescent and adult health systems, a lack of available adult clinicians, difficulties in breaking the bond with pediatric clinicians, lack of payment for transition support, a lack of training in childhood-onset conditions among adult clinicians, the failure of pediatric clinicians to prepare adolescents for an adult model of care, and a lack of communication between pediatric and adult clinicians and systems of care (NASEM, 2015). In terms of pediatric specialty care, only 17 percent of youth with special health care needs and 14 percent of youth without special health care needs receive anticipatory guidance on transition preparation from their health care providers (Lebrun-Harris et al., 2018).

While the transition of care to adult clinicians is complex and requires the cooperation of patients and their families, clinicians play an essential role in successful transition (White et al., 2018). Got Transition's *Six Core Elements of Health Care Transition™ 3.0* is the widely adopted approach based on a report from a coalition that included the Academy of Pediatrics, the American Academy of Family Physicians, and the American College of Physicians (White et al., 2020). The *Six Core Elements* define the basic components of a structured transition process and include customizable sample tools for each core element, with tailoring to the type of practice facilitating the health care transition and type of condition (see Table 2-1).

Many well-described barriers to transition of care exist at the clinician level, particularly the lack of coordination between pediatric and adult clinicians at the time of transition. The list of potential clinician-level barriers to transition is extensive (see Box 2-2).

TABLE 2-1 Summary of *Six Core Elements* approach for pediatric and adult practices

Practice or Provider	#1: Transition and/or care policy	#2: Tracking and monitoring	#3: Transition readiness and/or orientation to adult practice	#4: Transition planning and/or integration into adult approach to care or practice	#5: Transfer of care and/or initial visit	#6: Transition completion or ongoing care
Pediatric	Create and discuss with youth and/or family	Track progress of youth and/or family transition preparation and transfer	Conduct transition readiness assessments	Develop transition plan, including needed readiness assessment skills and medical summary, prepare youth for adult approach to care, and communicate with new clinician	Transfer of care with information and communication including residual pediatric clinician's responsibility	Obtain feedback on the transition process and confirm young adult has been seen by the new clinician
Adult	Create and discuss with young adult and guardian, if needed	Track progress of young adult's integration into adult care	Share and discuss welcome and FAQs with young adult and guardian, if needed	Communicate with previous clinician, ensure receipt of transfer package	Review transfer package, address young adult's needs and concerns at initial visit, update self-care assessment and medical summary	Confirm transfer completion with previous clinician, provide ongoing care with self-care skill building and link to needed specialists

NOTE: Clinicians who care for youth and/or young adults throughout the lifespan can use both the pediatric and adult sets of core elements without the transfer process components.

SOURCES: White et al., 2020. Copyright ©2014–2023 GOT TRANSITION®.

Certain types of pediatric patients face additional barriers. For example, an analysis of 2017 National Electronic Health Records Survey data found that pediatricians are more likely to accept Medicaid insurance than adult clinicians (MACPAC, 2021). This raises questions about how difficult it is for pediatric patients with Medicaid insurance to transition to adult care. Understanding these use patterns is critical when implementing transition of care programs.

USE OF SUBSPECIALTY CARE

Use of subspecialty care indicates whether a service is received; it does not say whether the service was needed or the quality of that service provision. Pediatric subspecialists assist children and their families by attending to health problems referred to them, providing advice, performing procedures, and sharing in the care of patients with unstable health conditions. Four types of referrals encapsulate these responsibilities: (1) short-term non-procedural consultation for diagnostic or treatment advice; (2) short-term procedural consultation for a specific diagnostic evaluation (e.g., echocardiogram, allergy testing) or management (e.g., endoscopy for a gastrointestinal bleed); (3) longer term co-management in which they share care for the health problem with primary care clinicians; and (4) principal care, which involves co-management with the specialist providing all the care for a given problem (Forrest, 2009). See Chapter 3 for data analyses on the use of pediatric subspecialty care and Chapter 7 for more on the primary care–subspecialist interface, including referral.

OUTCOMES OF SUBSPECIALTY CARE

Advances in pediatric care in general have led to dramatic improvements in the health and well-being of children (see Chapter 1). Measuring quality of care, including clinical outcomes, can be difficult in subspecialty pediatrics given the low prevalence of many of the conditions addressed by subspecialists, the impact of different developmental stages among pediatric patients, and the challenges of demonstrating long-term impact of care (Schuster, 2015). Evidence from small studies of individual subspecialties suggests that pediatric subspecialists are more likely to perform comprehensive assessments and adhere to evidence-based guidelines of care for a particular disorder, compared with care by non-specialists (Cloutier et al., 2018; Conway et al., 2006; Feldman et al., 2015; Hudgins et al., 2021; McCulloh et al., 2012). Evidence on clinical outcomes from subspecialty care (as compared to non-specialty care or no care) is limited. Specific examples from individual studies include:

> **BOX 2-2**
> **Transition Barriers between Pediatric and Adult Clinicians**
>
> **Communication and/or Consultation Gaps**
> - Lack of communication, coordination, guidelines, and protocols between the pediatric and adult systems
> - Inadequate communication from pediatric clinicians, often with a lack of medical records and follow-up recommendations
> - Lack of long-term follow-up guidelines with children and youth with special health care needs
> - Gap in consultation with pediatric clinicians
> - Adult clinicians' concerns about not enough adult subspecialty or mental health care clinicians to care for young adults
>
> **Training Limitations**
> - Lack of knowledge and/or training in pediatric-onset conditions and adolescent development and behavior
> - Difficulty meeting psychosocial needs of young adults with pediatric-onset conditions
> - Caring for adult patients reliant on caregivers
>
> **Care Delivery, Care Coordination, and/or Staff Support Gaps**
> - Lack of care coordination and follow-up
> - Lack of mental health and supportive services
> - Unfamiliarity with local and regional resources for young adults with chronic conditions
> - Lack of adequate infrastructure and training
> - Administrative constraints and lack of time and reimbursement
> - Lack of insurance coverage for young adults

- Survival from pediatric non-traumatic cardiac arrest in pediatric emergency departments was higher than in general emergency departments (Michelson et al., 2018).
- Five-year survival rates for pediatric leukemias were significantly lower (46.4 percent versus 75.1 percent) for patients not treated at a pediatric cancer center (Howell et al., 2007).
- Lung transplantation in children was associated with better survival when performed at pediatric centers as opposed to adult centers, even if the volume at the adult centers (including adult transplantation) was higher (Khan et al., 2015).
- There is some evidence of better outcomes when surgery is performed by a pediatric surgeon as compared to general surgeons (Borenstein et al., 2005; Evans and van Woerden, 2011).

Lack of Patient Knowledge and Engagement
- Young adults' lack of knowledge about disease treatments, medications, and medical history
- Lack of information about community resources and/or support groups
- Dependency on parents or guardians
- Lack of self-advocacy, decision-making skills, and self-care skills
- Poor adherence to care
- Unrealistic expectations of youth or young adult knowledge of adult medical system and lack of readiness for adult care

Lack of Comfort with Adult Care
- Unrealistic youth, young adult, and family expectations of time and attention
- Concerns regarding loss of strong relationships with previous clinicians (patient, parent, and/or staff)
- Pediatric clinicians' lack of confidence in adult clinician and in the stylistic differences between pediatric and adult care, particularly for some youth and young adults with intellectual or developmental disabilities or behavioral health conditions
- Parents' reluctance to relinquish responsibility
- Parents unaware of changes in privacy issues/changes in privacy requirements among clinicians, caregivers, and young adult patients

SOURCE: Adapted from White et al., 2018. Reproduced with permission from *Pediatrics*. Copyright © 2018 by the AAP.

Medical advances in the twentieth century and more recently have resulted in more children with complex medical needs surviving past infancy, increasing the need for timely access to pediatric subspecialty care (Lonetti et al., 2019; Oh et al., 2022; Siegel et al., 2020). For example, between 2002 and 2016, death rates decreased for some childhood cancers such as pediatric leukemias and lymphomas (Siegel et al., 2020). Survival rates for children with acute myeloid leukemia are now at 70 percent (Lonetti et al., 2019). Yet despite these gains, the impact on survival varies by type of disorders, type of treatment, and sociodemographic characteristics. For example, from 2001 to 2015, survival from pediatric cancers were highest among females, those aged 15 to 19 years, non-Hispanic Whites, and those residing in counties in the top 25 percent by economic status (Siegel et al., 2020). According to Yohe et al. (2019), "overall survival rates for pediatric patients with high-risk or relapsed rhabdomyosarcoma have not improved significantly since the 1980s." Advanced heart failure in children with congenital heart disease is uncommon but increasing and is associated with significant morbidity, mortality, and resource use, with approximately one in five affected children not surviving to hospital discharge (Burstein et al., 2019). Moreover, children's all-cause mortality rates in the United States are increasing, although much of this is attributable to increases in injury-related deaths, including gun violence (Woolf et al., 2023).

KEY FINDINGS AND CONCLUSIONS

Key Findings

Finding #2-1: There have been significant changes in the physical, mental, and behavioral health status of the U.S. pediatric population, which drives need and demand for subspecialty care.

Finding #2-2: Children's health needs are becoming increasingly more complex.

Finding #2-3: There are factors beyond provider supply that impact access to needed pediatric subspecialty care, including patient/family factors (e.g., insurance and out-of-pocket costs, time availability, broadband access, and transportation), subspecialty provider factors (e.g., provider network, care model), and health system-level factors (e.g., reimbursement model, geospatial distribution of clinicians, and equity).

Finding #2-4: Demand for subspecialty care is driven by patients and families (including self-referral), primary care clinicians (for short-term consultation or long-term co-management), and subspecialists themselves (for return visits or for cross-referral to other subspecialists).

Finding #2-5: Children covered by Medicaid, rural children, and children with chronic illness or special health care needs often face increased access barriers to pediatric subspecialty care.

Finding #2-6: The financial viability to support a practice in some locations, such as rural areas (given the lower prevalence of many disorders cared for by subspecialists), contributes to the geographic distribution of subspecialists.

Finding #2-7: The increase in closings of both rural and urban hospitals, and diminished pediatric services within non-children's hospitals, further exacerbates the problem of limited access to pediatric subspecialty care.

Finding #2-8: High-volume experience with children is associated with improved health outcomes.

Finding #2-9: Demographic and cultural factors such as racial/ethnic concordance, language, and immigration status can influence access to care.

Conclusions

Conclusion #2-1: Pediatric medical subspecialists play a pivotal role in enhancing the survival and health of children with chronic conditions and complex health care needs.

Conclusion #2-2: Children's use of subspecialty care is influenced by a complex and interconnected mix of patient, family, community, provider, and health system factors.

Conclusion #2-3: Regionalization of medical subspecialty care is logical given the lower prevalence of conditions requiring subspecialty care and the technologies and resources available in centralized centers of care.

Conclusion #2-4: The pediatric workforce and the health care system more generally need to be nimble in their ability to be responsive to the changing health care needs of infants, children, and adolescents.

Conclusion #2-5: A systematic approach to monitoring children's changing health needs and access to pediatric primary and subspecialty care is needed to inform interventions to improve equity in subspecialty care as well as to prepare the optimal workforce to be able to address those needs.

RECOMMENDATION

The needs of children in the twenty-first century differ from the needs of those in the twentieth century. More attention is needed to ensure optimal access, coordination, and impact on the health and well-being of infants, children, and adolescents. The Agency for Healthcare Research and Quality (AHRQ) produces an annual report on health care quality and disparities (AHRQ, 2023). Similarly, improved monitoring of children's changing health needs and demands, access to care, disparities, and trends in the pediatric workforce are all essential to inform future workforce planning efforts. Understanding these trends will help determine the appropriate education and training needed to prepare the pediatric workforce to work collaboratively toward meeting children's health care needs and which subspecialties should be prioritized for different interventions or programs (e.g. loan repayment) and inform innovative models of care to improve access. Therefore, in order to achieve a goal of **promoting collaboration and effective use of services between pediatric primary care clinicians and subspecialty physicians,** the committee provides the following recommendation:

> RECOMMENDATION 2-1 The Agency for Healthcare Research and Quality should submit a biennial report to the Secretary of the Department of Health and Human Services summarizing the changing demands and needs for pediatric primary and subspecialty care, status of access to that care, and disparities in receipt of those services. This report should include information on the pediatric generalist and subspecialist workforce broadly (including data on clinicians from backgrounds underrepresented in medicine).

REFERENCES

ABP (American Board of Pediatrics). 2023. *Estimated driving distance to visit a pediatric subspecialist.* https://www.abp.org/content/estimated-driving-distance-visit-pediatric-subspecialist (accessed April 21, 2023).

AECD (Annie E. Casey Foundation). 2022. *2022 KIDS COUNT data book.* https://www.aecf.org/resources/2022-kids-count-data-book (accessed December 22, 2022).

Aetna. 2023. *HMO, POS, PPO, EPO and HDHP with HSA: What's the difference?* https://www.aetna.com/health-guide/hmo-pos-ppo-hdhp-whats-the-difference.html (accessed July 14, 2023).

AHRQ (Agency for Healthcare Research and Quality). 2017. *Anxiety in children.* https://effectivehealthcare.ahrq.gov/products/anxiety-children/research-2017 (accessed May 2, 2023).

AHRQ. 2022. *Attention deficit hyperactivity disorder: Diagnosis and treatment in children and adolescents.* https://effectivehealthcare.ahrq.gov/products/attention-deficit-hyperactivity-disorder/protocol (accessed May 2, 2023).

AHRQ. 2023. *National Healthcare Quality and Disparities Reports.* https://www.ahrq.gov/research/findings/nhqrdr/index.html (accessed May 5, 2023).

Alberto, C. K., J. Kemmick Pintor, R. M. McKenna, D. H. Roby, and A. N. Ortega. 2019. Racial and ethnic disparities in provider-related barriers to health care for children in California after the ACA. *Global Pediatric Health* 6:1-9.

Alberto, C. K., J. Kemmick Pintor, A. Martinez-Donate, L. P. Tabb, B. Langellier, and J. P. Stimpson. 2021. Association of maternal-clinician ethnic concordance with Latinx youth receipt of family-centered care. *JAMA Network Open* 4(11):e2133857.

Amminger, G. P., L. P. Henry, S. M. Harrigan, M. G. Harris, M. Alvarez-Jimenez, H. Herrman, H. J. Jackson, and P. D. McGorry. 2011. Outcome in early-onset schizophrenia revisited: Findings from the early psychosis prevention and intervention centre long-term follow-up study. *Schizophrenia Research* 131(1-3):112-119.

Anderson, G., and J. Horvath. 2002. *Chronic conditions: Making the case for ongoing care.* http://www.partnershipforsolutions.org/DMS/files/chronicbook2002.pdf (accessed April 13, 2023).

Arakelyan, M. S. Freyleue, D. Avula, J. L. McLaren, A. J. O'Malley, and J. K. Leyenaar. 2023. Pediatric mental health hospitalizations at acute care hospitals in the U.S., 2009-2019. *JAMA* 329(12):1000-1011.

Aristizabal, P., J. Singer, R. Cooper, K. J. Wells, J. Nodora, M. Milburn, S. Gahagan, D. E. Schiff, and M. E. Martinez. 2015. Participation in pediatric oncology research protocols: Racial/ethnic, language and age-based disparities. *Pediatric Blood & Cancer* 62(8):1337-1344.

Baio, J., L. Wiggins, D. L. Christensen, M. J. Maenner, J. Daniels, Z. Warren, M. Kurzius-Spencer, W. Zahorodny, C. R. Rosenberg, and T. White. 2018. Prevalence of autism spectrum disorder among children aged 8 years—Autism and Developmental Disabilities Monitoring Network, United States, 2014. *MMWR Surveillance Summaries* 67(6):1.

Bardach, N. S., T. R. Coker, B. T. Zima, J. M. Murphy, P. Knapp, L. P. Richardson, G. Edwall, and R. Mangione-Smith. 2014. Common and costly hospitalizations for pediatric mental health disorders. *Pediatrics* 133(4):602-609.

Berg, A. T., H. H. Altalib, and O. Devinsky. 2017. Psychiatric and behavioral comorbidities in epilepsy: A critical reappraisal. *Epilepsia* 58(7):1123-1130.

Berry, J. G., M. Hall, D. E. Hall, D. Z. Kuo, E. Cohen, R. Agrawal, K. D. Mandl, H. Clifton, and J. Neff. 2013. Inpatient growth and resource use in 28 children's hospitals: A longitudinal, multi-institutional study. *JAMA Pediatrics* 167(2):170-177.

Bisgaier, J., and K. V. Rhodes. 2011. Auditing access to specialty care for children with public insurance. *New England Journal of Medicine* 364(24):2324-2333.

Bisgaier, J., D. Polsky, and K. V. Rhodes. 2012. Academic medical centers and equity in specialty care access for children. *Archives of Pediatrics and Adolescent Medicine* 166(4):304-310.

Bitsko, R. H., A. H. Claussen, J. Lichstein, L. I. Black, S. E. Jones, M. L. Danielson, J. M. Hoenig, S. P. Davis Jack, D. J. Brody, S. Gyawali, M. J. Maenner, M. Warner, K. M. Holland, R. Perou, A. E. Crosby, S. J. Blumberg, S. Avenevoli, J. W. Kaminski, and R. M. Ghandour. 2022. Mental health surveillance among children—United States, 2013-2019. *Morbidity and Mortality Weekly Report* 71(Suppl 2):1-42.

Bitzer, E. M., S. Volkmer, M. Petrucci, N. Weissenrieder, and M.-L. Dierks. 2012. Patient satisfaction in pediatric outpatient settings from the parents' perspective—the child zap: A psychometrically validated standardized questionnaire. *BMC Health Services Research* 12(1):347.

Blackwell, C. K., A. J. Elliott, J. Ganiban, J. Herbstman, K. Hunt, C. B. Forrest, and C. A. Carmago, Jr. 2019. General health and life satisfaction in children with chronic illness. *Pediatrics* 143(6):e20182988.

Borenstein, S. H., T. To, A. Wajja, and J.C. Langer. 2005. Effect of subspecialty training and volume on outcome after pediatric inguinal hernia repair. *Journal of Pediatric Surgery* 40(1):75-80.

Bright, M. A., C. Knapp, M. S. Hinojosa, S. Alford, and B. Bonner. 2016. The comorbidity of physical, mental, and developmental conditions associated with childhood adversity: A population based study. *Maternal and Child Health Journal* 20:843-853.

Brunkhorst-Kanaan, N., B. Libutzki, A. Reif, H. Larsson, R. V. McNeill, and S. Kittel-Schneider. 2021. ADHD and accidents over the life span—a systematic review. *Neuroscience & Biobehavioral Reviews* 125:582-591.

Burdick, K. J., L. K. Lee, R. Mannix, M. C. Monuteaux, M. P. Hirsh, and E. W. Fleegler. 2023. Racial and ethnic disparities in access to pediatric trauma centers in the United States: A geographic information systems analysis. *Annals of Emergency Medicine* 81(3):325-333.

Burstein, D. S., P. Shamszad, D. Dai, C. S. Almond, J. F. Price, K. Y. Lin, M. J. O'Connor, R. E. Shaddy, C. E. Mascio, and J. W. Rossano. 2019. Significant mortality, morbidity and resource utilization associated with advanced heart failure in congenital heart disease in children and young adults. *American Heart Journal* 209:9-19.

Butwicka, A., W. Fendler, A. Zalepa, A. Szadkowska, M. Zawodniak-Szalapska, A. Gmitrowicz, and W. Mlynarski. 2016. Psychiatric disorders and health-related quality of life in children with type 1 diabetes mellitus. *Psychosomatics* 57(2):185-193.

CAHMI (Child and Adolescent Health Measurement Initiative). 2023a. *2020 National Survey of Children's Health (NSCH) data query: Indicator 1.9: Does this child have current or lifelong health conditions?* https://www.childhealthdata.org/browse/survey/results?q=8838&r=1 (accessed April 21, 2023).

CAHMI. 2023b. *2020 National Survey of Children's Health (NSCH) data query: Indicator 4.5: During the past 12 months, did this child see a specialist other than a mental health professional?* https://www.childhealthdata.org/browse/survey/results?q=9391&r=1&g=1000 (accessed April 21, 2023).

CDC (Centers for Disease Control and Prevention). 2020. *QuickStats: Percentage of children aged <18 years who received a well-child checkup in the past 12 months, by age group and year—National Health Interview Survey, United States, 2008 and 2018.* https://www.cdc.gov/mmwr/volumes/69/wr/mm6908a5.htm (accessed April 20, 2023).

CDC. 2021. *Children and youth with special healthcare needs in emergencies.* https://www.cdc.gov/childrenindisasters/children-with-special-healthcare-needs.html#:~:text=Children%20and%20youth%20with%20special%20healthcare%20needs%20(CYSHCN)%2C%20also,than%20their%20typically%20developing%20peers (accessed April 21, 2023).

CDC. 2022. *Diseases you almost forgot about (thanks to vaccines).* https://www.cdc.gov/vaccines/parents/diseases/forgot-14-diseases.html (accessed December 22, 2022).

CDC. 2023. *Data and statistics on children's mental health.* https://www.cdc.gov/childrensmentalhealth/data.html (accessed May 5, 2023).

CHA (Children's Hospital Association). 2017. *Pediatric workforce shortages persist* https://glin.com/files/documents/bulletin_board/chgme_workforce_shortage_fact_sheet.pdf (accessed April 21, 2023).

Chang, H.-K., J.-W. Hsu, J.-C. Wu, K.-L. Huang, H.-C. Chang, Y.-M. Bai, T.-J. Chen, and M.-H. Chen. 2018a. Traumatic brain injury in early childhood and risk of attention-deficit/hyperactivity disorder and autism spectrum disorder: A nationwide longitudinal study. *The Journal of Clinical Psychiatry* 79(6):21226.

Chang, L. V., A. N. Shah, E. R. Hoefgen, K. A. Auger, H. Weng, J. M. Simmons, S. S. Shah, and A. F. Beck on behalf of the H2O Study Group. 2018b. Lost earnings and nonmedical expenses of pediatric hospitalizations. *Pediatrics* 142(3):e20180195.

Chang, W. W. 2018. *The rapidly disappearing community pediatric inpatient unit.* https://www.the-hospitalist.org/hospitalist/article/170115/pediatrics/rapidly-disappearing-community-pediatric-inpatient-unit (accessed April 13, 2023).

Charpignon, M.-L., J. Ontiveros, S. Sundaresan, A. Puri, J. Chandra, K. D. Mandl, and M. S. Majumder. 2022. Evaluation of suicides among U.S. adolescents during the COVID-19 pandemic. *JAMA Pediatrics* 176(7):724-726.

Chavira, D. A., A. F. Garland, S. Daley, and R. Hough. 2008. The impact of medical comorbidity on mental health and functional health outcomes among children with anxiety disorders. *Journal of Developmental and Behavioral Pediatrics* 29(5):394-402.

Chen, A., S. Demaestri, K. Schweiberger, J. Sidani, R. Wolynn, D. Chaves-Gnecco, R. Hernandez, S. Rothenberger, E. Mickievicz, J. D. Cowden, and M. I. Ragavan. 2023. Inclusion of non-English speaking participants in pediatric research: A review. *JAMA Pediatrics* 177(1):81-88.

Cheung, A. H., N. Kozloff, and D. Sacks. 2013. Pediatric depression: An evidence-based update on treatment interventions. *Current Psychiatry Reports* 15:1-8.

Cloutier, M. M., P. M. Salo, L. J. Akinbami, R. D. Cohn, J. C. Wilkerson, G. B. Diette, S. Williams, K. S. Elward, J. M. Mazurek, J. R. Spinner, T. A. Mitchell, and D. C. Zeldin. 2018. Clinician agreement, self-efficacy, and adherence with the guidelines for the diagnosis and management of asthma. *Journal of Allergy and Clinical Immunology: In Practice* 6(3):886-894.e4.

CMS (Centers for Medicare & Medicaid Services). 2021. *Guidance on coordinating care provided by out-of-state providers for children with medically complex conditions.* https://www.medicaid.gov/federal-policy-guidance/downloads/cib102021.pdf (accessed April 18, 2023).

CMS. 2022. *Re: Health homes for children with medically complex conditions.* https://www.medicaid.gov/federal-policy-guidance/downloads/smd22004.pdf (accessed April 18, 2023).

Cohen, A. L., and D. A. Christakis. 2006. Primary language of parent is associated with disparities in pediatric preventive care. *The Journal of Pediatrics* 148(2):254-258.

Coker, T. R., M. N. Elliott, S. L. Toomey, D. C. Schwebel, P. Cuccaro, S. Tortolero Emery, S. L. Davies, S. N. Visser, and M. A. Schuster. 2016. Racial and ethnic disparities in ADHD diagnosis and treatment. *Pediatrics* 138(3):e20160407.

Connolly, M. D., M. J. Zervos, C. J. Barone II, C. C. Johnson, and C. L. M. Joseph. 2016. The mental health of transgender youth: Advances in understanding. *Journal of Adolescent Health* 59(5):489-495.

Conway, P. H., S. Edwards, E. R. Stucky, V. W. Chiang, M. C. Ottolini, and C. P. Landrigan. 2006. Variations in management of common inpatient pediatric illnesses: Hospitalists and community pediatricians. *Pediatrics* 118(2):441-447.

Cortelyou-Ward, K. D., N. Atkins, A. Noblin, T. Rotarius, Ph. White, and C. Carey. 2020. Navigating the digital divide: Barriers to telehealth in rural areas. *Journal of Health Care for the Poor and Underserved* 31(4):1546-1556.

Cree, R. A., R. H. Bitsko, L. R. Robinson, J. R. Holbrook, M. L. Danielson, C. Smith, J. W. Kaminski, M. K. Kenney, and G. Peacock. 2018. Health care, family, and community factors associated with mental, behavioral, and developmental disorders and poverty among children aged 2-8 years—United States, 2016. *Morbidity and Mortality Weekly Report* 67(50):1377-1383.

Curtin, S. 2020. State suicide rates among adolescents and young adults aged 10-24: United States, 2000–2018. *National Vital Statistics Reports* 69(11):1-10.

Danielson, M. L., R. H. Bitsko, R. M. Ghandour, J. R. Holbrook, M. D. Kogan, and S. J. Blumberg. 2018. Prevalence of parent-reported ADHD diagnosis and associated treatment among U.S. children and adolescents, 2016. *Journal of Clinical Child & Adolescent Psychology* 47(2):199-212.

Darby, J. B., N. Tamaskar, S. Kumar, K. Sexson, M. de Guzman, M. E. M. Rocha, and S. T. Shulman. 2019. Variability in Kawasaki disease practice patterns: A survey of hospitalists at pediatric hospital medicine 2017. *Hospital Pediatrics* 9(9):724-728.

Davidoff, A., G. Kenney, and L. Dubay. 2005. Effects of the State Children's Health Insurance Program expansions on children with chronic health conditions. *Pediatrics* 116(1):e34-e42.

Drewry, J., B. Sen, M. Wingate, J. Bronstein, E. M. Foster, and M. Kotelchuck. 2015. The impact of the State Children's Health Insurance Program's unborn child ruling expansions on foreign-born Latina prenatal care and birth outcomes, 2000–2007. *Maternal and Child Health Journal* 19(7):1464-1471.

Dunlap, J. L., J. D. Jaramillo, R. Koppolu, R. Wright, F. Mendoza, and M. Bruzoni. 2015. The effects of language concordant care on patient satisfaction and clinical understanding for Hispanic pediatric surgery patients. *Journal of Pediatric Surgery* 50(9):1586-1589.

DVHA (Department of Vermont Health Access). 2023. *Provider network info.* https://dvha.vermont.gov/providers/provider-network-info (accessed July 14, 2023).

Elixhauser, A. 2008. *Statistical Brief #56: Hospital stays for children, 2006.* https://hcup-us.ahrq.gov/reports/statbriefs/sb56.jsp (accessed April 20, 2023).

Epstein, J. N., K. J. Kelleher, R. Baum, W. B. Brinkman, J. Peugh, W. Gardner, P. Lichtenstein, and J. Langberg. 2014. Variability in ADHD care in community-based pediatrics. *Pediatrics* 134(6):1136-1143.

Evans, C., and H. C. van Woerden. 2011. The effect of surgical training and hospital characteristics on patient outcomes after pediatric surgery: A systematic review. *Journal of Pediatric Surgery* 46(11):2119-2127.

Fegert, J. M., B. Vitiello, P. L. Plener, and V. Clemens. 2020. Challenges and burden of the Coronavirus 2019 (COVID-19) pandemic for child and adolescent mental health: A narrative review to highlight clinical and research needs in the acute phase and the long return to normality. *Child and Adolescent Psychiatry and Mental Health* 14(20). https://doi.org/10.1186/s13034-020-00329-3.

Feldman, H. M., N. J. Blum, A. E. Gahman, and J. Shults. 2015. Diagnosis of attention-deficit/hyperactivity disorder by developmental pediatricians in academic centers: A DBPnet study. *Academic Pediatrics* 15(3):282-288.

Finning, K., O. C. Ukoumunne, T. Ford, E. Danielsson-Waters, L. Shaw, I. R. De Jager, L. Stentiford, and D. A. Moore. 2019. The association between child and adolescent depression and poor attendance at school: A systematic review and meta-analysis. *Journal of Affective Disorders* 245:928-938.

FitzGerald, C. and S. Hurst. 2017. Implicit bias in healthcare professionals: A systematic review. *BMC Medical Ethics* 18:19.

Flores, G., and Lin, H. 2013. Trends in racial/ethnic disparities in medical and oral health, access to care, and use of services in U.S. children: Has anything changed over the years? *International Journal for Equity in Health* 12(10). https://doi.org/10.1186/1475-9276-12-10.

Flower, K. B., S. Wurzelmann, C. Tucker, C. Rojas, M. E. Díaz-González de Ferris, and F. Sylvester. 2021. Spanish-speaking parents' experiences accessing academic medical center care: Barriers, facilitators and technology use. *Academic Pediatrics* 21(5):793-801.

Forrest, C. B. 2009. A typology of specialists' clinical roles. *Archives of Internal Medicine* 169(11):1062-1068.

Forrest, C. B., J. Schuchard, C. Bruno, S. Amaral, E. D. Cox, K. E. Flynn, P. S. Hinds, I. Huang, M. D. Kappelman, J. A. Krishnan, R. B. Kumar, J. Lai, A. S. Paller, W. Phipatanakul, L. E. Schanberg, K. Sumino, E. R. Weitzman, and B. B. Reeve. 2022. Self-reported health outcomes of children and youth with 10 chronic diseases. *Journal of Pediatrics* 246:207-212.e.1. https://doi.org/10.1016/j.jpeds.2022.02.052.

França, U. L., and M. L. McManus. 2017. Availability of definitive hospital care for children. *JAMA Pediatrics* 171(9):e171096.

França, U. L., and M. L. McManus. 2018. Trends in regionalization of hospital care for common pediatric conditions. *Pediatrics* 141(1):e20171940.

Franks, P. W., R. L. Hanson, W. C. Knowler, M. L. Sievers, P. H. Bennett, and H. C. Looker. 2010. Childhood obesity, other cardiovascular risk factors, and premature death. *New England Journal of Medicine* 362:485-493.

Freed, G. L. 2021. Editorial: The pediatric subspecialty workforce is more complex than meets the eye. *JAMA Pediatrics* 175(10):1006-1008.

Fristad, M. A., and H. A. MacPherson. 2014. Evidence-based psychosocial treatments for child and adolescent bipolar spectrum disorders. *Journal of Clinical Child & Adolescent Psychology* 43(3):339-355.

Fuentes-Afflick, E., N. A. Hessol, T. Bauer, M. J. O'Sullivan, V. Gomez-Lobo, S. Holman, T. E. Wilson, and H. Minkoff. 2006. Use of prenatal care by Hispanic women after welfare reform. *Obstetrics and Gynecology* 107(1):151-160.

Gans, D., M. Battistelli, M. Ramirez, L. Cabezas, and N. Pourat. 2013. *Assuring children's access to pediatric subspecialty care in California*. Los Angeles, CA: UCLA Center for Health Policy Research.

GAO (U.S. Government Accountability Office). 2019. *CMS oversight should ensure state implementation of screening and enrollment requirements*. Report no. GAO-20-8. Washington, DC: GAO. https://www.gao.gov/products/GAO-20-8 (accessed July 14, 2023).

Gerteis, J., D. Izrael, D. Deitz, L. LeRoy, R. Ricciardi, T. Miller, and J. Basu. 2014. *Multiple chronic conditions chartbook*. Rockville, MD: Agency for Healthcare Research and Quality. pp. 7-14.

Ghandour, R. M., L. J. Sherman, C. J. Vladutiu, M. M. Ali, S. E. Lynch, R. H. Bitsko, and S. J. Blumberg. 2019. Prevalence and treatment of depression, anxiety, and conduct problems in U.S. children. *The Journal of Pediatrics* 206:256-267.e3.

Greenwood, B. N., R. R. Hardeman, L. Huang, and A. Sojourner. 2020. Physician–patient racial concordance and disparities in birthing mortality for newborns. *Proceedings of the National Academy of Sciences* 117(35):21194-21200.

Gutman, C. K., L. Cousins, J. Gritton, E. J. Klein, J. C. Brown, J. Scannell, and K. C. Lion. 2018. Professional interpreter use and discharge communication in the pediatric emergency department. *Academic Pediatrics* 18(8):935-943.

Hoagwood, K., and S. S. Olin. 2002. The NIMH Blueprint for Change Report: Research priorities in child and adolescent mental health. *Journal of the American Academy of Child and Adolescent Psychiatry* 41(7):760-767.

Hogan, M. F. 2003. The President's New Freedom Commission: Recommendations to transform mental health care in America. *Psychiatric Services* 54(11):1467-1474.

Horak, R. V., J. F. Griffin, A. Brown, S. T. Nett, L. M. Christie, M. L. Forbes, S. Kubis, S. Li, M. N. Singleton, J. T. Verger, B. P. Markovitz, J. P. Burns, S. A. Chung, A. G. Randolph, and the Pediatric Acute Lung Injury and Sepsis Investigator's (PALISI) Network. 2019. Growth and changing characteristics of pediatric intensive care 2001–2016. *Critical Care Medicine* 47(8):1135-1142.

Howell, D. L., K. C. Ward, H. D. Austin, J. L. Young, and W. G. Woods. 2007. Access to pediatric cancer care by age, race, and diagnosis, and outcomes of cancer treatment in pediatric and adolescent patients in the state of Georgia. *Journal of Clinical Oncology* 25(29):4610-4615.

HRSA (Health Resources and Services Administration). 2022. *Children and youth with special health care needs: NSCH data brief June 2022*. https://mchb.hrsa.gov/sites/default/files/mchb/programs-impact/nsch-data-brief-children-youth-special-health-care-needs.pdf (accessed December 22, 2022).

Hsiang, W. R., A. Lukasiewicz, M. Gentry, C.-Y. Kim, M. P. Leslie, R. Pelker, H. P. Forman, and D. H. Wiznia. 2019. Medicaid patients have greater difficulty scheduling health care appointments compared with private insurance patients: A meta-analysis. *INQUIRY: The Journal of Health Care Organization, Provision, and Financing* 56:0046958019838118.

Hsueh, L., A. T. Hirsh, G. Maupome, and J. C. Stewart. 2021. Patient–provider language concordance and health outcomes: A systematic review, evidence map, and research agenda. *Medical Care Research and Review* 78(1):3-23.

Hudgins, J. D., M. I. Neuman, M. C. Monuteaux, J. Porter, and K. A. Nelson. 2021. Provision of guideline-based pediatric asthma care in U.S. emergency departments. *Pediatric Emergency Care* 37(10):507-512.

Jaramillo, J., E. Snyder, J. L. Dunlap, R. Wright, F. Mendoza, and M. Bruzoni. 2016. The Hispanic clinic for pediatric surgery: A model to improve parent–provider communication for Hispanic pediatric surgery patients. *Journal of Pediatric Surgery* 51(4):670-674.

Kalb, L. G., E. K. Stapp, E. D. Ballard, C. Holingue, A. Keefer, and A. Riley. 2019. Trends in psychiatric emergency department visits among youth and young adults in the U.S. *Pediatrics* 143(4):e20182192.

Kaul, S., A. C. Kirchhoff, N. E. Morden, C. S. Vogeli, and E. G. Campbell. 2015. Physician response to patient request for unnecessary care. *American Journal of Managed Care* 21(11):823-832.

Kern-Goldberger, A. S., N. M. Money, J. S. Gerber, and C. P. Bonafide. 2021. Inpatient subspecialty consultations: A new target for high-value pediatric hospital care? *Hospital Pediatrics* https://doi.org/10.1542/hpeds.2021-006165.

Kern-Goldberger, A. S., E. M. Dalton, I. R. Rasooly, M. Congdon, D. Gunturi, L. Wu, Y. Li, J. S. Gerber, and C. P. Bonafide. 2023. Factors associated with inpatient subspecialty consultation patterns among pediatric hospitalists. *JAMA* 6(3):e232648.

Kessler, R. C., P. Berglund, O. Demler, R. Jin, K. R. Merikangas, and E. E. Walters. 2005. Lifetime prevalence and age-of-onset distributions of DSM-IV disorders in the national comorbidity survey replication. *Archives of General Psychiatry* 62(6):593-602.

Khan, M. S., W. Zhang, R. A. Taylor, E. D. McKenzie, G. B. Mallory, M. G. Schecter, D. L. S. Morales, J. S. Heinle, and I. Adachi. 2015. Survival in pediatric lung transplantation: The effect of center volume and expertise. *The Journal of Heart and Lung Transplantation* 34(8):1073-1081.

Krugman, S. D., and D. Rauch. 2022. *An unexpected shortage: Hospital beds for children.* https://www.healthaffairs.org/do/10.1377/forefront.20220615.615247 (accessed April 13, 2023).

Kunin, M., E. Turbitt, S. A. Gafforini, L. A. Sanci, N. A. Spike, and G. L. Freed. 2018. General practitioner referrals to paediatric specialist outpatient clinics: Referral goals and parental influence. *Journal of Primary Health Care* 10(1):76-80.

Kuriyan, A. B., W. E. Pelham, B. S. Molina, D. A. Waschbusch, E. M. Gnagy, M. H. Sibley, D. E. Babinski, C. Walther, J. Cheong, and J. Yu. 2013. Young adult educational and vocational outcomes of children diagnosed with ADHD. *Journal of Abnormal Child Psychology* 41:27-41.

Kyu, H. H., C. Pinho, J. A. Wagner, J. C. Brown, A. Bertozzi-Villa, F. J. Charlson, L. E. Coffeng, L. Dandona, H. E. Erskine, and A. J. Ferrari. 2016. Global and national burden of diseases and injuries among children and adolescents between 1990 and 2013: Findings from the Global Burden of Disease 2013 study. *JAMA Pediatrics* 170(3):267-287.

Lange, S. J., L. Kompaniyets, D. S. Freedman, E. M. Kraus, R. Porter, H. M. Blanck, and A. B. Goodman. 2021. Longitudinal trends in body mass index before and during the COVID-19 pandemic among persons aged 2–19 years—United States, 2018–2020. *Morbidity and Mortality Weekly Reports* 70(37):1278-1283.

Larson, K., E. A. Gottschlich, W. L. Cull, and L. M. Olson. 2021. High-deductible health plans for U.S. children: Trends, health service use, and financial barriers to care. *Academic Pediatrics* 21(8):1345-1354.

Lasswell, S. M., W. D. Barfield, R. W. Rochat, and L. Blackmon. 2010. Perinatal regionalization for very low-birth-weight and very preterm infants: A meta-analysis. *JAMA* 304(9):992-1000.

Lawrence, J. M., J. Divers, S. Isom, S. Saydah, G. Imperatore, C. Pihoker, S. M. Marcovina, E. J. Mayer-Davis, R. F. Hamman, L. Dolan, D. Dabelea, D. J. Pettitt, and A. D. Liese for the SEARCH for Diabetes in Youth Study Group. 2021. Trends in prevalence of type 1 and type 2 diabetes in children and adolescents in the U.S., 2001–2017. *Journal of the American Medical Association* 326(8):717-727.

Lebrun-Harris, L. A., M. A. McManus, S. M. Ilango, M. Cyr, S. B. McLellan, M. Y. Mann, and P. H. White. 2018. Transition planning among U.S. youth with and without special health care needs. *Pediatrics* 142(4):e20180194.

Lebrun-Harris, L. A., R. M. Ghandour, M. D. Kogan, and M. D. Warren. 2022. Five-year trends in U.S. children's health and well-being, 2016-2020. *JAMA Pediatrics* 176(7):e220056. https://doi.org/10.1001/jamapediatrics.2022.0056.

Leiba, A., B. Fishman, G. Twig, D. Gilad, E. Derazne, A. Shamiss, T. Shohat, O. Ron, and E. Grossman. 2019. Association of adolescent hypertension with future end-stage renal disease. *JAMA Internal Medicine* 179(4):517-523.

Leibowitz, A., W. G. Manning, Jr., E. B. Keeler, N. Duan, K. N. Lohr, and J. P. Newhouse. 1985. Effect of cost-sharing on the use of medical services by children: Interim results from a randomized controlled trial. *Pediatrics* 75(5):942-951.

Little, P., M. Dorward, G. Warner, K. Stephens, J. Senior, and M. Moore. 2004. Importance of patient pressure and perceived pressure and perceived medical need for investigations, referral, and prescribing in primary care: Nested observational study. *BMJ* 328(7437):444.

Loe, I. M., and H. M. Feldman. 2007. Academic and educational outcomes of children with ADHD. *Journal of Pediatric Psychology* 32(6):643-654.

Lonetti, A., A. Pession, and R. Masetti. 2019. Targeted therapies for pediatric AML: Gaps and perspective. *Frontiers in Pediatrics* 7:463.

Lor, M., and G. A. Martinez. 2020. Scoping review: Definitions and outcomes of patient–provider language concordance in healthcare. *Patient Education and Counseling* 103(10):1883-1901.

MACPAC (Medicaid and CHIP Payment and Access Commission). 2017. *State Medicaid fee-for-service physician payment policies.* https://www.macpac.gov/publication/states-medicaid-fee-for-service-physician-payment-policies (accessed January 4, 2023).

MACPAC. 2020. Medicaid payment policy for out-of-state hospital services. https://www.macpac.gov/wp-content/uploads/2020/01/Medicaid-Payment-Policy-for-Out-of-State-Hospital-Services.pdf (accessed July 12, 2023).

MACPAC. 2021. *Physician acceptance of new Medicaid patients: Findings from the National Electronic Health Records Survey.* https://www.macpac.gov/wp-content/uploads/2021/06/Physician-Acceptance-of-New-Medicaid-Patients-Findings-from-the-National-Electronic-Health-Records-Survey.pdf (accessed April 13, 2023).

Maenner, M. J., Z. Warren, A. R. Williams, E. Amoakohene, A. V. Bakian, D. A. Bilder, M. S. Durkin, R. T. Fitzgerald, S. M. Furnier, M. M. Hughes, C. M. Ladd-Acosta, D. McArthur, E. T. Pas, A. Salinas, A. Vehorn, S. Williams, A. Esler, A. Grzybowski, J. Hall-Lande, R. H. N. Nguyen, K. Pierce, W. Zahorodny, A. Hudson, L. Hallas, K. C. Mancilla, M. Patrick, J. Shenouda, K. Sidwell, M. DiRienzo, J. Gutierrez, M. H. Spivey, M. Lopez, S. Pettygrove, Y. D. Schwenk, A. Washington, and K. A. Shaw. 2023. Prevalence and characteristics of autism spectrum disorder among children aged 8 years—Autism and Developmental Disabilities Monitoring Network, 11 sites, United States, 2020. *Morbidity and Mortality Weekly Report* 72(2):1-14.

Manetto, N., J. Greenberg, and C. Reddy. 2020. Policies to enhance care of out-of-state pediatric Medicaid beneficiaries. In *Health Affairs Blog.* https://www.healthaffairs.org/content/forefront/policies-enhance-care-out-of-state-pediatric-medicaid-beneficiaries (accessed July 12, 2023).

Marcin, J. P., U. Shaikh, and R. H. Steinhorn. 2016. Addressing health disparities in rural communities using telehealth. *Pediatric Research* 79(1):169-176.

Mayer, M. L. 2006. Are we there yet? Distance to care and relative supply among pediatric medical subspecialties. *Pediatrics* 118(6):2313-2321.

McCulloh, R. J., S. Smitherman, S. Adelsky, M. Congdon, J. Librizzi, K. Koehn, and B. Alverson. 2012. Hospitalist and nonhospitalist adherence to evidence-based quality metrics for bronchiolitis. *Hospital Pediatrics* 2(1):19-25.

McManus, M., P. White, A. Schmidt, M. Barr, C. Langer, K. Barger, and A. Ware. 2020. Health care gap affects 20% of United States population: Transition from pediatric to adult health care. *Health Policy OPEN* 1:100007.

McPherson, M., P. Arango, H. Fox, C. Lauver, M. McManus, P. W. Newacheck, J. M. Perrin, J. P. Shonkoff, and B. Strickland. 1998. A new definition of children with special health care needs. *Pediatrics* 102(1):137-139.

Merikangas, K. R., M. E. Calkins, M. Burstein, J. He, R. Chiavacci, T. Lateef, K. Ruparel, R. C. Gur, T. Lehner, H. Hakonarson, and R. E. Gur. 2015. Comorbidity of physician and mental disorders in the Neurodevelopmental Genomics Cohort Study. *Pediatrics* 135(4):e927-e938.

Meyer, H. 2021. Families with sick kids on Medicaid seek easier access to out-of-state hospitals. *NPR*.

Michelson, K. A., J. D. Hudgins, M. C. Monuteaux, R. G. Bachur, and J. A. Finkelstein. 2018. Cardiac arrest survival in pediatric and general emergency departments. *Pediatrics* 141(2):e20172741. https://doi.org/10.1542/peds.2017-2741.

Ming, D. Y., K. A. Jones, M. J. White, J. E. Pritchard, B. G. Hammill, C. Bush, G. L. Jackson, and S. R. Raman. 2022. Healthcare utilization for Medicaid-insured children with medical complexity: Differences by sociodemographic characteristics. *Maternal and Child Health Journal* 26:2407-2418.

Mosquera, R. A., E. B. C. Avritscher, C. Pedroza, C. S. Bell, C. L. Samuels, T. S. Harris, J. C. Eapen, A. Yadav, M. Poe, R. L. Parlar-Chun, J. Berry, and J. E. Tyson. 2021. Hospital consultation from outpatient clinicians for medically complex children: A randomized clinical trial. *JAMA Pediatrics* 175(1):e205026.

Müller, H., S. Laier, and A. Bechdolf. 2014. Evidence-based psychotherapy for the prevention and treatment of first-episode psychosis. *European Archives of Psychiatry and Clinical Neuroscience* 264:17-25.

Muskens, J. B., F. P. Velders, and W. G. Staal. 2017. Medical comorbidities in children and adolescents with autism spectrum disorders and attention deficit hyperactivity disorders: A systematic review. *European Child & Adolescent Psychiatry* 26(9):1093-1103.

Myers, S. R., C. C. Branas, B. French, M. L. Nance, and B. G. Carr. 2019. A national analysis of pediatric trauma care utilization and outcomes in the United States. *Pediatric Emergency Care* 35(1):1-7.

NASEM (National Academies of Sciences, Engineering, and Medicine). 2015. *Investing in the health and well-being of young adults*. Washington, DC: The National Academies Press.

NASEM. 2023. *Addressing the long-term effects of the COVID-19 pandemic on children and families*. Edited by T. R. Coker, J. A. Gootman, and E. P. Backes. Washington, DC: The National Academies Press.

Nguengang Wakap, S., D. M. Lambert, A. Olry, C. Rodwell, C. Gueydan, V. Lanneau, D. Murphy, Y. Le Cam, and A. Rath. 2020. Estimating cumulative point prevalence of rare diseases: Analysis of the Orphanet database. *European Journal of Human Genetics* 28(2):165-173.

NRC and IOM (National Research Council and Institute of Medicine). 2004. *Children's health, the nation's wealth: Assessing and improving child health*. Washington, DC: The National Academies Press.

Oh, S. H., I. S. Jeong, D. Y. Kim, J. M. Namgoong, W. K. Jhang, S. J. Park, D. H. Jung, D. B. Moon, G. W. Song, G. C. Park, T. Y. Ha, C. S. Ahn, K. H. Kim, S. Hwang, S. G. Lee, and K. M. Kim. 2022. Recent improvement in survival outcomes and reappraisal of prognostic factors in pediatric living donor liver transplantation. *Liver Transplantation* 28(6):1011-1023.

Perreira, K. M., and J. M. Pedroza. 2019. Policies of exclusion: Implications for the health of immigrants and their children. *Annual Review of Public Health* 40:147-166.

Pho, K. 2012. *Why more primary care doctors are referring patients to specialists*. https://www.kevinmd.com/2012/01/primary-care-doctors-referring-patients-specialists.html (accessed April 20, 2023).

Pollitz, K. 2022. *Network adequacy standards and enforcement*. https://www.kff.org/health-reform/issue-brief/network-adequacy-standards-and-enforcement/ (accessed July 10, 2023).

Price-Feeney, M., A. E. Green, and S. Dorison. 2020. Understanding the mental health of transgender and nonbinary youth. *Journal of Adolescent Health* 66(6):684-690.

Rankin, J., L. Matthews, S. Cobley, A. Han, R. Sanders, H. D. Wiltshire, and J. S. Baker. 2016. Psychological consequences of childhood obesity: Psychiatric comorbidity and prevention. *Adolescent Health, Medicine and Therapeutics* 7:125-146.

Ray, K. N., L. E. Ashcraft, J. M. Kahn, A. Mehrotra, and E. Miller. 2016. Family perspectives on high-quality pediatric subspecialty referrals. *Academic Pediatrics* 16(6):594-600.

Reardon, J. L., P. Lembeck, T. Murray, and P. Weiss. 2020. Mental health in the pediatric subspecialties: Physicians' beliefs and confidence in providing care. *Academic Pediatrics* 20(7):E53-E54.

Rimes, K. A., N. Goodship, G. Ussher, D. Baker, and E. West. 2019. Non-binary and binary transgender youth: Comparison of mental health, self-harm, suicidality, substance use and victimization experiences. *International Journal of Transgenderism* 20(2-3):230-240.

Rimsza, M. E., H. S. Ruch-Ross, C. J. Clemens, W. B. Moskowitz, and H. J. Mulvey. 2018. Workforce trends and analysis of selected pediatric subspecialties in the United States. *Academic Pediatrics* 18(7):805-812.

Ringberg, U., N. Fleten, and O. H. Førde. 2014. Examining the variation in GPs' referral practice: A cross-sectional study of GPs' reasons for referral. *British Journal of General Practice* 64(624):e426-e433.

Rodgers, C. R. R., M. W. Flores, O. Bassey, J. M. Augenblick, and B. Le Cook. 2022. Racial/ethnic trends in children's mental health care access and expenditures from 2010–2017: Disparities remain despite sweeping policy reform. *Journal of the American Academy of Child & Adolescent Psychiatry* 61(7):915-925.

Rodriguez Santana, I., A. Mason, N. Gutacker, P. Kasteridis, R. Santos, and N. Rice. 2023. Need, demand, supply in health care: Working definitions, and their implications for defining access. *Health Economics, Policy and Law* 18(1):1-13.

Romano, I., C. Buchan, L. Baiocco-Romano, and M. A. Ferro. 2021. Physical–mental multimorbidity in children and youth: A scoping review. *BMJ Open* 11:e043124.

Rubinstein, T. B., A. M. Davis, M. Rodriguez, and A. M. Knight. 2018. Addressing mental health in pediatric rheumatology. *Current Treatment Options in Rheumatology* 4:55-72.

Sanyaolu, A., C. Okorie, X. Qi, J. Locke, and S. Rehman. 2019. Child and adolescent obesity in the United States: A public health concern. *Global Pediatric Health* https://doi.org/10.1177/2333794X19891305.

Schimmelmann, B. G., P. Conus, S. Cotton, P. D. McGorry, and M. Lambert. 2007. Pretreatment, baseline, and outcome differences between early-onset and adult-onset psychosis in an epidemiological cohort of 636 first-episode patients. *Schizophrenia Research* 95(1-3):1-8.

Schuster, M. A. 2015. Measuring quality of pediatric care: Where we've been and where we're going. *Pediatrics* 135(4):748-751.

Shear, K., R. Jin, A. M. Ruscio, E. E. Walters, and R. C. Kessler. 2006. Prevalence and correlates of estimated DSM-IV child and adult separation anxiety disorder in the national comorbidity survey replication. *American Journal of Psychiatry* 163(6):1074-1083.

Siegel, D. A., L. C. Richardson, S. J. Henley, R. J. Wilson, N. F. Dowling, H. K. Weir, E. W. Tai, and N. Buchanan Lunsford. 2020. Pediatric cancer mortality and survival in the United States, 2001–2016. *Cancer* 126(19):4379-4389.

Siffel, C., M. DerSarkissian, K. Kponee-Shovein, W. Spalding, Y. M. Gu, M. Cheng, and M. S. Duh. 2020. Suicidal ideation and attempts in the United States of America among stimulant-treated, non-stimulant-treated, and untreated patients with a diagnosis of attention-deficit/hyperactivity disorder. *Journal of Affective Disorders* 266:109-119.

Skinner, A. C., and M. L. Mayer. 2007. Effects of insurance status on children's access to specialty care: A systematic review of the literature. *BMC Health Services Research* 7(1):194.

Slocum, T. A., R. Detrich, S. M. Wilczynski, T. D. Spencer, T. Lewis, and K. Wolfe. 2014. The evidence-based practice of applied behavior analysis. *The Behavior Analyst* 37:41-56.

St. Amant, H. G., S. M. Schrager, C. Peña-Ricardo, M. E. Williams, and D. L. Vanderbilt. 2018. Language barriers impact access to services for children with autism spectrum disorders. *Journal of Autism and Developmental Disorders* 48(2):333-340.

Stark, A. R., D. M. Pursley, L. Papile, E. C. Eichenwald, C. T. Hankins, R. K. Buck, T. J. Wallace, P. G. Bondurant, and N. E Faster. 2023. Standards for levels of neonatal care: II, III, and IV. *Pediatrics* 151(6):e2023061957.

Stephens, M. R., A. S. Murthy, and P. J. McMahon. 2019. Wait times, health care touchpoints, and nonattendance in an academic pediatric dermatology clinic. *Pediatric Dermatology* 36(6):893-897.

Stierman, B., J. Afful, M. D. Carroll, T. Chen, O. Davy, S. Fink, C. D. Fryar, Q. Gu, C. M. Hales, J. P. Hughes, Y. Ostchega, R. J. Storandt, and L. J. Akinlami. 2021. National Health and Nutrition Examination Survey 2017–March 2020 prepandemic data files—Development of files and prevalence estimates for selected health outcomes. *National Health Statistics Reports* No. 158.

Stroul, B. A., and R. M. Friedman. 1986. *A system of care for severely emotionally disturbed children and youth.* https://www.ojp.gov/pdffiles1/Digitization/125081NCJRS.pdf (accessed May 1, 2023).

Sump, C. A., T. L. Marshall, A. J. Ipsaro, S. J. Patel, D. C. Warner, P. W. Brady, and P. A. Hagedorn. 2020. Uncertain diagnoses in a children's hospital: Patient characteristics and outcomes. *Diagnosis* 8(3):353-357.

Takeshita, J., S. Wang, A. W. Loren, N. Mitra, J. Shults, D. B. Sin, and D. L. Sawinski. 2020. Association of racial/ethnic and gender concordance between patients and physicians with patient experience ratings. *JAMA Open Network* 3(11):2024583.

Timbie, J. W., A. M. Kranz, A. Mahmud, and C. L. Damberg. 2019. Specialty care access for Medicaid enrollees in expansion states. *American Journal of Managed Care* 25(3):e83-e87.

Tolbert, J., P. Drake, and A. Damico. 2022. *Key facts about the uninsured population.* https://www.kff.org/uninsured/issue-brief/key-facts-about-the-uninsured-population/#:~:text=1%20Nonelderly%20adults%20are%20more%20likely%20to%20be,risk%20of%20being%20uninsured%20than%20White%20people.%20 (accessed May 2, 2023).

Turner, A., T. Ricketts, and L. K. Leslie. 2020. Comparison of number and geographic distribution of pediatric subspecialists and patient proximity to specialized care in the U.S. between 2003 and 2019. *JAMA Pediatrics* 174(9):852-860.

Turner, A., T. Ricketts, and L. K. Leslie. 2022. Revisiting complexities in the pediatric subspecialty workforce. *JAMA Pediatrics* 176(1):98-99.

U.S. Census Bureau. 2020. *The next generation—percent change among the under 18 population: 2010 to 2019.* https://www.census.gov/library/visualizations/2020/comm/map-popest-under-18.html (accessed April 21, 2023).

Valderas, J. M., B. Starfield, C. B. Forrest, L. Rajmil, M. Roland, and B. Sibbald. 2009. Routine care provided by specialists to children and adolescents in the United States (2002–2006). *BMC Health Services Research* 9(1):221.

Van Cleave, J., S. L. Gortmaker, and J. M. Perrin. 2010. Dynamics of obesity and chronic health conditions among children and youth. *Journal of the American Medical Association* 303(7):623-630.

Vernacchio, L., J. M. Muto, G. Young, and W. Risko. 2012. Ambulatory subspecialty visits in a large pediatric primary care network. *Health Services Research* 47(4):1755-1769.

Visser, S. N., M. L. Danielson, R. H. Bitsko, J. R. Holbrook, M. D. Kogan, R. M. Ghandour, R. Perou, and S. J. Blumberg. 2014. Trends in the parent-report of health care provider-diagnosed and medicated attention-deficit/hyperactivity disorder: United States, 2003–2011. *Journal of the American Academy of Child & Adolescent Psychiatry* 53(1):34-46.e2.

VonAchen, P., M. M. Davis, J. Cartland, A. D'Arco, and K. Kan. 2022. Closure of licensed pediatric beds in health care markets within Illinois. *Academic Pediatrics* 22(3):431-439.

White, P. H., W. C. Cooley, Transitions Clinical Report Authoring Group, American Academy of Pediatrics, American Academy of Family Physicians, American College of Physicians, A. D. A. Boudreau, M. Cyr, B. E. Davis, D. E. Dreyfus, E. Forlenza, A. Friedland, C. Greenlee, M. Mann, M. McManus, A. I. Meleis, and L. Pickler. 2018. Supporting the health care transition from adolescence to adulthood in the medical home. *Pediatrics* 142(5):e20182587.

White, P., A. Schmidt, J. Shorr, S. Ilango, D. Beck, and M. McManus. 2020. *Six Core Elements of Health Care Transition 3.0.* https://www.gottransition.org/6ce/?integrating-full-package (accessed April 28, 2023).

Whitney, D. G., and M. D. Peterson. 2019. U.S. national and state-level prevalence of mental health disorders and disparities of mental health care use in children. *JAMA Pediatrics* 173(4):389-391.

Wise, P. H. 2007. The future pediatrician: The challenge of chronic illness. *The Journal of Pediatrics* 151(5 Suppl):S6-S10.

Witt, W. P., A. J. Weiss, and A. Elixhauser. 2014. *Statistical Brief #187: Overview of hospital stays for children in the United States, 2012.* https://www.hcup-us.ahrq.gov/reports/statbriefs/sb187-Hospital-Stays-Children-2012.jsp (accessed April 20, 2023).

Wojcik, M. H., M. Bresnahan, M. C. del Rosario, M. M. Ojeda, A. Kritzer, and Y. S. Fraiman. 2023. Rare diseases, common barriers: Disparities in pediatric clinical genetics outcomes. *Pediatric Research* 93(1):110-117.

Wolfe, M. K., N. C. McDonald, and G. M. Holmes. 2020. Transportation barriers to health care in the United States: Findings from the National Health Interview Survey, 1997–2017. *American Journal of Public Health* 110(6):815-822.

Woolf, S. H., E. R. Wolf, and F. P. Rivara. 2023. The new crisis of increasing all-cause mortality in U.S. children and adults. *Journal of the American Medical Association* 329(12):975-976.

Woolford, S. J., M. Sidell, X. Li, V. Else, D. R. Young, K. Resnicow, and C. Koebnick. 2021. Changes in body mass index among children and adolescents during the COVID-19 pandemic. *Journal of the American Medical Association* 326(14):1434-1436.

Xu, W. Y., Y. Li, C. Song, S. Bose-Brill, and S. M. Retchin. 2022. Out-of-network care in commercially insured pediatric patients according to medical complexity. *Medical Care* 60(5):375-380.

Yang, L., C. G. Magnussen, L. Yang, P. Bovet, and B. Xi. 2020. Elevated blood pressure in childhood or adolescence and cardiovascular outcomes in adulthood: A systematic review. *Hypertension* 75:948-955.

Yang, K. G., M. W. Flores, N. J. Carson, and B. Le Cook. 2022. Racial and ethnic disparities in childhood ADHD treatment access and utilization: Results from a national study. *Psychiatric Services* https://doi.org/10.1176/appi.ps.202100578.

Yard, E., L. Radhakrishnan, M. F. Ballesteros, M. Sheppard, A. Gates, Z. Stein, K. Hartnett, A. Kite-Powell, L. Rodgers, J. Adjemian, D. C. Ehlman, K. Holland, N. Idaikkadar, A. Ivey-Stephenson, P. Martinez, R. Law, and D. M. Stone. 2021. Emergency department visits for suspected suicide attempts among persons aged 12–25 years before and during the COVID-19 pandemic—United States, January 2019–May 2021. *Morbidity and Mortality Weekly Report* 70(24):888-894.

Yohe, M. E., C. M. Heske, E. Stewart, P. C. Adamson, N. Ahmed, C. R. Antonescu, E. Chen, N. Collins, A. Ehrlich, R. L. Galindo, B. E. Gryder, H. Hahn, S. Hammond, M. E. Hatley, D. S. Hawkins, M. N. Hayes, A. Hayes-Jordan, L. J. Helman, S. Hettmer, M. S. Ignatius, C. Keller, J. Khan, D. G. Kirsch, C. M. Linardic, P. J. Lupo, R. Rota, J. F. Shern, J. Shipley, S. Sindiri, S. J. Tapscott, C. R. Vakoc, L. H. Wexler, and D. M. Langenau. 2019. Insights into pediatric rhabdomyosarcoma research: Challenges and goals. *Pediatric Blood & Cancer* 66(10):e27869.

Yu, S. M., R. M. Nyman, M. D. Kogan, Z. J. Huang, and R. H. Schwalberg. 2004. Parent's language of interview and access to care for children with special health care needs. *Ambulatory Pediatrics* 4(2):181-187.

Zablotsky, B., L. I. Black, M. J. Maenner, L. A. Schieve, M. L. Danielson, R. H. Bitsko, S. J. Blumberg, M. D. Kogan, and C. A. Boyle. 2019. Prevalence and trends of developmental disabilities among children in the United States: 2009–2017. *Pediatrics* 144(4):e20190811.

Zima, B. T., R. Bussing, L. Tang, L. Zhang, S. Ettner, T. R. Belin, and K. B. Wells. 2010. Quality of care for childhood attention-deficit/hyperactivity disorder in a managed care Medicaid program. *Journal of the American Academy of Child & Adolescent Psychiatry* 49(12):1225-1237. e1-e11.

Zima, B. T., J. Rodean, M. Hall, N. S. Bardach, T. R. Coker, and J. G. Berry. 2016. Psychiatric disorders and trends in resource use in pediatric hospitals. *Pediatrics* 138(5):e20160909.

Zima, B. T., J. B. Edgcomb, J. Rodean, S. D. Cochran, C. A. Harle, J. Pathak, C.-H. Tseng, and R. Bussing. 2022. Use of acute mental health care in U.S. children's hospitals before and after statewide COVID-19 school closure orders. *Psychiatric Services* 73(11):1202-1209.

3

Pediatric Subspecialty Use Data Analyses

After the committee reviewed the existing literature, it learned that there are no recent data (i.e., within the past 10 years) that comprehensively describe patterns of children's medical subspecialty physician use. To fill this gap, the committee examined data analyses that used three complementary data sources.[1] The first analysis by Carelon Research (formerly HealthCore), the only analysis commissioned by the committee, examined commercially insured individuals enrolled in Elevance Health (formerly Anthem, Inc.).[2] The second analysis was submitted to this committee (by multiple researchers, including three members of this committee) and examined electronic health records from individuals obtaining care from eight of the nation's largest pediatric academic medical centers that participated in PEDSnet,[3] a national pediatric learning health system. The third analysis, submitted to the committee by researchers at The George Washington University (including one member of this committee), used the Transformed

---

[1] All three data analyses submitted to this committee can be found at https://nap.edu/27207.

[2] Carelon Research contributed aggregated data on trends in the use of pediatric subspeciality care by children receiving private health insurance coverage through Elevance Health. Carelon Research was not able to confirm the National Academies' interpretation of Carelon Research data and the accuracy of secondary analyses performed by the National Academies committee presented in this report. Statements herein do not necessarily represent the views and stance of Carelon Research or Elevance Health.

[3] For more information on PEDSnet, see https://pedsnet.org (accessed May 16, 2023).

Medicaid Statistical Information System (T-MSIS),[4] a national administrative dataset of beneficiaries insured by Medicaid or the Children's Health Insurance Program (CHIP). Each of these three data sources provides a different assessment of children's use of subspecialty care: rates for those enrolled in commercial insurance products (Elevance Health), for those who obtain care from large pediatric academic medical centers (PEDSnet), and for those enrolled in Medicaid/CHIP. Our a priori expectation was that the patterns would differ by each of these data sources, but as a collection, they provide a detailed assessment of children's use of subspecialty care in the United States.

METHODS

The following sections provide an overview of the methods for each of the three data analyses considered by the committee.[5]

Data Sources

As noted above, the committee examined three separate analyses of pediatric medical subspecialty use that used different data sources.

Elevance Health Data

Elevance Health data were from the Healthcare Integrated Research Database (HIRD®), a large health plan administrative database. Claims data were submitted for payment by health care clinicians for services to individuals enrolled in Elevance Health commercial (i.e., private) plans. The HIRD contains member enrollment, medical care (professional and facility claims), outpatient prescription drug events, and outpatient laboratory test results. All medical claims have associated diagnosis and procedure codes. Claims are subject to the quality control, inspection, and validation procedures performed by the individual health plans for payment processing purposes. The analysis used enrollment files and fully adjudicated claims with service dates between January 2011 and December 2021.

---

[4] For more information on T-MSIS, see https://www.medicaid.gov/medicaid/data-systems/macbis/transformed-medicaid-statistical-information-system-t-msis/index.html (accessed May 16, 2023).

[5] More information on the methods of each data analysis can be found within the full submissions to the committee; see https://nap.edu/27207.

PEDSnet Data

PEDSnet data are imported from individual hospital electronic health record systems and standardized to a common data model. Participating institutions included: Ann & Robert H. Lurie Children's Hospital of Chicago, Children's Hospital Colorado, Children's Hospital of Philadelphia, Cincinnati Children's Hospital Medical Center, Nationwide Children's Hospital, Nemours Children's Health, Seattle Children's Hospital, and Stanford Children's Health. Within the PEDSnet database, the study cohort included patients with at least one outpatient visit where the clinician specialty was general pediatrics in one of the academic pediatric medical centers during the time period of January 2010 to December 2021, and where the patient age was less than 21 years old at the end of the calendar year. The PEDSnet data also provided information on payer and patient race and ethnicity. For analyses that examined any subspecialty use across the full study period, insurance was defined as public insurance (i.e., Medicaid or CHIP) if at any time that was their payment for outpatient visits; otherwise, if they ever listed as private/commercial insurance in their general outpatient visits, they are listed as "commercial," and all others are listed as "unknown/self-pay." To reduce the number of patients with missing race and ethnicity data, we used the recommended CDC approach for a combined race/ethnicity variable in which "ethnicity" was used to define the Hispanic category and race was used if non-Hispanic (Yoon et al., 2021).

T-MSIS Data

The T-MSIS is a national dataset of Medicaid and CHIP data from states, territories, and the District of Columbia. T-MSIS data included enrollment, service use, and clinician information. The first available year of T-MSIS is 2016; the analysis used data from 2016 through 2019. Data characteristics of the T-MSIS are reported by the Centers for Medicare & Medicaid Services.[6] The analysis included data from 44 states, DC, and Puerto Rico, and excluded Arkansas, California, Delaware, Indiana, Minnesota, and Pennsylvania.[7]

Subspecialty Use Rate

To evaluate children's use of pediatric subspecialty care, subspecialty use was defined as the annual number of children with at least one completed visit to any subspecialist in an outpatient setting per population. This

---

[6] For more information, see https://www.medicaid.gov/dq-atlas/welcome (accessed May 4, 2023).

[7] Six states were excluded due to high percentages of missing data.

measure excludes patients for whom a referral to a subspecialist was made but the visit was not completed. These use rates excluded visits to subspecialists in emergency department or inpatient settings. The PEDSnet analysis included annual rates of patients seeing multiple types of subspecialties, defined as having at least one visit with more than one subspecialty type in that year. Both Elevance Health and PEDSnet cohorts were comprised of children and youth aged less than 21 years and computed annual specialty use rates from 2011 to 2021. The PEDSnet analysis provided contrasts of children insured by Medicaid/CHIP versus children who are commercially insured children as well as differences by race/ethnicity. The subspecialty use rate calculation for these analyses was any subspecialty use across the observation period.

The Elevance Health denominators required that individuals over one year of age have at least 6 months of plan enrollment in a given year; individual calendar year denominators ranged from 4,998,694 to 5,439,618. The PEDSnet denominator included individuals with a visit to a general pediatrician and was therefore a use-based sample of primary care users at the 8 hospitals; calendar year denominators rose every year, increasing from 493,628 in 2011 to 858,551 in 2021. The T-MSIS analysis included beneficiaries less than 19 years old in calendar years 2016 through 2019 only who were insured by Medicaid/CHIP at any point in a given year. The age range for this cohort was chosen to align with the Medicaid/CHIP eligibility group—that is, children younger than 19 years. The analysis identified children insured by Medicaid/CHIP in each calendar year with any outpatient visit and computed the annual number of children less than 19 years old insured by Medicaid/CHIP with at least one visit to a subspecialist in an outpatient setting per 1,000 total children less than 19 years insured by Medicaid/CHIP using each specialty or profession in a year. For primary care physicians and advanced practice clinicians, reported in Chapter 4, a similar use rate was calculated. The T-MSIS analysis further included pediatric and adult medical subspecialties and examined subspecialist use rates by beneficiary age range (i.e., less than 1 year, 1 to 11 years, and 12 to 18 years). The calendar year denominators for total children insured by Medicaid/CHIP ranged from 32,545,218 to 33,585,419.

Subspecialties

For the commissioned analysis done by Carelon Research, the committee identified 25 pediatric medical subspecialties to be analyzed. This included 14 pediatric subspecialties for which the American Board of Pediatrics (ABP) provides board certification: adolescent medicine, pediatric cardiology, child abuse pediatrics, pediatric critical care medicine, developmental-behavioral pediatrics, pediatric emergency medicine, pediatric endocrinology, pediatric gastroenterology, pediatric hematology/oncology, pediatric infectious diseases, neonatal-perinatal medicine, pediatric nephrology, pediatric pulmonology, and pediatric rheumatology. Pediatric critical care medicine, pediatric emergency medicine, neonatal-perinatal medicine were included in overall outpatient specialist use rates, but because these specialties provide so few outpatient services, they were excluded from specialty-specific calculations. Pediatric hospital medicine was excluded because it does not typically provide care in outpatient settings. The committee included the five subspecialties that the ABP co-sponsors for which board certification is administered by other specialty boards: hospice and palliative medicine, medical toxicology, sleep medicine, sports medicine, and pediatric transplant hepatology. Finally, the committee identified an additional six subspecialties that are included in combined training programs, have certifications by specialty boards that are not co-sponsored by ABP, or do not have formal certification programs, but are commonly recognized as pediatric medical subspecialties: pediatric allergy and immunology, child neurology, obesity medicine, pediatric dermatology, clinical genetics, and pediatric rehabilitation medicine. The PEDSnet and T-MSIS analyses examined the same 23 subspecialties. The T-MSIS analysis also examined adult medical subspecialties that corresponded to the included pediatric subspecialties, excluding those with no adult counterpart (i.e., adolescent medicine, child abuse pediatrics, clinical genetics, developmental-behavioral pediatrics, and neonatal-perinatal medicine) as well as psychiatry, family medicine, internal medicine, obstetrics and gynecology, advanced practice nurses, and physician assistants. (This chapter will focus on the T-MSIS results for pediatric subspecialty care. See Chapter 4 for analysis of other clinicians.)

RESULTS

The following sections include the committee's analysis of the results of the three data analyses, including temporal trends, use rates by subspecialty type, subspecialist use by payer and race/ethnicity, the most common diagnoses by subspecialty, and an analysis of the adult subspecialty workforce providing care to children. It is important to note that not all of the analyses examined all of the same variables, and so the sources are indicated for each set of results.

Temporal Trends

Among children in the Elevance Health cohort, annual rates of subspecialist use rose from 7.9 percent in 2011 to 10.4 percent in 2021, an absolute increase of 2.5 percentage points and a relative increase of 31.6 percent (see Figure 3-1). Rates of subspecialist use in the four years of T-MSIS data were slightly lower than those of the commercially insured Elevance Health population (ranging from 7.9 percent to 9.2 percent), and stable across the observation period.

Subspecialist use rates for children in the PEDSnet academic medical center cohort across the study period ranged from 18 to 21 percent, while the number of children with at least one general pediatrician visit at that center (i.e., eligible denominator for the rates) rose markedly (see Figure 3-2). Because the number of children in the denominator rose each year, the absolute number of children with a subspecialist visit increased from 97,596 to 172,104. Within the PEDSnet cohort, children with visits to two or more types of subspecialists increased by 1.2 percentage points (from 4.7 percent in 2011 to 5.9 percent in 2021), a relative rise of 25.5 percent over

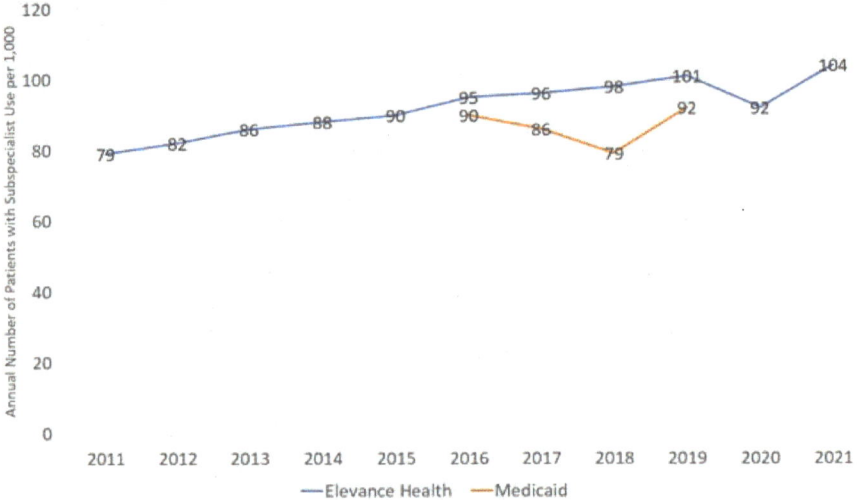

FIGURE 3-1 Temporal trends in annual outpatient pediatric subspecialist use rates in commercially insured and publicly insured cohorts.
NOTES: The commercially insured data is based on the Carelon Research data analysis; the publicly insured data is based on the T-MSIS Medicaid/CHIP cohorts. The chart shows trends across an 11-year period from 2011 to 2021 for the commercially insured Elevance Health cohort and a 4-year period from 2016 to 2019 for the national Medicaid/CHIP cohort. A child was categorized as having subspecialist use if they had one or more visits in an outpatient setting with one of the 25 pediatric medical subspecialties in that year. Denominators for Elevance Health included children enrolled for at least 6 months for a given calendar year. Denominators for T-MSIS include children enrolled at any time over the course of a year.

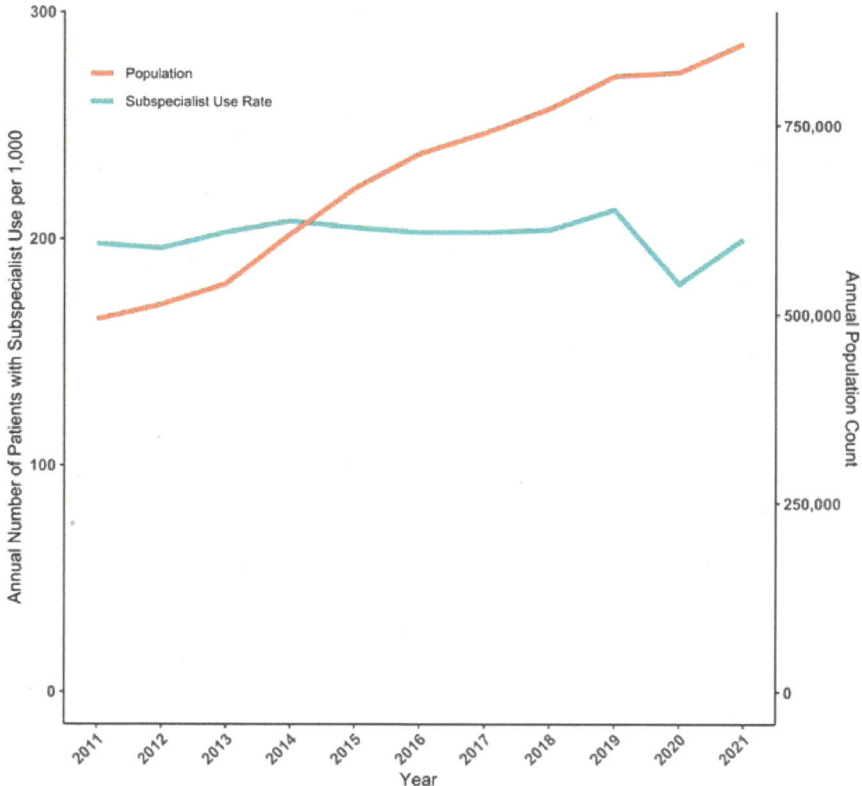

FIGURE 3-2 Temporal trends in annual outpatient pediatric subspecialist use rates and counts of patients seen by a general pediatrician within the academic medical health systems. Data are from the PEDSnet cohort.
NOTES: The chart shows trends in annual subspecialty use rates and the size of the eligible population (i.e., at least one visit to a general pediatrician at the academic medical health system in the index or prior year) across an 11-year period from 2011 to 2021 for children less than 21 years in the PEDSnet academic medical center cohort. A child was categorized as having any subspecialist use if they had one or more visits in an outpatient setting with one of the pediatric medical subspecialties.

this time period. Although rates dropped in calendar year 2020 due to the pandemic, they returned to prepandemic levels in 2021.

Use Rates by Subspecialty Type

The change over time in annual subspecialist use rates varied markedly by type of subspecialist and by cohort. For the Elevance Health cohort (see Table 3-1), 20 of the 21 subspecialities with sufficient sample size for estimation experienced an increase. In the PEDSnet academic medical center cohort (see Table 3-2), 14 of 22 subspecialties experienced increases. In both data sources, child neurology, pediatric cardiology, pediatric endocrinology, and pediatric gastroenterology were among the subspecialties with the highest use rates. In the Elevance Health data, the use rate for pediatric infectious diseases was stable until 2021 when it doubled, likely a result of care for children with COVID-19.

TABLE 3-1 Change in the Annual Outpatient Subspecialist Use Rates, 2011 versus 2021, by Pediatric Medical Subspecialty, Elevance Health Data

Pediatric Medical Subspecialty	Subspecialty Use Rate per 1,000 Children		Percentage Relative Change
	2011	2021	
Adolescent Medicine	34.2	35.6	4
Child Abuse Pediatrics	<0.1	<0.1	n/a
Child Neurology	7.2	9.9	38
Clinical Genetics	1.1	1.3	18
Developmental-Behavioral Pediatrics	2.8	2.4	−14
Hospice and Palliative Medicine	0.2	0.2	−27
Medical Toxicology	<0.1	<0.1	n/a
Obesity Medicine	<0.1	<0.1	n/a
Pediatric Allergy/Immunology	2.2	2.5	14
Pediatric Cardiology	10.6	15.2	43
Pediatric Dermatology	1.8	2.5	39
Pediatric Endocrinology	6.0	8.9	48
Pediatric Gastroenterology	7.0	10.4	49
Pediatric Hematology/Oncology	2.2	3.7	64
Pediatric Infectious Diseases	0.9	2.3	144
Pediatric Nephrology	1.2	1.9	58
Pediatric Pulmonology	4.0	5.0	25
Pediatric Rehabilitation Medicine	0.3	0.6	100
Pediatric Rheumatology	0.9	3.6	300
Pediatric Transplant Hepatology	<0.1	<0.1	n/a
Sleep Medicine	0.6	0.7	17
Sports Medicine	1.2	2.8	133

NOTES: Carelon Research data are from beneficiaries enrolled in an Elevance Health (formerly Anthem, Inc.) health plan (i.e., commercial insurance). Annual use rates were computed as the number of children with one or more visits to a pediatric subspecialist per 1,000 beneficiaries.

TABLE 3-2 Change in the Annual Outpatient Subspecialist Use Rates, 2011 versus 2021, by Pediatric Medical Subspecialty, PEDSNet

	Subspecialist Use Rate per 1,000 Children		
Pediatric Medical Subspecialty	2011	2021	Percentage Relative Change
Adolescent Medicine	14.5	17.0	18
Child Abuse Pediatrics	1.1	0.5	−53
Child Neurology	20.9	24.1	15
Dermatology	11.0	17.8	61
Developmental-Behavioral Pediatrics	19.4	27.4	41
Genetics	4.2	5.7	36
Hospice and Palliative Medicine	0.6	0.4	−35
Medical Toxicology	<0.1	<0.1	n/a
Obesity	<0.1	<0.1	n/a
Pediatric Allergy and Immunology	19.9	22.0	10
Pediatric Cardiology	28.7	32.1	12
Pediatric Endocrinology	17.6	22.0	25
Pediatric Gastroenterology	26.3	36.9	40
Pediatric Hematology/Oncology	11.4	12.4	9
Pediatric Infectious Diseases	3.2	2.5	−21
Pediatric Nephrology	5.6	12.8	127
Pediatric Pulmonology	15.7	18.3	17
Pediatric Rheumatology	4.0	5.0	26
Pediatric Transplant Hepatology	<0.1	0.6	n/a
Rehabilitation	15.1	10.8	−29
Sleep Medicine	1.5	1.0	−34
Sports Medicine	3.5	7.7	118

NOTES: PEDSnet data are from eight large pediatric academic medical centers. Annual subspecialist use rates were computed as the number of children with one or more visits to a pediatric subspecialist per 1,000 individuals with a general pediatrician visit during the index or prior calendar year.

Although the T-MSIS data are limited to 2016 through 2019 (see Table 3-3), similar to the Elevance Health and PEDSnet cohorts, child neurology, pediatric cardiology, pediatric endocrinology, and pediatric gastroenterology had some of the highest subspecialist use rates. However, pediatric dermatology and pediatric emergency medicine also experienced high rates of beneficiary use. The committee notes that these data are restricted to

TABLE 3-3 Change in the Annual Outpatient Subspecialist Use Rates, 2016 vs. 2019, by Pediatric Medical Subspecialty, T-MSIS

	Subspecialist Use Rate per 1,000 Children with Medicaid/CHIP		
Pediatric Medical Subspecialty	2016	2019	Percentage Relative Change
Adolescent Medicine	28.2	26.6	−6%
Child Abuse Pediatrics	0.4	0.4	−4%
Child Neurology	6.4	7.2	13%
Clinical Genetics	1.3	1.3	−2%
Developmental-Behavioral Pediatrics	3.6	3.7	5%
Pediatric Hospice and Palliative Medicine	0.3	0.3	−14%
Pediatric Medical Toxicology	<0.1	<0.1	n/a
Pediatric Obesity Medicine	0.1	<0.1	n/a
Pediatric Allergy/Immunology	0.8	1.0	26%
Pediatric Cardiology	7.4	8.4	13%
Pediatric Dermatology	8.3	8.7	5%
Pediatric Endocrinology	5.8	6.4	11%
Pediatric Gastroenterology	6.3	7.6	20%
Pediatric Hematology/Oncology	4.2	4.5	6%
Pediatric Infectious Diseases	2.2	2.3	8%
Pediatric Nephrology	2.0	2.2	13%
Pediatric Pulmonology	4.7	5.1	9%
Pediatric Rehabilitation Medicine	0.3	0.4	5%
Pediatric Rheumatology	0.7	0.9	26%
Pediatric Transplant Hepatology	<0.1	<0.1	n/a
Pediatric Sleep Medicine	0.2	0.3	74%
Pediatric Sports Medicine	0.8	1.1	28%

NOTE: T-MSIS is a national dataset of Medicaid/CHIP claims. Annual subspecialist use rates were computed as the number of beneficiaries less than 19 years old insured by Medicaid/CHIP with one or more visits to a pediatric subspecialist per 1,000 beneficiaries less than 19 years old insured by Medicaid/CHIP.

outpatient clinics and excluded visits to emergency departments or inpatient care settings. The high rate of pediatric emergency medicine may be due to the inclusion of urgent care visits in the T-MSIS analysis, which are not included in the other two dataset analyses.

A few patterns of use emerge across the three cohorts. For example, children insured by Medicaid/CHIP had higher subspecialist use rates to developmental-behavioral pediatrics compared with individuals in the commercially insured Elevance Health cohort, but lower use rates compared with the academic medical center PEDSnet cohort. Pediatric cardiology rates were lower for the population insured by Medicaid/CHIP in comparison with both the Elevance Health and PEDSnet cohorts.

Subspecialist Use by Payer and Race/Ethnicity Groups, PEDSnet Data Only

On average, patients in the PEDSnet cohort were 5.5 years old on cohort entry. The cohort was 49 percent female, 13.6 percent Hispanic, 26.2 percent non-Hispanic Black/African-American, 39.6 percent non-Hispanic White, 5.7 percent Asian/Pacific Islander, 3.2 percent Multiple Race, and 11.8 percent other or unknown. The payer status was 43.3 percent commercial, 46.7 percent Medicaid/CHIP, and 10.0 percent unknown/self-pay. Across the full duration of the 11-year study period, patients averaged 4 years (SD 3.4 years) of follow-up care, and 43.3 percent of patients had at least one subspecialist visit during that time period (see Figure 3-3). This proportion varied by payer, with nearly half of patients insured by Medicaid/CHIP experiencing use of at least one subspecialist. In additional analyses (data not shown), the committee found that annual rates of subspecialist use were consistently higher for patients with Medicaid insurance versus commercial insurance. In addition, the proportion of patients insured by Medicaid/CHIP that had visits with multiple types of subspecialists was nearly twice as high as those with commercial insurance.

As seen in Figure 3-4, Hispanic, non-Hispanic Black/African-American patients and multiple-race patients were more likely than other race/ethnicity groups to have a subspecialist visit or multiple types of subspecialist visits at some point during the study period. Following patients in the other/unknown category, Asian/Pacific Islanders were least likely to use subspecialty care. The differences across the race/ethnicity groups were smaller than the differences found between the payer categories.

Most Common Diagnoses by Subspecialty, PEDSnet Data Only

For the PEDSnet analysis, diagnosis codes assigned by the subspecialists were extracted for each subspecialist visit. Clinically similar codes were aggregated into a single category to obtain a rank-ordered list of the three most common diagnoses recorded by subspecialists (see Table 3-4).

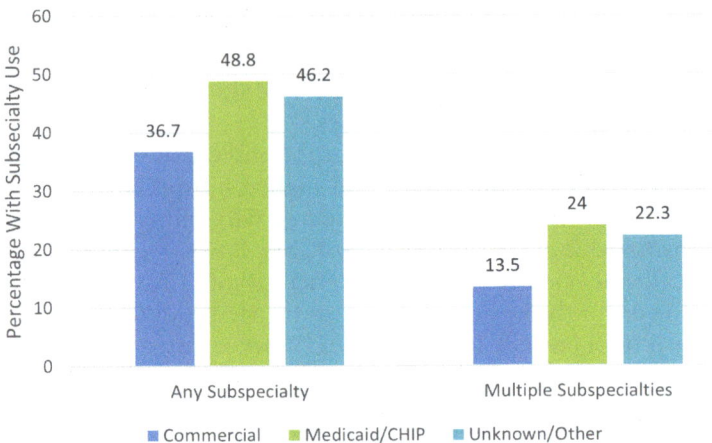

FIGURE 3-3 Proportion of any or multiple subspecialties use by payer, 2011-2021, PEDSnet.
NOTES: PEDSnet data are from eight large pediatric academic medical centers. Proportions represent the share of children with at least one visit to a subspecialist during the study period. Children on average had 4 years of follow-up. Children insured by Medicaid/CHIP at any time during their follow-up period were classified as having that type of insurance.

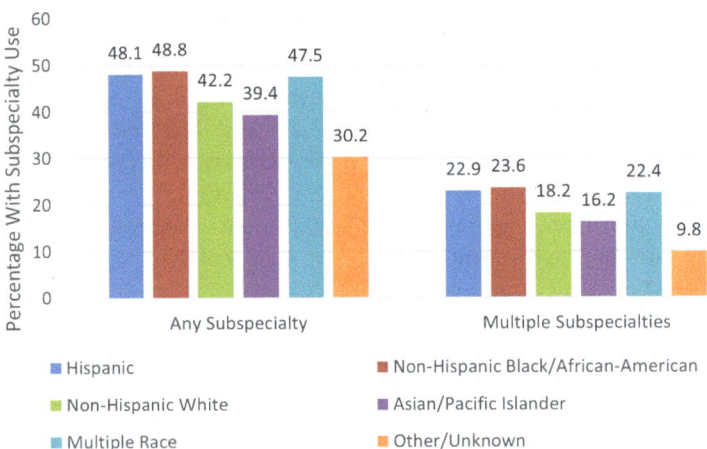

FIGURE 3-4 Proportion of any or multiple types of subspecialist use by race and ethnicity, 2011–2021.
NOTES: PEDSnet data are from eight large pediatric academic medical centers. Proportions for any subspecialist use represent the share of children with at least one visit to a subspecialist across the full study period. The proportion of children with multiple subspecialties use included the share of children who saw two or more types of subspecialists across the full study period. Children on average had 4 years of follow-up. Children with Hispanic ethnicity were categorized as Hispanic race/ethnicity, otherwise their race category was used.

TABLE 3-4 Pediatric Medical Subspecialists' Three Most Commonly Diagnosed Health Conditions in Outpatient Settings, 2011–2021, PEDSnet

Pediatric Subspecialty	Three Most Common Health Conditions Rank Ordered
Adolescent Medicine	Obesity Sexually transmitted infection Contraception
Child Abuse Pediatrics	Child sexual abuse Foster care Possible victim of child abuse
Child Neurology	Seizure/epilepsy Headache, including migraine Developmental delay
Clinical Genetics	Developmental delay Autism spectrum disorder Poor muscle tone
Developmental-Behavioral Pediatrics	Developmental delay Autism spectrum disorder Attention deficit hyperactivity disorder
Hospice and Palliative Medicine	Palliative care Pain Hospice care
Medical Toxicology	Lead poisoning Abnormal blood chemistry Iron-deficiency anemia
Obesity Medicine	Obesity Obstructive sleep apnea, including snoring History of bariatric surgery
Pediatric Allergy/Immunology	Allergic rhinitis Allergies, including food allergies Atopic dermatitis
Pediatric Cardiology	Heart murmur Chest pain Palpitations
Pediatric Dermatology	Atopic dermatitis Warts and molluscum contagiosum Inflammatory dermatitis
Pediatric Endocrinology	Obesity Short stature Type 1 diabetes mellitus
Pediatric Gastroenterology	Constipation Gastroesophageal reflux Feeding problem

(continued)

TABLE 3-4 Continued

Pediatric Subspecialty	Three Most Common Health Conditions Rank Ordered
Pediatric Hematology/Oncology	Anemia, including iron-deficiency anemia Acute lymphoid leukemia Thrombocytopenia
Pediatric Infectious Diseases	Positive tuberculin test Fever Upper respiratory infection
Pediatric Nephrology	Hypertension Chronic kidney disease Proteinuria
Pediatric Pulmonology	Asthma Obstructive sleep apnea, including snoring Cough
Pediatric Rehabilitation Medicine	Muscle weakness Abnormal gait Developmental delay
Pediatric Rheumatology	Joint pain Antinuclear-antibody positive Hypermobility syndrome
Pediatric Transplant Hepatology	Depression, including suicidal ideation Postoperative state Liver disease
Sleep Medicine	Obstructive sleep apnea, including snoring Sleep disorder Trisomy 21
Sports Medicine	Pain Patellofemoral stress syndrome Ankle sprain

NOTES: All diagnosis codes were from outpatient clinics. Data from urgent care centers, emergency departments, and inpatient settings were excluded.

For example, multiple codes for hypertension (i.e., elevated blood pressure, essential hypertension, hypertensive disorder, and secondary hypertension) were combined into a single cluster. Perhaps the most remarkable result that emerges from this list is the number of diagnoses that are common conditions or health problems that are usually managed in primary care settings. It is possible that some patients with common diagnoses such as constipation on further evaluation were diagnosed with an uncommon disorder, such as congenital aganglionic megacolon. It is also possible that common diagnoses like headache represent severe cases that have been intransigent to standard primary care treatment.

Adult Subspecialty Workforce, T-MSIS Data Only

The data presented above may underrepresent use rates of subspecialty care by children, as some children may receive subspecialty care from adult clinicians. To examine the extent to which this happens, T-MSIS data were used to investigate the adult subspecialty workforce providing service to the pediatric population insured by Medicaid/CHIP. Table 3-5 provides the subspecialist use rates for 2019 by adult and pediatric medical subspecialty physicians for beneficiaries younger than 19 years old insured by Medicaid/CHIP and by age range (i.e., less than 1 year, 1–11 years, and 12–18 years).

Overall, for most subspecialties, children were more likely to have an outpatient visit to a pediatric subspecialist than an adult subspecialist. Generally, pediatric patients in the adolescent years were more likely to be treated by adult medical subspecialty physicians than those in the younger age ranges. Some additional patterns of care are also notable. For example, a high rate of outpatient pediatric patients insured by Medicaid/CHIP saw adult allergy and immunology specialists compared with pediatric allergy and immunology specialists. This may be related to the small number of pediatric allergy and immunology specialists concentrating on the smaller number of children with serious immunologic diseases.

WHAT THESE DATA MEAN

Across the data sources, approximately 10 to 20 percent of children less than 21 years saw a pediatric medical subspecialist each year. The rate estimates vary widely across and within datasets, which may be due to differences in access to subspecialty care by type of payer, geographic accessibility differences across regions of the United States, type of health system, and a range of other factors (see Chapter 2 for full discussion on access to subspecialty care). Wide variation (but consistent among datasets) in use of different types of subspecialties points to the need for subspecialty workforce development and access initiatives to analyze these trends and consider prioritizing some subspecialties over others in order to decrease disparities in access.

The analyses show weak evidence for rising rates per 1,000 population of subspecialty use from 2011 to 2021. However, the PEDSnet academic medical center data make it clear that these institutions have experienced an increase in demand for subspecialty care since 2010 due largely to an overall increased number of children receiving most of their care (primary and subspecialty) within their systems; that is, the rate per 1000 children has not increased, but the denominator has. Moreover, the need for multiple subspecialties for the same child has increased even more, pointing toward an increase in complexity among patients served.

TABLE 3-5 Adult and Pediatric Medical Subspecialty Outpatient Subspecialist Use Rates for Children Less Than 19 Years Covered by Medicaid/Children's Health Insurance Program, T-MSIS Calendar Year 2019

Medical Subspecialty	Use Rate per 1,000 Children Insured by Medicaid/CHIP Age: All <19 Years	Use Rate per 1,000 Children Insured by Medicaid/CHIP, by Age		
		<1 Year	1–11 Years	12–18 Years
Adult Neurology	2.8	0.9	2.4	3.9
Child Neurology	7.2	3.5	7.5	7.5
Adult Hospice and Palliative Medicine	0.3	0.4	0.3	0.3
Pediatric Hospice and Palliative Medicine	0.3	0.3	0.3	0.2
Adult Medical Toxicology	<0.1	<0.1	<0.1	<0.1
Pediatric Medical Toxicology	<0.1	<0.1	<0.1	<0.1
Adult Obesity Medicine	0.2	0.2	0.2	0.2
Pediatric Obesity Medicine	<0.1	<0.1	<0.1	<0.1
Adult Allergy/Immunology	10.8	2.3	11.8	10.4
Pediatric Allergy/Immunology	1.0	0.5	1.2	0.8
Adult Cardiology	0.6	0.4	0.4	1.0
Pediatric Cardiology	8.4	16.1	8.0	7.9
Adult Dermatology	1.9	1.4	1.7	2.3
Pediatric Dermatology	8.7	3.4	6.5	13.4
Adult Emergency Medicine	18.7	12.5	20.0	17.3
Pediatric Emergency Medicine	6.9	10.0	8.1	4.4
Adult Endocrinology	0.3	0.1	0.2	0.7
Pediatric Endocrinology	6.4	3.0	5.0	9.3
Adult Gastroenterology	0.4	0.1	0.1	0.9
Pediatric Gastroenterology	7.6	8.5	7.7	7.3
Adult Hematology/Oncology	0.2	0.1	0.2	0.3
Pediatric Hematology/Oncology	4.5	4.7	4.7	4.2
Adult Infectious Disease	0.4	0.4	0.3	0.6
Pediatric Infectious Disease	2.3	4.5	2.6	1.6
Adult Nephrology	0.3	0.1	0.2	0.5
Pediatric Nephrology	2.2	2.4	2.1	2.4

TABLE 3-5 Continued

Medical Subspecialty	Use Rate per 1,000 Children Insured by Medicaid/CHIP	Use Rate per 1,000 Children Insured by Medicaid/CHIP, by Age		
	Age: All <19 Years	<1 Year	1–11 Years	12–18 Years
Adult Pulmonology	0.2	0.1	0.2	0.3
Pediatric Pulmonology	5.1	3.6	6.1	3.6
Adult Rehabilitation Medicine	1.1	0.3	0.9	1.6
Pediatric Rehabilitation Medicine	0.4	0.2	0.4	0.3
Adult Rheumatology	0.2	<0.1	0.1	0.3
Pediatric Rheumatology	0.9	0.5	0.7	1.2
Adult Transplant Hepatology	<0.1	<0.1	<0.1	<0.1
Pediatric Transplant Hepatology	<0.1	<0.1	<0.1	<0.1
Adult Sleep Medicine	0.8	0.4	0.8	0.7
Pediatric Sleep Medicine	0.3	0.3	0.3	0.2
Adult Sports Medicine	2.8	2.0	1.9	4.5
Pediatric Sports Medicine	1.1	0.8	0.9	1.5

NOTES: T-MSIS is a national dataset of Medicaid/CHIP claims. Annual subspecialist use rates were computed as the number of beneficiaries less than 19 years old insured by Medicaid/CHIP with one or more evaluation and management visits to a pediatric subspecialist per 1,000 beneficiaries less than 19 years old insured by Medicaid/CHIP.

All datasets used in these analyses are national in scope, but none were fully nationally representative. Furthermore, they were intentionally chosen to provide a set of complementary approaches for understanding patterns of subspecialist use. Carelon Research included data from one multistate health insurance company and was restricted to beneficiaries with commercial insurance. PEDSnet included patients insured by different commercial insurance plans as well as beneficiaries with Medicaid/CHIP insurance, but the analysis was limited to patients within eight large, pediatric academic medical centers. T-MSIS includes only the population insured by Medicaid/CHIP.

There are several reasons why the subspecialty use rates were lower in the Carelon Research and T-MSIS cohorts compared with the PEDSnet cohort. First, Carelon Research and T-MSIS were based on children enrolled in health plans, which included both users and non-users of health care, while PEDSnet was a use-based cohort that did not contain information on primary or specialty care that occurred outside the academic medical care system. Second, Carelon Research and T-MSIS included children who sought care from all types of settings, both community and academic institutions, while PEDSnet included children obtaining care from academic medical centers only. Children receiving care in academic medical centers may have higher acuity and thus more intense service use. Third, PEDSnet has devoted extensive effort to validating physician subspecialty, working with each member institution to examine and improve the quality of this data element. It is possible that Carelon Research's rates were lower because some subspecialty care may have been billed as a pediatric medical group rather than a specific subspecialty group practice. The T-MSIS analysis relied on primary specialty in the National Plan and Provider Enumeration System dataset, which may not fully capture physician subspecialties. Fourth, Carelon Research data just include beneficiaries with commercial insurance only and T-MSIS only includes beneficiaries insured by Medicaid/CHIP, while PEDSnet patients are not limited based on insurance type (with 40 percent having Medicaid/CHIP coverage). Finally, the T-MSIS data are also limited in the years of available data, from 2016 through 2019.

As diagnoses seen by subspecialties are often those that can be managed to some extent by primary care, innovations to improve the primary care-subspecialty interface might be promoted and incentivized as a way to improve access to appropriate care for these problems. (See Chapter 7 for more on the pediatric primary–subspecialty care interface, including optimizing referrals.)

KEY FINDINGS AND CONCLUSIONS

Key Findings

<u>Finding 3-1</u>: Each year about 10 to 20 percent of children less than 21 years of age obtain care from a pediatric medical subspecialist.

<u>Finding 3-2</u>: Although the rates of subspecialist use in academic medical centers remained constant, the absolute number of children seeing a subspecialist increased markedly because of the larger total population of children cared for in these institutions.

<u>Finding 3-3</u>: Overall annual rates of use of multiple types of subspecialists (i.e., patients seeing more than one type of subspecialist) increased in pediatric academic medical centers.

Finding 3-4: The change in subspecialist use rates between 2011 and 2021 varied by type of pediatric medical subspecialist.

Finding 3-5: Within academic medical center practices, children insured by Medicaid/CHIP insurance were more likely to have at least one pediatric medical subspecialty visit than those with commercial insurance. For the general population with Medicaid/CHIP insurance, use rate varied across the pediatric subspecialties.

Finding 3-6: For many pediatric medical subspecialties, the most commonly managed health conditions are those that may be able to be managed in primary care settings.

Finding 3-7: The data across the three analyses showed similar variations in use of different types of pediatric medical subspecialties.

Finding 3-8: Adult subspecialists provide a share of health care services to the pediatric population with Medicaid/CHIP insurance. More adult subspecialists see adolescent age patients than younger children.

Conclusions

Conclusion 3-1: The share of children using pediatric medical subspecialty care increased somewhat from 2011 to 2021, but temporal trends varied significantly by subspecialty type and payer.

Conclusion 3-2: In a select group of the nation's large pediatric academic medical centers, growth in the number of children cared for increased markedly from 2011 to 2021, although the share of children requiring pediatric medical subspecialty care remained constant.

Conclusion 3-3: In a select group of the nation's large pediatric academic medical centers, children enrolled in Medicaid/CHIP compared with those who are commercially insured had a higher use of pediatric medical subspeciality care.

Conclusion 3-4: Some portion of subspecialty use may be amenable to substitution with primary care services.

Conclusion 3-5: Adult subspecialists are important parts of the workforce that provide care to the pediatric population.

REFERENCE

Yoon, P., J. Hall, J. Fuld, S. L. Mattocks, B. C. Lyons, R. Bhatkoti, J. Henley, A. D. McNaghten, D. Daskalakis, and S. K. Pillai. 2021. Alternative methods for grouping race and ethnicity to monitor COVID-19 outcomes and vaccination coverage. *Morbidity and Mortality Weekly Report* 70:1075-1080.

4

The Pediatric Health Care Workforce Landscape

A range of practitioners are responsible for the health care of children. General pediatricians and pediatric subspecialty physicians focus exclusively on the health and development of infants, children, adolescents, and young adults. General pediatricians often form continuous relationships with children and their families to support their development into adulthood with unique understandings of all the factors that affect their well-being. Pediatric subspecialty physicians often also have long-term relationships with patients, especially those children who have chronic illness. In addition, many other health and social care practitioners provide high-quality care and services for children and youth and are critical to the pediatric health care workforce, especially for team-based care.

This chapter focuses primarily on ABP-certified pediatric subspecialty physicians, including their demographics and work profiles. Additionally, a brief overview of general pediatricians and many of the other health care professionals that provide pediatric care is presented to give a sense of the broader workforce that cares for children and often work together with pediatric subspecialty physicians. Chapter 7 further explores the interface between primary care clinicians and pediatric subspecialty physicians.

THE PATHWAY TO BECOMING A PEDIATRIC SUBPECIALTY PHYSICIAN

The design and maintenance of the pathway to becoming a certified pediatric subspecialist in the United States is a joint responsibility largely shared by the Accreditation Council for Graduate Medical Education

(ACGME) and the American Board of Pediatrics (ABP) or the American Osteopathic Board of Pediatricians (AOBP).

The committee recognizes that individuals need to make multiple decisions in the course of the pathway to becoming a pediatric subspecialist. The typical pediatric subspecialty workforce pathway, and key decision points, are exemplified in Figure 4-1. (For more on the specific factors along this pathway that influence an individual's choice to pursue pediatric subspecialty training throughout this pathway, see Chapter 5.)

The committee first recognizes that life experiences even before high school can contribute to the choice to pursue pediatrics and ultimately, subspecialty training. In general, a student proceeds from high school, to college, and then medical school. Potential subspecialty trainees are lost at each of these points if they do not choose to pursue higher education

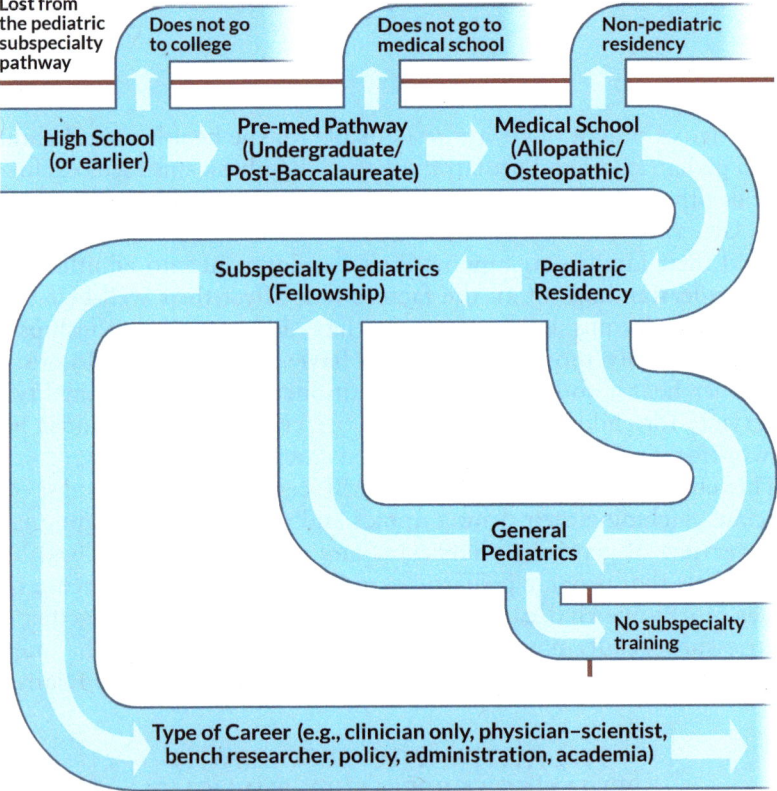

FIGURE 4-1 The typical pediatric subspecialty workforce pathway.
NOTE: This figure does not reflect all the alternative pathways and combined training programs available for some pediatric subspecialties.
SOURCE: Committee generated.

or enter a non-pediatric residency program. Typically, fourth year medical students with an interest in pursuing pediatrics apply to pediatric residency programs through the National Residency Match Program (NRMP), but some residents will be accepted into fellowship training programs outside of the NRMP process. (See discussion later in this chapter.) After choosing to enter a pediatric residency, the trainee next needs to make a choice about pursuing subspecialty training as opposed to remaining a general pediatrician. Figure 4-1 recognizes that individuals who choose to pursue general pediatrics may later return for subspecialty training (as opposed to entering a fellowship immediately after residency). Finally, pediatric subspecialists need to make decisions about the type of career they would like to pursue, including as a clinician, physician–scientist, bench researcher, policy maker, administrator, and/or educator. Many subspecialists participate in more than one of these focus areas. The following sections give a brief overview of the education and training requirements along this pathway.

Overview of Education and Training Requirements

As of May 2023,[1] in addition to a number of basic requirements regarding the structure and content of residency programs, ABP-certified pediatric residency programs are required to have faculty members with subspecialty board certification in adolescent medicine, developmental-behavioral pediatrics, neonatal-perinatal medicine, pediatric critical care medicine, pediatric emergency medicine, and subspecialists from at least five other distinct pediatric medical disciplines (ACGME, 2022a). Exposure to a variety of pediatric subspecialists may help influence decisions to enter those career paths.

As described in Chapter 1, requirements for subspecialty training evolved over the past several decades. In the late 1980s, an expectation for in-depth research experiences became a requirement (Stevenson et al., 2014). In 1996, the Federation of Pediatric Organizations issued a policy statement emphasizing that the goal of fellowship training was to create academic pediatricians by fostering competence in clinical care, education and research (FOPO, 2001). The statement included guidelines for fellowship, including the development of clinical skills, opportunities for scholarly activities, training to ensure graduates are effective teachers, and the presence of mentors. In 2004, the Subspecialties Committee of ABP affirmed this commitment to creating academic subspecialists and noted:

---

[1] As of the writing of this report, several changes have been proposed for residency training. However, those changes have not been approved or finalized.

In discussing optional pathways for fellowship training, the question was raised whether a "third-tier," clinical-only, fellowship training pathway should be established...the Subspecialties Committee concluded that additional clinical training in lieu of a scholarly activity experience was not consistent with the principal goal of fellowship training being preparation for a career in academic pediatrics. (ABP, 2004, p.10)

Today, with the exception of pediatric hospital medicine, ACGME requires all pediatric subspecialty fellowships to be 36 months in length with a requirement for scholarly activity included (ACGME, 2022a). Although there are multiple, specific alternate training pathways for fellows interested in a career focused on research, no similar pathway for a career focused on clinical care remains. For more on the research requirements of fellowship and alternate training pathways, see Chapter 5.

Preparation of Pediatric Subspecialists to Care for Today's Children

Entrustable professional activities (EPAs) are the "observable, routine activities that a pediatric subspecialist should be able to perform safely and effectively to meet the needs of their patients" (ABP, 2023a). The ABP worked with the pediatrics community to develop a core set of seven EPAs (for all subspecialties), with three or more additional EPAs specific to the subspecialty. Similarly, EPAs exist for general pediatrics. However, questions have been raised about the preparation of the pediatric subspecialty workforce to fully meet the needs of today's children in light of their evolving health needs (see Chapter 2).

In part, lack of preparation in some key areas may lie in residency training. As noted by Hilgenberg et al. (2021): "While the ACGME and [ABP] periodically publish residency program curricular changes, programs have limited resources and time in which to design, adapt, individualize, and/or implement changes and may struggle to respond, resulting in curricular gaps." In fact, Hilgenberg et al. (2021) found that 59 percent of graduating pediatrics residents planning for careers in primary care and 49 percent of graduating pediatrics residents planning for careers in subspecialty care desired additional clinical training. Among program directors and associate program directors, 21 percent identified additional clinical training as most needed in their curricula. Some smaller studies have suggested specific training needs in residency for cultural competence (Rule et al., 2018) and the care of working with transgender and gender non-conforming patients (Barber Doucet et al., 2021). Furthermore, pediatric residents and subspecialty fellows may not be fully prepared to address or refer for mental health and substance use disorders (Green et al., 2019, 2022). For example, while nearly two-thirds of pediatric subspecialty fellows believe they should be responsible for the emotional and mental health concerns of children with chronic medical conditions, few feel competent to do so (Green et al., 2022). Just 53 percent of graduating general pediatrics residents from 2015 to 2018 demonstrated achieving the level of competence for behavioral and mental health care needed to provide care independently (Schumacher et al., 2020). Hadland and colleagues (2016) suggested that all pediatric clinicians should be trained to prevent and treat addiction, and that "residency programs should develop specific training in [medication-assisted treatment] and offer robust clinical experiences in youth addiction medicine" (Hadland et al., 2016).

GENERAL PEDIATRICIANS

The following section gives a brief overview of actively practicing general pediatricians, residents in general pediatrics, and pediatric residency programs.

Demographics

As of July 2023, 56,882 pediatricians are actively maintaining their certification with ABP in general pediatrics only (not including those who are actively maintaining certification in general pediatrics as well as certifications in one or more pediatric subspecialties) (ABP, 2023b). However, this number does not recognize pediatricians who are trained and practicing, but not certified by ABP. For example, while most physicians with degrees as doctors of osteopathic medicine (D.O.s) pursue primary specialty certification through ABP, a number of D.O.s pursue primary specialty certification through AOBP. As of December 31, 2017, 648 D.O. pediatricians had active AOBP specialty board certificates, with 42 D.O.s certified in a pediatric subspecialty (Wieting et al., 2018). An analysis by the Association of American Medical Colleges of the American Medical Association Physician Masterfile estimated that in 2021, there were 60,305 actively practicing general pediatricians in the United States, or 1,720 individuals under age 24 per pediatrician (AAMC, 2023). This estimate includes physicians who were not certified by ABP, but who indicated that pediatrics was their primary area of work.

Among pediatricians who are currently maintaining their certification in general pediatrics, nearly 81 percent are American medical graduates and 71 percent are female (ABP, 2023c). As shown in Figure 4-2, general and subspecialty pediatricians are predominantly White/Non-Hispanic, but those who are in training, recently graduated, and/or not yet certified are increasingly diverse. (See later in this chapter for more specific demographic data on the pediatric subspecialties.)

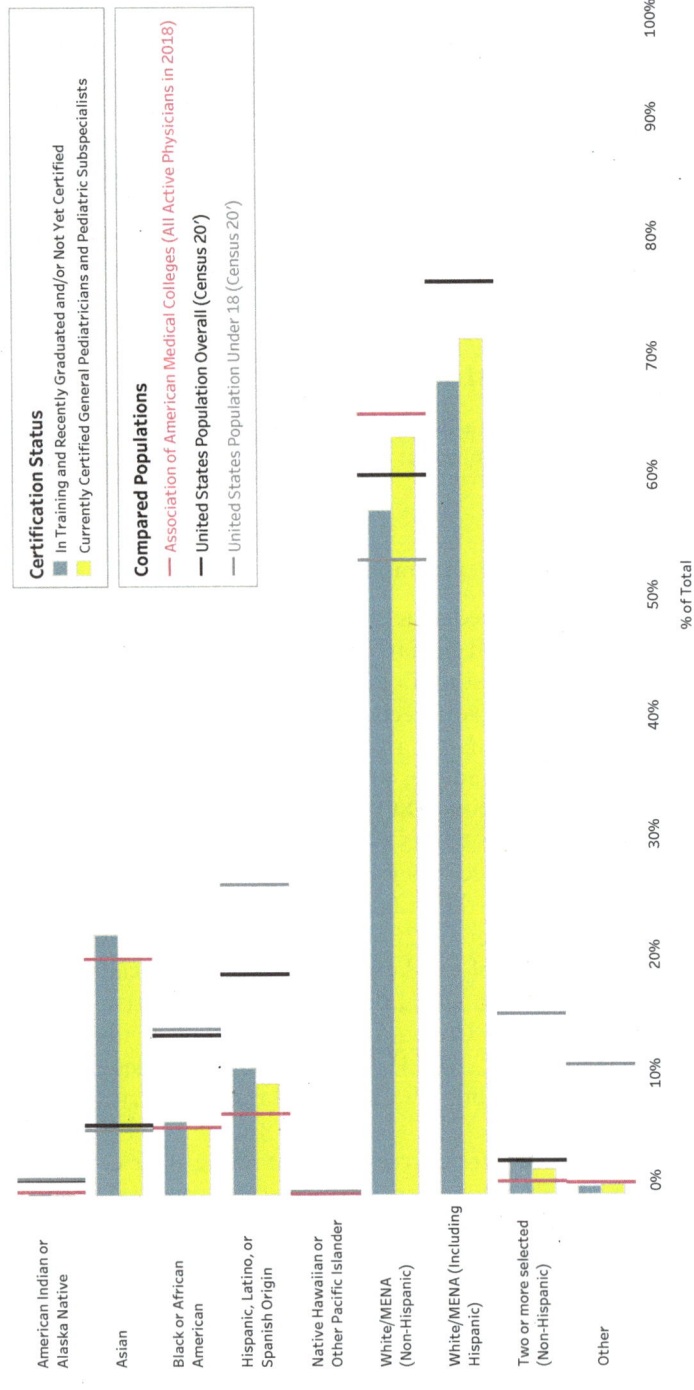

FIGURE 4-2 Comparisons of estimated race and ethnicity percentages among pediatricians, all physicians, and U.S. populations (under 18 and overall).
NOTE: MENA = Middle East and North Africa
SOURCE: ABP, 2023d. Reprinted with permission from the American Board of Pediatrics.

Pediatric Residents and Training Programs

In 2022, there were 11,930 residents (including all years of residency and residents in combined programs and alternate pathways) in general pediatrics (an 11.6 percent increase over the previous 10 years) (ABP, 2023e). Eighteen percent of these residents were training in a combined program or alternate pathway. Twenty-one percent[2] of the 9,801 general pediatrics residents not in combined programs or alternate pathways are international medical graduates. Data from 2019[3] show that 14.5[4] percent of residents not in a combined program or alternative pathway had a D.O. (ABP, 2023e). Like currently certified pediatricians, the majority of first year general pediatrics residents (73 percent) are female (up from 70.2 percent in 2008) (ABP, 2023f). Pediatrics is second only to obstetrics and gynecology for the largest percentage of active female residents (ACGME, 2021). This is significant as female pediatricians are more likely to work part time than male pediatricians (Freed et al., 2016, 2017). In 2022, 53.1 percent of all general pediatrics residents were White; 21.4 percent were Asian; 7.5 percent were Hispanic, Latino, or of Spanish origin; and 6.3 percent were Black or African American (ABP, 2023g). Nearly 19 percent of residents were identified as having a background that is underrepresented in medicine (URiM). The number of residency positions in pediatrics increases every year, and those positions are rarely unfilled (see Table 4-1). Residency and fellowship training programs have a wide geographic distribution, but with large areas of the country not being represented (see Figure 4-3).

PEDIATRIC SUBSPECIALTY FELLOWS

As noted earlier, some pediatrics residents pursue fellowship training in more specialized areas of pediatric care beyond the required training for general pediatrics. This section includes a discussion of pediatric fellows, including their basic demographics, and focuses primarily on the ABP-certified subspecialties.

---

[2] Calculated on the ABP dashboard by choosing to analyze by medical school location and choosing "categorical pediatrics" under the residency training pathway for all training levels and all training program locations (ABP, 2023e).

[3] 2019 is the most recent year for which data on degree are available.

[4] Calculated on the ABP dashboard by choosing to analyze by medical degree and choosing "categorical pediatrics" under the residency training pathway for all training levels and all training program locations (ABP, 2023e).

TABLE 4-1 Postgraduate Year 1 (PGY-1) Pediatrics (Categorical) Positions Offered and Percentage Filled, 2018–2023

Year	PGY-1 Positions Offered	Percentage Filled
2023	2,986	97.1%
2022	2,942	97.2%
2021	2,901	98.6%
2020	2,864	98.2%
2019	2,847	97.6%
2018	2,768	97.9%

NOTES: This table does not include positions offered through combined training programs or alternate pathways. It also may underestimate the percentage of positions filled as it does not include matches made outside the NRMP process.
SOURCES: NRMP, 2022, 2023a.

Demographics

In 2023, NRMP reported that there were 860 accredited programs in the 15 ABP-certified pediatric medical specialties participating in the match, offering 1,786 positions, ranging from 23 positions in child abuse pediatrics to 288 positions in neonatal-perinatal medicine (NRMP, 2023b). An important note is that while most fellows match to their programs through NRMP, some fellows will be accepted into accredited programs outside of the formal match process (ABP, 2023i; Freed and Wickham, 2023; Macy et al., 2021). As shown in Table 4-2, average position fill rates for accredited programs both through the formal NRMP process and the final fill rate (as calculated by ABP) show significant variation across pediatric subspecialties. These data show the average fill rate for each ABP subspecialty over the time period from 2014 to 2022. Given the small numbers for some subspecialties, fill rates may vary each year—therefore, examination of the average over a period of time presents a more complete picture of the challenges some subspecialties experience in filling available positions. Overall, however, these numbers and fill rates may not reflect the need for each of those subspecialties, and many factors influence the decision to pursue subspecialty training (see Chapter 5). For example, a high fill rate may not reflect the need for even more positions to meet the health care needs of children, and a low fill rate may reflect too many positions being available.

In addition to the variation in fill rates, as seen in Figure 4-4, there is wide variation in the number of first-year fellows by subspecialty (ABP, 2023j). Some subspecialties have had a steady increase in the number of first-year fellows (particularly among the more procedural subspecialties), while others have remained relatively stable (particularly among the

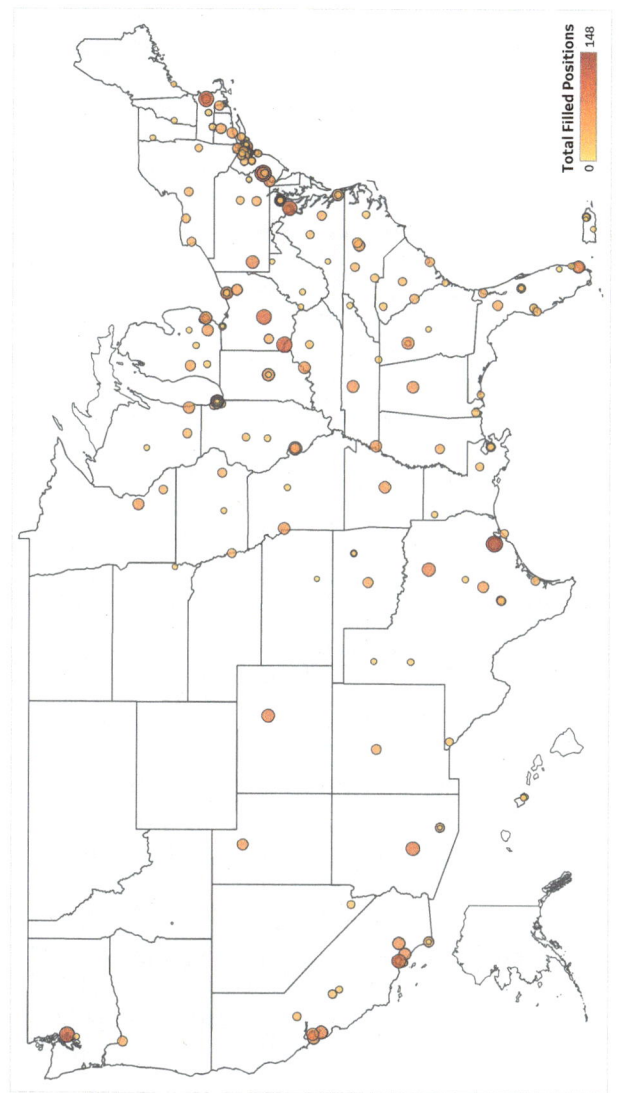

FIGURE 4-3 Pediatric residency and fellowship training programs, 2021–2022.
SOURCE: Modified from ABP, 2023h. Data retrieved by ABP based on academic year snapshot data from the ACGME. Reprinted with permission from the American Board of Pediatrics.

TABLE 4-2 ABP-Certified Subspecialty by Average NRMP-Reported Fellowship Match Fill Rate and Average ABP-Calculated Final Fill Rate, 2014–2022

Pediatric Subspecialty	NRMP-Reported Fill Rate	ABP-Calculated Final Fill Rate
Pediatric Gastroenterology	94.1%	108.3%
Pediatric Hospital Medicine	98.6%	107.9%
Pediatric Cardiology	96.0%	103.9%
Pediatric Critical Care Medicine	96.7%	103.8%
Neonatal-Perinatal Medicine	91.9%	103.4%
Pediatric Emergency Medicine	98.9%	103.3%
Adolescent Medicine	78.9%	98.6%
Pediatric Hematology/Oncology	90.0%	97.9%
Pediatric Pulmonology	63.0%	86.9%
Pediatric Endocrinology	64.7%	86.0%
Developmental-Behavioral Pediatrics	64.3%	82.8%
Pediatric Rheumatology	64.2%	79.2%
Pediatric Infectious Diseases	57.0%	79.0%
Child Abuse Pediatrics	58.7%	69.0%
Pediatric Nephrology	53.3%	65.7%

NOTE: Final fill rates may be over 100 percent, as some programs may ultimately accept more fellows than the number of positions reported in the NRMP process.
SOURCES: ABP, 2023i; NRMP, 2023b.

subspecialties that typically involve fewer procedures). The total number of first-year fellows has grown by more than 27 percent between 2012 and 2022, in part due to the establishment of certification for pediatric hospital medicine in 2019 (ABP, 2023k).

Similar to general pediatrics fellows, 12.6 percent[5] of first-year subspecialty fellows (in both U.S. and Canadian programs) in 2022 had a D.O. degree and 26.9 percent were international medical graduates (ABP, 2023k). Additionally, subspecialty fellows are predominantly female (70.3 percent of first-year fellows in 2022, up from 59.8 percent in 2008) and nearly 17 percent of residents were identified as having a URiM background (ABP, 2023k,l). (See later in this chapter for the percentage of women and

---

[5] Calculated on the ABP dashboard by choosing to analyze by medical degree and choosing "all" under the "training program location" filter (ABP, 2023k).

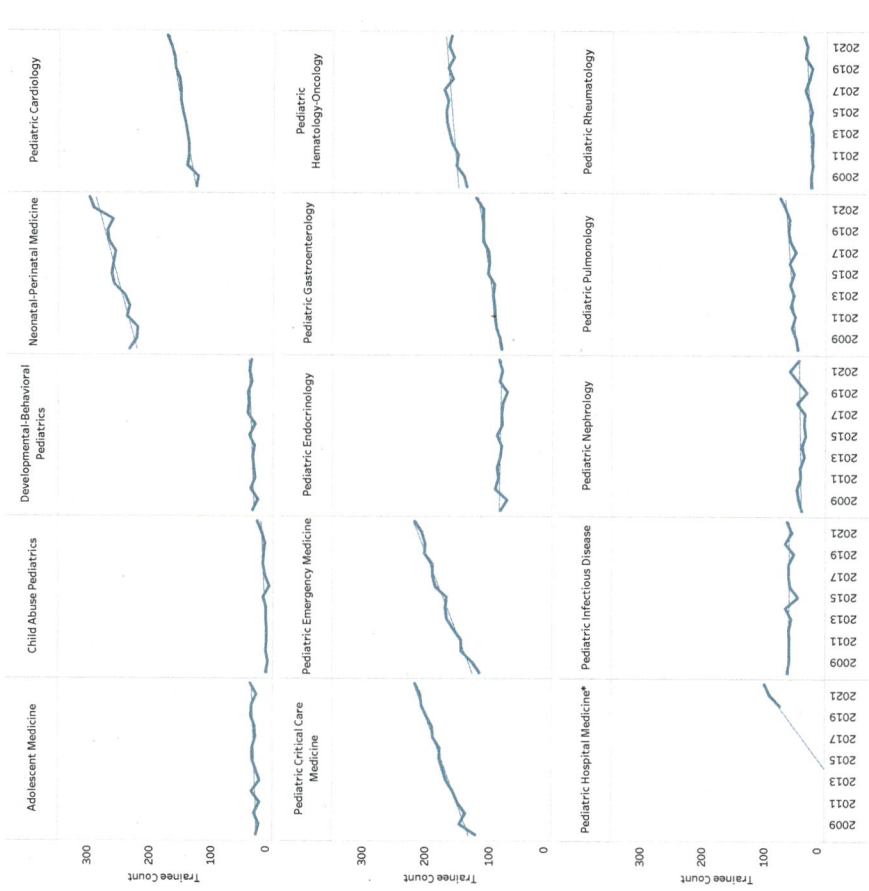

(continued)

FIGURE 4-4 Number of NRMP-matched first-year fellows by subspecialty, 2008–2022.
NOTES: Pediatric hospital medicine fellowships were first accredited and reported in 2020. NRMP match rate data reflect the positions offered and accepted within the NRMP match process and do not account for fellows who enroll in programs outside of the formal match process.
SOURCE: ABP, 2023j. Reprinted with permission from the American Board of Pediatrics.

the percentage of individuals from URiM backgrounds by subspecialty for pediatric subspecialty fellows as compared with practicing pediatric subspecialists.)

ABP Co-Sponsored Subspecialties, Alternative Pathways, and Combined Training Programs

As noted in Chapter 1, some pediatric subspecialists are certified by co-sponsoring ABMS boards, by the American Osteopathic Board of Pediatrics, or via several combined training programs and non-standard pathways for subspecialization. Each of these pathways have different education and training requirements and procedures, but they have not been extensively studied as a whole. In 2023, NRMP reported on the availability of first-year fellowship positions in the following subspecialties certified via non-standard pathways and combined training programs:

- Pediatrics—Medical Genetics: 25 positions
- Pediatrics—Physical Medicine and Rehabilitation: 4 positions
- Pediatrics—Psychiatry/Child Psychiatry: 26 positions
- Child Neurology—177 positions
- Medicine—Pediatrics: 392 positions
- Pediatrics—Anesthesiology: 7 positions
- Pediatrics—Emergency Medicine: 9 positions (NRMP, 2023a).

Pediatric Surgical Subspecialists

The number of pediatric surgery training programs has increased, and such programs are considered among the most competitive (Alaish et al., 2020; Farooqui et al., 2023; Yheulon et al., 2019). Several ABMS boards offer subspecialty certificates in pediatric surgical subspecialties. For example, the American Board of Thoracic and Cardiac Surgery certifies congenital heart surgeons to care for infants, children, and adolescents with congenital, acquired, or end-stage heart disease (Surgical Advisory Panel et al., 2014). While there may not be formal subspecialty certification, several other surgical specialties (e.g., ophthalmology, orthopedic surgery, and plastic surgery) offer additional training (including fellowships) in the care of pediatric patients (Surgical Advisory Panel et al., 2014). However, concerns have been raised about the quality of pediatric surgical training, resulting in calls for improvements in training and certification (Alaish and Garcia, 2019; Alaish et al., 2020; Drake et al., 2017; Farooqui et al., 2023), such as through the American Pediatric Surgical Association's Right Child/Right Surgeon initiative (Alaish et al., 2020).

ACTIVELY PRACTICING PEDIATRIC SUBSPECIALTY PHYSICIANS

As shown in Table 4-3, the number of ABP-certified pediatric subspecialists maintaining certification varies widely by subspecialty area (ABP, 2023m). Similarly, the number of physicians trained in subspecialties co-sponsored by ABP but certified by another ABMS board are shown in Table 4-4.

The following sections will give an overview of the work profiles and demographics of actively practicing pediatric subspecialists (primarily those physicians practicing in one of the 15 ABP-certified subspecialties).

TABLE 4-3 Numbers of Pediatric Subspecialists Ever Certified by ABP and Numbers Maintaining Certification by Subspecialty

Subspecialty	Ever Certified	Maintaining Certification
Adolescent Medicine	836	580
Child Abuse Pediatrics	425	363
Developmental-Behavioral Pediatrics	1,043	803
Neonatal-Perinatal Medicine	7,871	5,319
Pediatric Cardiology	4,117	3,096
Pediatric Critical Care Medicine	3,689	3,128
Pediatric Emergency Medicine	3,493	3,017
Pediatric Endocrinology	2,218	1,508
Pediatric Gastroenterology	2,232	1,882
Pediatric Hematology/Oncology	4,231	2,929
Pediatric Hospital Medicine	2,542	2,537
Pediatric Infectious Diseases	1,876	1,368
Pediatric Nephrology	1,199	729
Pediatric Pulmonology	1,585	1,254
Pediatric Rheumatology	626	508
Total	37,983	29,021

NOTES: Data are as of June 14, 2023. Calculated on the ABP dashboard by choosing to analyze each certification area (i.e., subspecialty) by "all, no breakout."
SOURCE: ABP, 2023m.

TABLE 4-4 Numbers of Pediatric Subspecialists Co-Sponsored by ABP and Ever Certified by other ABMS boards and Numbers Maintaining Certification by Subspecialty

Subspecialty	Ever Certified	Maintaining Certification
Hospice and Palliative Medicine	479	414
Medical Toxicology	51	34
Sleep Medicine	394	350
Sports Medicine	416	348
Transplant Hepatology	179	153
Total	1,519	1,299

NOTES: Data are as of June 14, 2023. Calculated on the ABP dashboard by choosing to analyze each certification area (i.e., subspecialty) by "all, no breakout."
SOURCE: ABP, 2023m.

Work Profiles and Settings

Based on data collected in 2018–2022 from maintenance of certification enrollment surveys, 89 percent[6] of respondents from the ABP-certified subspecialties indicated that they worked full time (84.6 percent of women and 93.9 percent of men)[7] (ABP, 2023n). Eighty-five percent reported working 40 or more hours a week, and 24 percent reported working 60 or more hours a week.[7] A larger percentage of men reported working more than 50 hours per week as compared with women.[8] Given that women represent an increasing proportion of the subspecialty workforce, these practice patterns may have implications for future workforce planning. That is, if women work fewer hours, more subspecialists may be needed to provide the same amount of care. (See Chapter 5 for more on lifestyle influences on careers for female subspecialists.)

As seen in Figure 4-5, ABP-certified pediatric subspecialists report spending the bulk of their professional time on direct or consultative patient care. Less than 8 percent of subspecialists reported spending more than 50 percent of their time doing research, and nearly half (48.3 percent) reported not being involved in any research activities (ABP, 2023n).

---

[6] Calculated on the ABP dashboard by choosing "none (no breakout)" under "select to crosstab results" and by choosing the 15 ABP-certified subspecialties under "GP/subspecialty certification" filter (ABP, 2023n).

[7] Calculated on the ABP dashboard by choosing "gender" under the "select to crosstab results" filter and by choosing the 15 ABP-certified subspecialties under "GP/subspecialty certification" filter (ABP, 2023n).

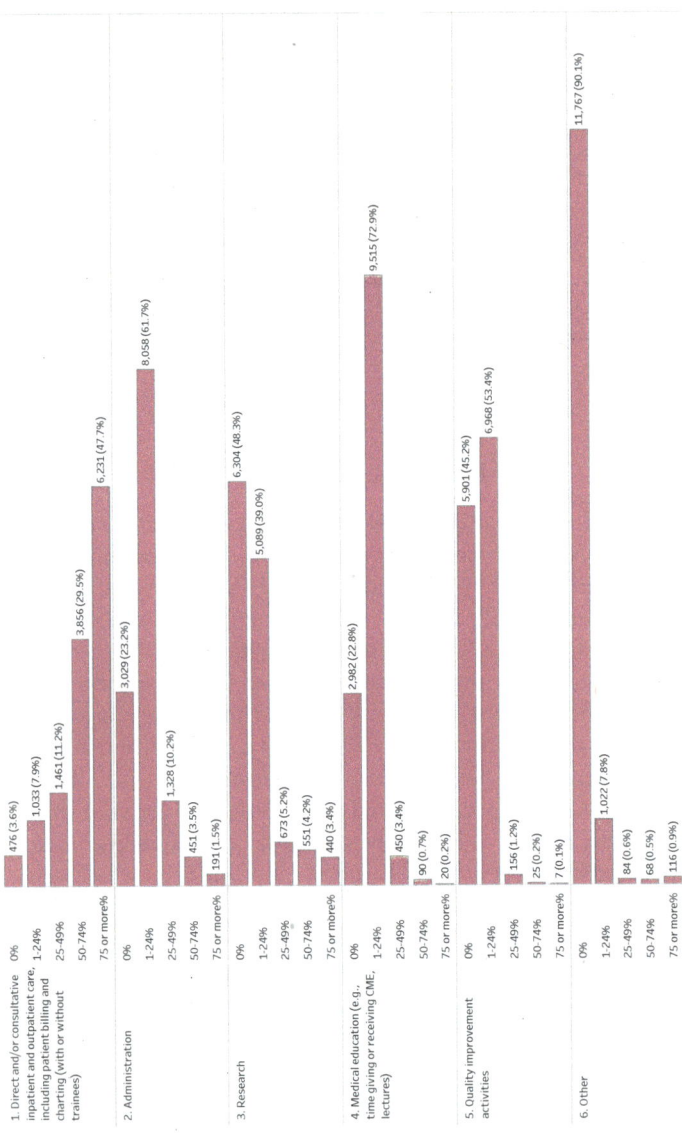

FIGURE 4-5 Proportion of Professional Time Spent on Patient Care, Administration, Research, Medical Education, Quality Improvement Activities, and Other.
NOTE: CME = continuing medical education.
SOURCE: ABP, 2023n. Reprinted with permission from the American Board of Pediatrics.

ABP-certified pediatric subspecialists are most likely to have their primary work setting in a medical school or parent university (32 percent), a non-government hospital or clinic (22 percent), or a pediatric or multispecialty group practice (26 percent) (ABP, 2023o).[8] The majority (78.5 percent) of subspecialists report some form of academic faculty appointment. One setting of care that is unique to children are children's hospitals. As noted by Colvin and colleagues (2016a), "[c]hildren's hospitals (whether freestanding or within a general hospital) provide a wide range of pediatric specialty care or are dedicated solely to specific disease states (e.g., pediatric cancer)." The authors noted that while children's hospitals only accounted for 3.4 percent of all hospitals, they represented about one third of all pediatric hospital discharges and almost half (42.5 percent) of discharges for children with medical complexity and high severity of illness (Colvin et al., 2016b).

Geographic Distribution

Most ABP-certified pediatric subspecialists report working primarily in an urban setting (76 percent), with 20 percent practicing primarily in suburban settings and 3 percent primarily in rural settings[9] (ABP, 2023o). Comparatively, approximately 19 percent of children (aged 17 years and younger) live in rural areas (KidsData, 2018). Among pediatricians who completed training in 2012 through 2021, nearly 31 percent of subspecialists (on average) report practicing in a medically underserved area (AAMC, 2022a). Furthermore, on average, nearly 60 percent of subspecialists are practicing in the state where they completed their training (AAMC, 2022b). As noted in Chapter 2, regionalization of these subspecialists is logical "given that highly specialized physicians would be unlikely to have enough patients to attend to in any single community" and that access to technologies and other resources for care will be more available in centralized care centers (Gans et al., 2013). According to Rimsza et al. (2018):

> There are many factors besides supply that can affect the geographic distribution of subspecialists, including location of training [see Figure 4-3], financial viability of practice location, limited availability of other physicians to share call and provide consultative services, and lack of employment opportunities for other family members. In addition, a subspecialist who is interested in teaching and research is likely to have limited opportunities to pursue these interests outside of an urban academic center.

---

[8] Calculated on the ABP dashboard by choosing "overall specialty status" under the "select to crosstab results" filter and by choosing the 15 ABP-certified subspecialties under "GP/subspecialty certification" filter (ABP, 2023o).

[9] Total is less than 100 percent due to rounding.

For all types of physicians, there are significant associations between physician practice location and their racial and ethnic composition. Physicians identifying as American Indian, Alaska Native, or Hawaiian/Pacific Islander; black or African American; and/or Hispanic/Latino are more likely to practice in impoverished areas, and areas federally designated as medically underserved or experiencing health professional shortages (Xierali et al., 2014). In general, URiM trainees are more likely to establish a practice in underserved areas (Walker et al., 2012).

Race, Ethnicity, and Sex

There is some evidence that racial concordance between patient and physician is associated with reduction in health disparities and increased patient satisfaction (Alberto et al., 2021; Greenwood et al., 2020; Takeshita et al., 2020). However, the pediatric workforce does not reflect the diversity of its patients (Lopez and Fuentes-Afflick, 2022; Mehta et al., 2019). In 2021, 26 percent of children under age 18 were Hispanic, Latino, or of Spanish origin (as compared with 6.2 percent of certified general pediatricians and 5.8 percent of certified pediatric subspecialists);[10] 14 percent of children under age 18 were Black or African American (as compared with 6.4 percent of certified general pediatricians and 4.4 percent of certified pediatric subspecialists) (ABP, 2023p,q). Although the pediatrics workforce overall does not reflect the diversity of U.S. children, recently graduated and/or not yet certified pediatricians are slightly more diverse than currently certified general pediatricians and subspecialists (see Table 4-5).

As shown in Figure 4-6, similar patterns are seen within the individual pediatric medical subspecialties. The pediatric subspecialty workforce has as few as 2.3 percent of pediatric pulmonologists and 2.4 percent of pediatric cardiologists and pediatric rheumatologists identifying as Black or African American and 4.0 percent of child abuse specialists identifying as Hispanic, Latino, or of Spanish descent (ABP, 2023q).[11]

Overall, pediatric medical subspecialists are becoming increasingly female and from URiM backgrounds. As seen in Table 4-6, the vast majority of subspecialties show an increased percentage of women and individuals who are URiM among subspecialty fellows as compared with certified subspecialists.

---

[10] Percentages for certified general pediatricians and certified subspecialists were calculated on the ABP dashboard by choosing "certification status with trainee type" under the "crosstab" filter and by choosing "no merging" under the "race and ethnicity groupings" filter (ABP, 2023q).

[11] Calculated on the ABP dashboard by choosing "GP/subspecialty" under the "crosstab" filter and by choosing "no merging" under the "race and ethnicity groupings" filter (ABP, 2023q).

TABLE 4-5 Estimated Percentages of Race and Ethnicity Groups and URiM Status by Certification Status

Certification Status	Black or African American	Hispanic, Latino, or Spanish Origin	White	URiM
Recently Graduated and/or Not Yet Certified	7.0	7.7	49.5	18.7
Certified General Pediatricians	6.4	6.2	61.0	15.9
Certified Pediatric Subspecialists	4.4	5.8	60.6	13.0

NOTES: Counts for URiM include categories of: American Indian or Alaska Native; Black or African American; Hispanic, Latino, or Spanish Origin; and Native Hawaiian or Other Pacific Islander. Individuals who indicated two or more race and ethnicity categories are not included in URiM.
Percentages for Black or African American; Hispanic, Latino, or Spanish Origin, and White were calculated on the ABP dashboard by choosing "certification status with trainee type" under the "crosstab" filter and by choosing "no merging" under the "race and ethnicity groupings" filter. For URiM, "merge to display URIM category" was chosen under the "race and ethnicity groupings" filter.
SOURCE: ABP, 2023q.

MODELING THE FUTURE SUBSPECIALTY WORKFORCE

In a committee webinar on November 2, 2022,[12] Laurel Leslie, vice president of research for ABP, and Colin Orr, assistant professor in the Division of General Pediatrics and Adolescent Medicine at The University of North Carolina at Chapel Hill, gave a presentation on a workforce model under development to estimate the future supply of the pediatric subspecialty physician workforce. The model is a partnership between ABP and The University of North Carolina at Chapel Hill's Cecil G. Sheps Center for Health Services Research (AMSPDC, 2020). The model will use historical data for the supply of 14 of the ABP-certified subspecialties,[13] and then apply different scenarios to see what the impact would be on future supply. The model intends to look not just at absolute numbers, but also to consider changing work profiles (e.g., time spent in direct clinical care), geography (at multiple levels), age, and gender. The model is unique from other forecasting models in that it has separate forecasts for each subspecialty. The model does not make any assumptions about increased use of

---

[12] The webinar recording can be accessed at https://www.nationalacademies.org/event/11-02-2022/the-pediatric-subspecialty-workforce-and-its-impact-on-child-health-and-well-being-webinar-3.
[13] Hospital medicine was excluded due to a lack of sufficient data.

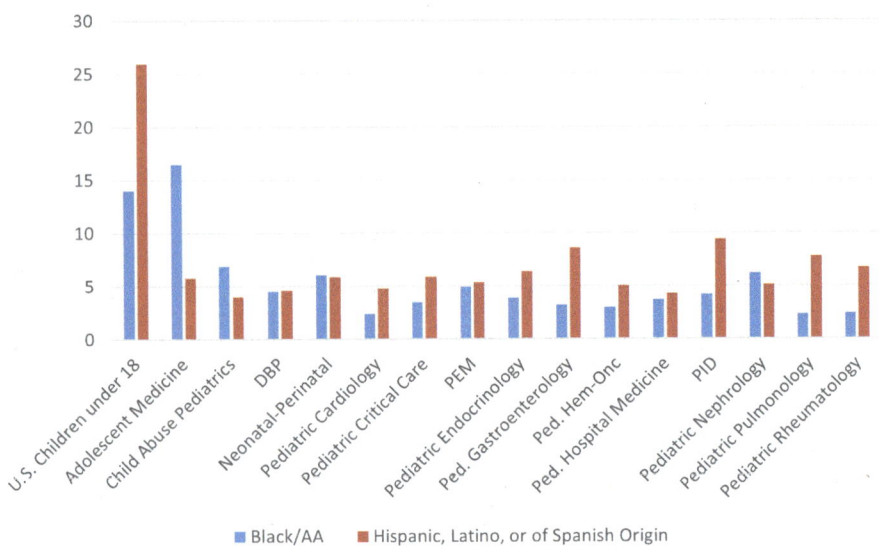

FIGURE 4-6 Diversity of the pediatric subspecialty physician workforce in comparison with U.S. children, 2021.
NOTES: DBP = developmental-behavioral pediatrics; Hem/Onc = hematology/oncology; PEM = pediatric emergency medicine; PID = pediatric infectious diseases. Percentages for the subspecialties were calculated on the ABP dashboard by choosing "GP/subspecialty" under the "crosstab" filter and by choosing "no merging" under the "race and ethnicity groupings" filter.
SOURCES: ABP, 2023p,q.

telehealth or advanced practice providers (e.g., advanced practice registered nurses [APRNs], physician assistants). Early results presented at the webinar indicate that growth (e.g., in absolute numbers, number of clinicians per 100,000 children) varies by subspecialty. Papers on the results of modeling by subspecialty are scheduled to be made public in 2023.

PRIMARY CARE CLINICIANS

Apart from pediatricians, a variety of primary care clinicians provide care for children, particularly in team-based models of care. These clinicians include nurses, physician assistants, and physicians (e.g., adult subspecialty physicians who care for children, family medicine physicians). Information on the use of primary care clinicians (apart from pediatricians) for subspecialty care is not well known.

TABLE 4-6 Pediatric Subspecialty Fellows in U.S. Fellowship Programs and Pediatricians Maintaining Certification in ABP-Certified Subspecialties by Sex and URiM Status, 2022

Subspecialty	Percentage Women		Percentage URiM*	
	Fellows	Certified	Fellows	Certified
Adolescent Medicine	79.6	76.8	27.9	26.8
Child Abuse Pediatrics	77.6	83.0	18.2	15.9
Developmental-Behavioral Pediatrics	89.7	76.6	20.8	14.0
Neonatal-Perinatal Medicine	72.4	58.3	20.1	14.8
Pediatric Cardiology	53.5	40.6	11.0	9.2
Pediatric Critical Care Medicine	65.2	48.6	13.0	12.0
Pediatric Emergency Medicine	67.2	60.8	18.0	12.5
Pediatric Endocrinology	80.3	73.6	19.4	14.2
Pediatric Gastroenterology	69.4	52.3	20.5	14.7
Pediatric Hematology/Oncology	68.5	60.3	13.0	10.0
Pediatric Hospital Medicine	73.1	72.8	16.5	11.0
Pediatric Infectious Diseases	68.9	58.8	17.4	17.8
Pediatric Nephrology	70.1	62.5	14.6	12.9
Pediatric Pulmonology	65.5	49.2	17.7	13.1
Pediatric Rheumatology	76.9	70.7	18.7	12.2
Overall	**68.8**	**58.8**	**16.8**	**13.0**

NOTES: Data for specialists maintaining certification reflect those who answered the survey as a part of maintenance of certification from 2018 to 2022, and are estimates given the response rate of 60.5 percent. The data overall do not include information regarding the small group of subspecialists who have completed fellowship training but are not yet certified. Counts for URiM include categories of: American Indian or Alaska Native; Black or African American; Hispanic, Latino, or Spanish Origin; and Native Hawaiian or Other Pacific Islander. Individuals who indicated two or more race and ethnicity categories are not included in URiM.

URiM percentages for fellows were calculated on the ABP dashboard by examining each subspecialty by choosing "merge to display URiM category" under the "race and ethnicity groupings" filter. The overall percentage was calculated by choosing "all" under the "subspecialty selection" filter (ABP, 2023l).

URIM percentages for certified subspecialists were calculated on the ABP dashboard by choosing "GP/subspecialty" under the "crosstab" filter and choosing "URiM" under the "race and ethnicity" filter and choosing "merge to display URiM category" under the "race and ethnicity groupings" filter. The overall percentage was calculated by choosing "certification status" under the "crosstab" filter (ABP, 2023q).

Female percentages for fellows were calculated on the ABP dashboard by examining each subspecialty by choosing to analyze data by gender and choosing "all" for the training level filter and choosing "U.S. programs" under the training location filter (ABP, 2023r). The overall percentage was calculated by choosing to analyze data by gender and choosing "all" for the training level filter and choosing "U.S. programs" under the training location filter (ABP, 2023k).

Female percentages calculated on the ABP dashboard by examining each subspecialty and by choosing to analyze data by gender and by choosing "maintaining their certification" under the "certification status for age tables" filter (ABP, 2023m). The overall percentage appears as a comparison for "all subspecialties combined." Data are as of June 14, 2023.
SOURCES: ABP, 2023k,l,m,q,r.

Analysis of Usage of Primary Care Clinicians for Pediatric Medical Subspecialty Care

As noted in Chapter 3, the committee received a data analysis[14] that examined subspecialty care using the Transformed Medicaid Statistical Information System (T-MSIS),[15] a national administrative dataset of Medicaid and Children's Health Insurance Program (CHIP) beneficiaries. The T-MSIS analysis relied on primary specialty in the National Plan and Provider Enumeration System (NPPES) dataset, which may not fully capture physician subspecialties. T-MSIS data included enrollment, service usage, and provider information. The analysis used data from 2016 (the first available year of T-MSIS) through 2019. T-MSIS has known data quality challenges, which are analyzed and reported by the Centers for Medicare & Medicaid Services.[16] The analysis included data from 44 states, DC, and Puerto Rico, and excluded Arkansas, California, Delaware, Indiana, Minnesota, and Pennsylvania.

The T-MSIS analysis examined adult medical subspecialties that corresponded to pediatric counterparts as well as primary care specialties, including pediatrics, family medicine, internal medicine, obstetrics and gynecology, APRNs (pediatric), and physician assistants (medical). The analysis also included the specialty of psychiatry and subspecialty of child and adolescent psychiatry. In the primary care and advanced practice provider workforce that cares for children insured by Medicaid/CHIP, use of nurse practitioners and physician assistants increased significantly from 2016 to 2019 (see Table 4-7) and the number of advanced practice providers providing care to the pediatric Medicaid population also increased (see Figure 4-7). A limitation to these data is that because advanced practice providers working in subspecialty care may not have a subspecialty designation, counts of advanced practice providers likely represent growth across both primary and subspecialty care.

Nurses

Registered nurses (RNs) and APRNs are critical members of the pediatric health care team who assume numerous roles to meet a variety of care needs across diverse care settings (ICN, 2022; NASEM, 2021a). APRNs include nurse practitioners (NPs), clinical nurse specialists (CNSs), certified registered nurse anesthetists, and certified nurse midwives. RNs and APRNs can assume essential responsibilities related to: (1) caring for children with

---

[14] All three data analyses submitted to this committee can be found at https://nap.edu/27207.

[15] For more information on T-MSIS, see https://www.medicaid.gov/medicaid/data-systems/macbis/transformed-medicaid-statistical-information-system-t-msis/index.html (accessed October 11, 2023).

[16] For more information, see https://www.medicaid.gov/dq-atlas/welcome (accessed May 4, 2023).

TABLE 4-7 Medicaid Outpatient Primary Care and Advanced Practice Provider Usage, T-MSIS 2016–2019

	Usage Rate per 1,000 Medicaid/CHIP Beneficiaries			
Specialty	2016	2017	2018	2019
Pediatrics	463.1	444.9	427.9	493.60
Family Medicine	23.8	19.2	18.1	19.49
Internal Medicine	137.0	129.2	121.6	128.91
Obstetrics-Gynecology	11.9	7.5	7.1	7.67
Advanced Practice Registered Nurses (Pediatrics)	45.8	52.5	54.7	67.45
Advanced Practice Registered Nurses	88.9	107.1	117.2	147.80
Physician Assistants	50.6	57.8	63.2	75.46
Adult Psychiatry	8.5	8.3	8.2	8.87
Child and Adolescent Psychiatry	2.7	2.7	2.7	3.01

NOTES: Annual usage rates were computed as the number of pediatric Medicaid/Children's Health Insurance Program (CHIP) beneficiaries with one or more evaluation and management visits to a pediatric subspecialist per 1,000 Medicaid beneficiaries less than 19 years old. Clinician specialty was determined using the primary specialty in the National Plan and Provider Enumeration System dataset and may overrepresent the number of clinicians in primary care, such as for internal medicine physicians.

special health care needs; (2) leading teams to improve the care and reduce the costs of high-need, high-cost patients; (3) coordinating the care of children with special health care needs between the primary and subspecialty clinicians; (4) assessing problems to educate and plan with patients and families; and (5) evaluating outcomes (NASEM, 2021a,b). RNs can also lead transition initiatives between pediatric and adult care.

In general, nurses cover a broad continuum of care—from health promotion and disease prevention to curative care and care coordination to palliative care (IOM, 2011). In the context of subspecialty care, the use of RNs and APRNs in outpatient settings (e.g., primary care and ambulatory care) may help increase the availability of specialty care clinicians for the pediatric patients with the most critical or complex health care needs (Laurant et al., 2018; NASEM, 2021a,b; Perloff et al., 2016). With appropriate education and training, RNs and APRNs may provide the same care traditionally delivered by other clinicians such as "diagnostics, treatment, referral to other services, health promotion, management of chronic diseases, or management of acute problems needing same-day consultations" (Laurant et al., 2018). In acute care settings, RNs and APRNs assume care management responsibilities supporting management of changing patient

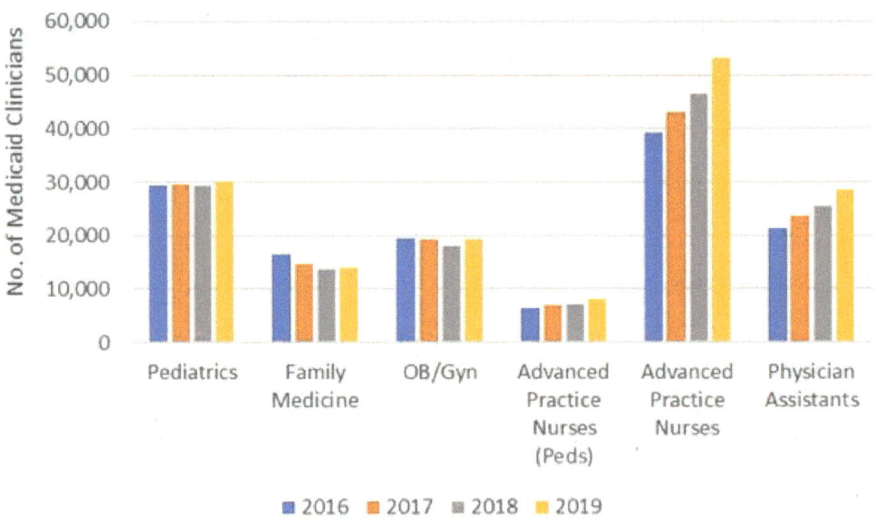

FIGURE 4-7 Medicaid outpatient primary care and advanced practice provider workforce, T-MSIS 2016–2019.
NOTES: The number of Medicaid clinicians is a count of the number of clinicians by specialty with at least one evaluation and management claim for a beneficiary less than 19 years old in the calendar year. Clinician specialty was determined using the primary specialty in the NPPES dataset and may overrepresent the number of clinicians in primary care. Advanced practice provider numbers likely represent practice in both primary and subspecialty care. OB/Gyn = obstetrics-gynecology; T-MSIS = Transformed Medicaid Statistical Information System.

conditions, preparing patients and families for discharge by providing education and self-management support, and facilitating transitions from acute to outpatient settings coordinating follow-up care and resources (Gonçalves et al., 2022; Semanco et al., 2022).

Nurse Practitioners

NPs are RNs who have additional education and clinical training in the care of a specific patient population that enables them to autonomously provide care to patients (NONPF, 2022). Since inception in the 1960s, the NP role and responsibilities evolved to meet patient health care needs and in response to evidence that they consistently provide high-quality care in diverse clinical settings (Aiken et al., 2021; Buerhaus, 2018; Gigli et al., 2021; NASEM, 2021a; Silver et al., 1968). While most NPs are trained in and practice in primary care settings, most NPs who provide pediatric care work in hospital and inpatient settings and one-third work in ambulatory and clinical settings, providing pediatric subspecialty care (AANP, 2022; Gigli et al., 2023). NPs increase children's access to care through their practice in settings that include: Federally Qualified Health Centers, retail clinics, home health, telehealth, schools and school-based health centers, nurse-managed health centers, ambulatory care clinics, as well as community and tertiary care hospitals (PNCB, 2022).

Although it is unclear how widely integrated NPs are in pediatric practices and hospitals, there is a demand for increased NP usage and expansion of the roles they play in care delivery (Freed et al., 2010a, 2011; Gigli et al., 2018; Merrit Hawkins Team, 2021). The NP workforce has more than doubled in the past decade and is expected to grow (Auerbach et al., 2018, 2020). NPs may be board certified in primary care pediatrics, acute care pediatrics, or both (AANP, 2023). There are more than 355,000 NPs in the United States, accounting for more than two-thirds of all APRN licenses (HRSA, 2019), but relatively few NPs choose to specialize in pediatrics (AANP, 2022; Freed et al., 2010a). Less than 4 percent of NPs specialize in pediatrics (2.4 percent primary care pediatric NPs, 0.6 percent acute care pediatric NPs) (AANP, 2022). A majority of NPs are family NPs (70.3 percent). Pediatric acute and primary care NPs report working in multiple subspecialties with pediatric patients, including adolescent care, cardiology, critical care, emergency care, gastroenterology, hematology/oncology, neonatology, and pulmonology (PNCB, 2022). A majority of the NP workforce who care for children are not certified specifically in pediatrics (e.g., family or psychiatric mental health NPs); the extent of their contribution to the delivery of pediatric subspecialty care is not well known (Gigli et al., 2023). There is no modeling for what types of services NPs provide, are needed for, or are best at providing in relation to pediatric subspecialty care. However, as noted earlier, the T-MSIS data analysis[17] submitted to this committee found that both NPs in general and pediatric NPs are increasingly caring for children insured by Medicaid/CHIP (see Table 4-7).

Education, certification, and licensure

The Consensus Model for APRN Regulation, Licensure, Accreditation, Certification and Education ("The Consensus Model") was developed in 2008 by a coalition of professional nursing organizations and established the framework for today's APRN workforce (see Figure 4-8). The Consensus Model defines six patient population foci for APRN education, certification, licensure, and practice. Education programs meet national accreditation standards, and graduates must pass a national certification exam prior to licensure as an NP. An NP education is broad in exposure

---

[17] All three data analyses submitted to this committee can be found at https://nap.edu/27207.

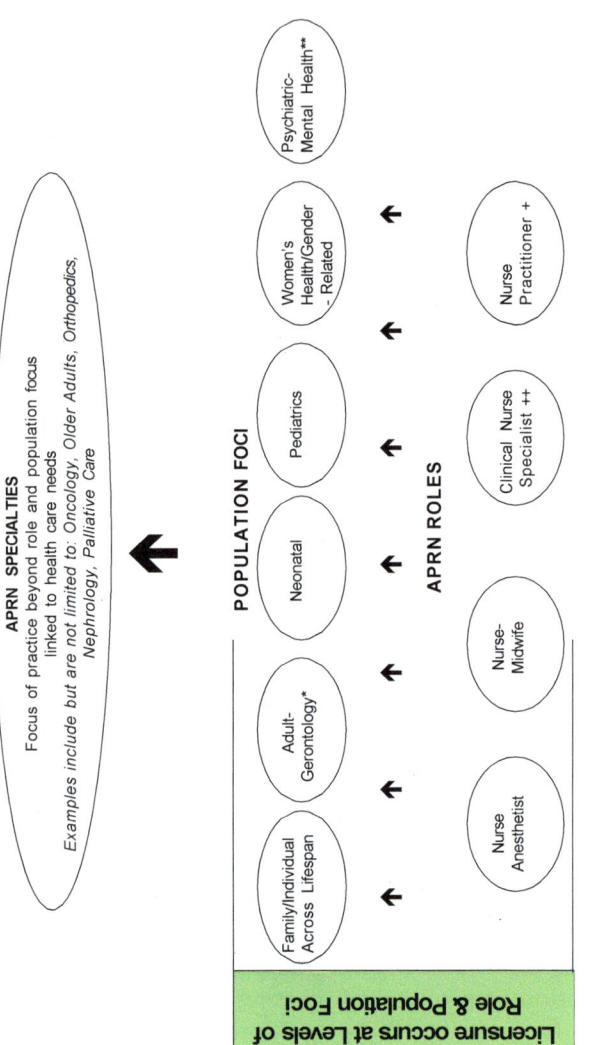

FIGURE 4-8 APRN Consensus Model.
SOURCE: APRN Joint Dialogue Group, 2008. Reprinted with the permission of the National Council of State Boards of Nursing (NCSBN).

to content across a population focus; as a result, specialty education (e.g., cardiology, oncology, critical care) predominantly occurs after completion of an NP program. There is no current mechanism or standardized process to evaluate or recognize an NP's specialty practice expertise.

The Consensus Model outlines expectations that an NP's practice aligns with their role in providing care (i.e., an NP working in a pediatric intensive care unit would be an acute care pediatric NP). According to a 2008 report on the Consensus Model:

> The certified nurse practitioner (CNP) is prepared with the acute care CNP competencies and/or the primary care CNP competencies. At this point in time the acute care and primary care CNP delineation applies only to the pediatric and adult-gerontology CNP population foci. Scope of practice of the primary care or acute care CNP is not setting specific but is based on patient care needs. Programs may prepare individuals across both the primary care and acute care CNP competencies. If programs prepare graduates across both sets of roles, the graduate must be prepared with the consensus-based competencies for both roles and must successfully obtain certification in both the acute and the primary care CNP roles. CNP certification in the acute or primary care roles must match the educational preparation for CNPs in these roles." (APRN, Joint Dialogue Group, 2008, p.10)

Over the ensuing decade since adoption of The Consensus Model, few states mandated such alignment (Gonzalez and Gigli, 2021), and no studies have examined the implications of alignment or misalignment between an NP's education and certification and practice on patient outcomes (Hoyt et al., 2022).

Clinical Nurse Specialists

Like NPs, CNSs have additional education and clinical training and follow requirements for licensure and certification. In 2018, CNSs accounted for almost 20 percent of APRN licenses, or approximately 86,000 licensed CNSs (HRSA, 2019). According to a 2008 report on the Consensus Model, "the CNS has a unique APRN role to integrate care across the continuum and through three spheres of influence: patient, nurse, system" (APRN Joint Dialogue Group, 2008, p.8). CNSs may provide direct patient care, but also collaborate with other professionals to promote evidence-based care and processes, particularly for patients with complex care needs, provide support and education to other health care workers, and promote quality improvement initiatives (Lewandowski and Adamle, 2009; Saunders, 2015; Valdivia, 2022).

CNSs may receive population-based certifications in adult/gerontology, pediatrics, and neonatal care (NACNS, 2023). In a study of the 9,470 CNSs who were registered with a National Provider Identifier,[18] most identified specialty areas of adult health (15.2 percent) and adult mental health (13.5 percent) (Reed et al., 2021). Only 6 percent indicated a specialty as oncology/pediatrics, pediatrics, perinatal, or neonatal and an additional 3 percent indicated a specialty in either child and adolescent or child and family psychiatric/mental health. The same study showed that the number of new CNSs specializing in pediatrics with a National Provider Identifier decreased from 2015 to 2019 (Reed et al., 2021).

School Nurses

An estimated 132,300 school nurses care for children in U.S. schools (Willgerodt et al., 2018). The 2021 National Academies report *The Future of Nursing 2020-2030* describes the importance of school nurses:

> School nurses are front-line health care providers, serving as a bridge between the health care and education systems. Hired by school districts, health departments, or hospitals, school nurses attend to the physical and mental health of students in school. As public health sentinels, they engage school communities, parents, and health care providers to promote wellness and improve health outcomes for children. School nurses are essential to expanding access to quality health care for students, especially in light of the increasing number of students with complex health and social needs. Access to school nurses helps increase health care equity for students. For many children living in or near poverty, the school nurse may be the only health care professional they regularly access. (NASEM, 2021a, p. 108)

Schools are increasingly being recognized not just as core educational institutions, but also as community-based assets that can be a central component of building healthy and vibrant communities (NASEM, 2017). Accordingly, schools and, by extension, school nurses are being incorporated into strategies for improving health care access, serving as hubs of health promotion and providers of population-based care (Maughan, 2018; NASEM, 2021a).

---

[18] A National Provider Identifier (NPI) is "a unique identification number for covered health care providers, created to help send health information electronically more quickly and effectively. Covered health care providers, all health plans, and health care clearinghouses must use NPIs in their administrative and financial transactions" (CMS, 2022).

Physician Assistants

Physician Assistants (PAs) have the potential to play an important role in the care of children in the United States, and the National Commission on the Certification of Physician Assistants (NCCPA) offers a certification of added qualifications in pediatrics (NCCPA, 2023). However, the impact of PAs is limited by their relative scarcity in pediatric practice (Freed et al., 2010a). According to a survey of 3,373 PAs who were certified for the first time (in 2019), 23.1 percent work in primary care (i.e., family medicine, internal medicine, general pediatrics) (NCCPA, 2020). However, only 59 (1.8 percent) reported a principal clinical practice area in general pediatrics and an additional 53 (1.6 percent) worked in the pediatric subspecialties; none reported a principal clinical practice area in adolescent medicine. Few studies exist on the actual or conceptual use of PAs in pediatrics (Doan et al., 2012; Doan et al., 2015; Freed et al., 2011; Mathur et al., 2005). As noted earlier, the T-MSIS data analysis[19] submitted to this committee found that usage rates of PAs for children insured by Medicaid/CHIP increased between 2016 and 2019 (see Table 4-7).

Primary Care Physicians

Some physicians who care for children may not necessarily complete a residency in general pediatrics, but instead are certified by another ABMS board. In fact, many ABMS boards apart from ABP offer subspecialty certificates related to the care of children and adolescents (see Table 4-8). Several of these subspecialties are included among the ABP non-standard pathways and combined training programs (see Chapter 1).

Adult-Trained Subspecialty Physicians Who Care for Children

Some children receive subspecialty care from adult-trained medical subspecialists (primarily internal medicine subspecialists). However, little is known about these practice patterns. In a study of children insured by Medicaid in Pennsylvania, Ray et al. (2016) found that adult subspecialists cared for 10 percent of children who received medical subspecialty care. The use of adult-trained subspecialists was higher (more than 18 percent) for children who lived farther away from a pediatric referral center. Similarly, one study of rheumatology referrals by primary care pediatricians in Minnesota, North Dakota, and South Dakota showed that 20 percent reported referring pediatric patients to adult rheumatologists, often because

---

[19] All three data analyses submitted to this committee can be found at https://nap.edu/27207.

TABLE 4-8 ABMS Boards with Subspecialty Certificates in the Care of Infants, Children, and Adolescents

ABMS Board	Subspecialty Certificates
American Board of Anesthesiology	Pediatric Anesthesiology
American Board of Dermatology	Pediatric Dermatology
American Board of Emergency Medicine	Pediatric Emergency Medicine
American Board of Family Medicine	Adolescent Medicine
American Board of Internal Medicine	Adolescent Medicine
American Board of Otolaryngology-Head and Neck Surgery	Complex Pediatric Otolaryngology
American Board of Pathology	Pathology-Pediatrics
American Board of Physical Medicine and Rehabilitation	Pediatric Rehabilitation
American Board of Psychiatry and Neurology*	Child and Adolescent Psychiatry Neurodevelopmental Disabilities
American Board of Radiology	Pediatric Radiology
American Board of Surgery	Pediatric Surgery
American Board of Thoracic and Cardiac Surgery	Congenital Cardiac Surgery
American Board of Urology	Pediatric Urology

NOTES: *This board offers specialty certificates in psychiatry, neurology, and neurology with special qualification in child neurology. ABMS = American Board of Medical Specialties.
SOURCE: ABMS, 2023.

of the shorter distance to the adult rheumatologist (as compared with a pediatric rheumatologist) (Correll et al., 2015). Ray et al. (2016) also found that other significant factors associated with a higher usage of adult-trained pediatric subspecialists were older age (i.e., 12 to 16 years old), minority race, lower neighborhood income, and managed care plan enrollment.

The T-MSIS data analysis[20] submitted to this committee found that not insignificant numbers of adult subspecialists are providing subspecialty care for pediatric patients insured by Medicaid/CHIP. For example, as shown in Table 3-5 in Chapter 3, adult-trained allergy and immunology specialists see a higher number of outpatient Medicaid/CHIP pediatric patients compared with pediatric allergy and immunology subspecialists.

---

[20] All three data analyses submitted to this committee can be found at https://nap.edu/27207.

Family Medicine Physicians

As part of their training, family physicians learn how to provide neonatal and routine newborn care, manage children who are acutely ill, and provide preventive health services to children (ACGME, 2022b). ACGME has program requirements for family medicine residency programs regarding the preparation of family medicine physicians in the care of children, but most program directors report challenges in meeting the required number of encounters (Krugman et al., 2023). Family physicians provide primary care, but typically do not address subspecialty care needs themselves (Bazemore et al., 2012; Makaroff et al., 2014; Phillips et al., 2006). However, as noted in Table 4-8, the American Board of Family Medicine (ABFM) does offer a certificate of added qualifications in adolescent medicine. The certification was first offered in 2001 and requires a 24-month fellowship in an ACGME-accredited fellowship in adolescent medicine (ABFM, 2023a); a search of the ABFM fellowship directory shows eight fellowship programs in the United States with a length of at least 24 months (ABFM, 2023b).

Previous studies have found that family medicine physicians provide 16 percent to 21 percent of physician visits by children (Jetty et al., 2021; Phillips et al., 2005). However, family physicians are decreasingly caring for children (Bazemore et al., 2012; Eden et al., 2020; Freed et al., 2004, 2010b; Wasserman et al., 2019), which could have significant repercussions on physician supply and access to care for children. For example, a recent cross-sectional survey showed a significant decline in the proportion of family medicine physicians caring for children under age five (from 92.5 percent to 87 percent) and ages 5 to 18 years (from 76.4 percent to 69.4 percent) between 2014 and 2018 (Eden et al., 2020). This trend was also seen with population-level data; using Vermont claims data, Wasserman et al. (2019) found that the percentage of children attending a family physician practice decreased from 2009 to 2016. In any given year, children were 5 percent less likely to see a family physician than a pediatrician compared with the year before (Wasserman et al., 2019). Most studies have found that children are more likely to see a family physician if they are female or have Medicaid, and are less likely to see a family physician if they live in an urban area. However, there have been mixed results about the more specific location (e.g., rural, suburban, area of the country) or age of children that are most likely to see family physicians (Cohen and Coco, 2010; Makaroff et al., 2014; Wasserman et al., 2019).

Jetty et al. (2021) found that scope of practice is often influenced by economic factors, geographic location, clinician age, and social factors, with pediatrician density also playing a role. In a qualitative study of family physicians, Russell et al. (2021) found that environmental, population, personal, and workplace factors all influence scope of practice, and addressing these factors could help family physicians maintain a broader scope of practice.

Hospice and Palliative Care Physicians

As noted in Chapter 1, hospice and palliative care is one of the subspecialties that is co-sponsored by the ABP along with multiple other specialty boards (ABP, 2022). Certification is available to pediatricians who have primary certification by ABP (along with certain other specialties) and is administered by the American Board of Internal Medicine; certification requires one year of fellowship training in an ACGME-accredited hospice and palliative medicine program (AAHPM, 2023). According to the National Hospice and Palliative Care Organization, "pediatric palliative and hospice care focuses on enhancing quality of life for the child and family, preventing and minimizing suffering, optimizing function, and providing opportunities for personal and spiritual growth. This care can be provided concurrently with life-prolonging care, curative care, or as the main focus of care" (NHPCO, 2023). Challenges to the receipt of hospice and palliative care include poor communication, ineffective models of care, reimbursement barriers, misalignment of state and federal policies, and a lack of understanding of (including training) and/or referral for hospice and palliative care (Bogetz et al., 2022; Johnson et al., 2021; Mack et al., 2021; Perales-Hull and Klein, 2022). Pediatric nurse practitioners also provide palliative care to children, and report challenges in their preparation for this role (Brock, 2021).

MENTAL HEALTH, BEHAVIORAL HEALTH, AND SOCIAL CARE PROFESSIONALS

While many clinicians are involved in addressing psychosocial needs of their patients, and a variety of professionals focus on psychosocial care, this section focuses on the care providers who focus their attention primarily on mental health, behavioral health, and psychosocial care needs—namely, psychiatrists, psychologists, and social workers. The committee recognizes that many APRNs and PAs focus on child and adolescent mental health, but they are not discussed in this section.

Child and Adolescent Psychiatrists

A child and adolescent psychiatrist (CAP) "specializes in the diagnosis and treatment of disorders of thinking, feeling, and/or behavior affecting children, adolescents, and their families" (AACAP, 2023a). CAPs work with patients and families to develop care plans that may include individual, group or family psychotherapy; medication; and/or consultation with other physicians or professionals from schools, juvenile courts, social agencies, or other community organizations. CAPs also act as advocates for the best interests of children and adolescents and perform consultations in a variety of settings (e.g., schools, juvenile courts, social agencies).

Estimations of the number of actively practicing CAPs are challenging because there is limited information about the proportion of time the average psychiatrist spends caring for children and adolescents. However, a 2018 analysis estimated that there were 9,956 actively practicing CAPs (approximately 15 CAPs per 100,000 children under 18 years) (Beck et al., 2018). CAPs were located in 28 percent of counties across the country, primarily in the northeastern United States as well as some counties on the West Coast.

Education and Training

CAP training includes 4 years of medical school; at least 3 years of residency training in medicine, neurology, and general psychiatry with adults; and 2 years of additional residency training in child and adolescent psychiatry (AACAP, 2023a). CAP residencies prioritize attention to "disorders that appear in childhood, such as pervasive developmental disorder, attention-deficit hyperactivity disorder (ADHD), learning disabilities, mental retardation, mood disorders, depressive and anxiety disorders, drug dependency and delinquency (conduct disorder)" (AACAP, 2023a). After completion of the CAP residency, CAPs are certified in general psychiatry by the American Board on Psychiatry and Neurology and may pursue subspecialty certification in child and adolescent psychiatry. In 2023, NRMP reported that 505 positions were offered in CAP in 127 programs, with an 82.4 percent match rate (NRMP, 2023b). Sixty-four percent of applicants were graduates of M.D. programs in the United States, 16 percent were graduates of osteopathic medical schools, and 20 percent were international medical graduates. The number of CAP positions and programs has increased since 2019; in 2019, 350 positions were offered in 108 programs.

As noted in Chapter 1, ABP has an agreement with the American Board of Psychiatry and Neurology wherein an applicant can complete requirements for certification in pediatrics, psychiatry, and CAP ("triple certification") at one of 11 combined training programs (ABP, 2023s). The combined program is 5 years in length and must include 24 months of training in pediatrics, 18 months of training in general psychiatry, and 18 months of training in CAP. Apart from ABP, child and adolescent psychiatrists may be trained through a variety of mechanisms such as traditional training programs, integrated training programs, and the Post Pediatric Portal Program (AACAP, 2023b).

Psychologists

Roberts and Steele (2017) define pediatric psychology as a multidisciplinary field that includes "both research and clinical practice that address a range of issues related to physical and psychosocial development, health, and illness among children, adolescents, and their families." (pg. 3). Psychologists possess the expertise and clinical proficiency to assist individuals in acquiring better coping strategies to manage mental health issues and various challenges in life through therapy (APA, 2023). Psychologists can be integrated in pediatric health care settings and systems (e.g., hospitals, pediatric subspecialty clinics, primary care) to help meet the needs of children and families facing chronic illnesses or disabilities (White and Belachew, 2022). (See Chapter 7 for more information on behavioral health integration.) Some pediatric health care subspecialty clinics have psychologists that are trained to care for children with comorbid medical and psychological conditions embedded in the practice, so that they can work collaboratively with the pediatric subspecialists (Apple and Clemente, 2022). Areas of expertise for pediatric psychologists include: "psychosocial, developmental and contextual factors contributing to the etiology, course and outcome of pediatric medical conditions; assessment and treatment of behavioral and emotional concomitants of illness, injury, and developmental disorders; prevention of illness and injury; promotion of health and health-related behaviors; education, training, and mentoring of psychologists and providers of medical care; improvement of health care delivery systems and advocacy for public policy that serves the needs of children, adolescents, and their families" (SPP, 2023). Psychologists can also receive specialty training in clinical child and adolescent psychology (Lin and Stamm, 2020).

Education and Training

The training pathway for pediatric psychologists typically involves completion of a Ph.D. or Psy.D. graduate program (generally 4–6 years of full-time study), including clinical practicum training. Some graduate programs offer specialized tracks in pediatric psychology. Prior to obtaining a doctoral degree, candidates must complete a one-year supervised internship. In most states, an additional year of supervised practice is required for licensure. Accredited pediatric psychology internships offer clinical exposure and research opportunities, leading to clinical competence. There are postdoctoral fellowships in pediatric psychology that typically last 1 to 2 years and provide additional training in pediatric clinical care and research. Many fellowships are based in hospitals and offer clinical experience with children facing acute and chronic disorders. Finally, psychologists must pass a national examination and additional state-specific examinations to obtain licensure (APA, 2023; Boat et al., 2016; Palermo et al., 2014).

Numbers of Pediatric Psychologists

Similar to CAPs, it is challenging to determine the exact number of practicing pediatric psychologists, partly because state boards grant licensure to psychologists in a general manner for both children and adults. Using data from the 2015 American Psychological Association Survey of Psychology Health Service Providers, the National Plan and Provider Enumeration System/National Provider Identifier Registry, and the American Board of Professional Psychology Board Certifications, Lin and Stamm (2020) found that nearly 6 percent of licensed doctoral-level psychologists self-reported a clinical child and adolescent specialty (4,012 out of 69,655) and approximately 6 percent of board-certified psychologists were certified in clinical child and adolescent psychology (268 out of 4,300) in the United States. However, the authors suggest that the number of psychologists that care for children and adolescents is likely higher than these data show, as the APA survey data show "23 percent of psychologists provide services to children frequently or very frequently and 34 percent provide services to adolescents frequently or very frequently" (Lin and Stamm, 2020). The data show that the distribution of clinical child and adolescent psychologists is uneven across the country, with the majority located in the Northeast and along the West Coast (Lin and Stamm, 2020).

Social Workers

The 2021 National Academies study *Implementing High-Quality Primary Care* identified social workers as an important part of the extended primary care team (NASEM, 2021b). For children, social workers can play a critical role on health care teams and can contribute to care coordination, the integration of behavioral health and primary care, and the provision of psychosocial support for inpatient and outpatient pediatric patients and their families (Children's National, 2023; Hospital for Special Surgery, 2023; Johns Hopkins Medicine, 2023; Jones et al., 2018; Ross et al., 2018). The National Association of Social Workers offers a Specialty Practice Section for supporting the development of "children, adolescents, and young adults" (NASW, 2023a). The section has a particular focus on physical, emotional, and behavior disorders as well as supporting transitions through young adulthood. Furthermore, social workers play a key role in children's well-being through their involvement in child welfare (e.g., child protective services, case management) (NASW, 2023b). In general, the inclusion of social workers in primary care settings has been associated with improved health outcomes (Cornell et al., 2020; Rehner et al., 2017).

OTHER RELATED HEALTH PROFESSIONALS

Many other professionals specialize in the care of children, such as dentists, pharmacists, podiatrists, and a broad array of therapists. While these members of the overall pediatric workforce are not the main focus of this study, many are active at the front lines of care and play an important role in referral and access to pediatric subspecialists. The following section highlight some of these professionals.

Care Coordinators

A variety of individuals with various titles and overlapping responsibilities help patients to coordinate their care needs across providers to and navigate the health care system overall. Some of the most common titles include care coordinators, care managers, case managers, and patient navigators. These roles are often filled by nurses or social workers. In these roles, the workers help to overcome barriers to care at the level of the patient, their socioeconomic environment, and the larger health care system. Activities may include patient education; assistance with insurance, transportation, or legal issues; referral to community resources; and encouragement to adhere to follow-up care (Joo and Huber, 2017; Kelly et al., 2015; Paskett et al., 2011; Woodward and Rice, 2015). While there are discrepancies in the definitions, scopes of practice, or qualifications for these individuals, there is evidence that care coordination contributes to improved outcomes in health care broadly (Berry et al., 2013; Gorin et al., 2017; NEJM Catalyst, 2018; Ruggiero et al., 2019).

Community Health Workers

Community health workers (CHWs) work within their communities to promote health and wellness; they are also known as outreach workers, community health advocates, community health representatives, and patient navigators (Rosenthal et al., 1998, 2010). There are more than 60,000 paid CHWs in the United States (BLS, 2023), as well as many volunteers (HRSA, 2023; Rosenthal et al., 2010). There is no standardized education or training, or scope of practice, for CHWs (Catalani et al., 2009). CHWs provide a wide range of services, including health education and coaching, medication adherence, care coordination, social support, outreach and engagement, health assessment and screenings, patient navigation, case management, program implementation, and referral management for medical and social services (BLS, 2023; HRSA, 2023; NASEM, 2020). CHWs also play an important role in addressing health disparities and improving health outcomes, particularly for underserved and marginalized populations

(Cosgrove et al., 2014; HRSA, 2023; Lewin et al., 2010; Vasan et al., 2020). Research has shown that CHWs increase disease knowledge, self-management, and health outcomes for children and youth with chronic diseases (Coutinho et al., 2020; Fox et al., 2007; Lewin et al., 2010; Randolph et al., 2021; Viswanathan et al., 2010). CHWs work collaboratively with clinicians, social workers, and other professionals to improve the health and well-being of the communities they serve, and may work in a variety of settings, such as community clinics, Federally Qualified Health Centers, hospitals, schools, and public health agencies.

KEY FINDINGS AND CONCLUSIONS

Key Findings

Finding #4-1: The current model of education and training for pediatric medical subspecialists focuses on the creation of academic pediatric specialists who demonstrate competency in core aspects of academic careers: clinical care, research, and education.

Finding #4-2: Limited resources and time may prevent training programs from adapting curricula quickly.

Finding #4-3: Pediatrics residents and fellows report feeling unprepared in key areas such as cultural competence and mental and behavioral health.

Finding #4-4: The ABP/ACGME requires all pediatric medical subspecialty fellowships to engage in scholarly activity (see also Chapter 5).

Finding #4-5: Fellowship position fill rates and numbers of first-year fellows show significant variation across the pediatric medical subspecialties.

Finding #4-6: A smaller percentage of female medical subspecialists report working full time or working 50 or more hours per week (as compared with male medical subspecialists).

Finding #4-7: Nearly half of actively practicing pediatric medical subspecialists do not participate in any research activities.

Finding #4-8: Most subspecialists practice in urban settings in a medical school or parent university, a non-government hospital or clinic, or a pediatric or multispecialty group practice.

Finding #4-9: Pediatric subspecialists are increasingly female and from URiM backgrounds. However, the pediatric workforce does not reflect the growing diversity of the U.S. population, particularly the pediatric population.

Finding #4-10: The health care usage of pediatricians, advanced practice nurses, and physician assistants providing outpatient care to the pediatric population insured by Medicaid increased from 2016 through 2019. However, there are not enough standard training programs or certifications for pediatric subspecialty NPs and PAs.

Finding #4-11: Adult-trained subspecialists provide a significant amount of care to children, but evidence about their numbers and patterns of care is scarce.

Finding #4-12: Family medicine physicians are decreasingly caring for children.

Finding #4-13: CAPs, child psychologists, and social workers provide crucial support for the mental health, behavioral health, and psychosocial care needs of children.

Finding #4-14: There is a paucity of data on the overall pediatric health care workforce, including both subspecialists and non-subspecialists.

Conclusions

Conclusion #4-1: The current model of education and training has not evolved substantially in response to the changing context of society and medicine, including the changing health needs of pediatric patients, changing practice patterns, and the changing needs of trainees.

Conclusion #4-2: Pediatric education and training needs to be more responsive to the changing needs of infants, children, and adolescents.

Conclusion #4-3: Advanced practice providers, adult-trained subspecialists, family medicine physicians, CAPs, child psychologists, social workers and many other health professionals are important parts of the workforce that provide overall care for the pediatric population, but there are variable levels of evidence for their numbers, patterns of care, and impact on child health and well-being.

RECOMMENDATION

As discussed in Chapter 2, the needs of children today are not the same as the needs of children from previous decades. The preparation of the subspecialty workforce has not evolved to fully meet the demands of the 21st century's population of infants, children, and adolescents, with limited ability to change education and training models quickly in response to emerging challenges. The committee notes that the biennial report called for in Recommendation 2-1 (see Chapter 2) could be used to help inform adjustments in curricula to meet these evolving needs. Therefore, to achieve a goal of **enhancing education, training, recruitment, and retention**, the committee provides the following recommendation:

RECOMMENDATION 4-1 The Association of Medical School Pediatric Department Chairs should periodically convene representatives from ABP and ACGME, all pediatric professional societies, and major pediatric education and training organizations (including, but not limited to, child and adolescent psychiatry, family medicine, and advanced practice providers) to review and adjust educational and training curricula (e.g., continuing education, standardized pediatric subspecialty training, and specialty recognition and certification) for pediatric residents and fellows. The goal of these convenings is to ensure that residency and fellowship programs are preparing a workforce that can address the evolving physical and mental health needs of the pediatric population.

The committee notes the importance of including a wide variety of training program representatives, including rural groups, to ensure that broad perspectives are included. Additionally, the inclusion of child psychiatry, family medicine, and advance practice providers is important both for their input as well as to allow them to bring back ideas and best practices to their own organizations.

REFERENCES

AACAP (American Academy of Child and Adolescent Psychiatry). 2023a. *What is child and adolescent psychiatry.* https://www.aacap.org/aacap/Medical_Students_and_Residents/Medical_Students/What_is_Child_and_Adolescent_Psychiatry.aspx (accessed April 24, 2023).

AACAP. 2023b. *How do I enter the field of child and adolescent psychiatry?* https://www.aacap.org/AACAP/Medical_Students_and_Residents/Medical_Students. How_do_I_enter_the_field_of_Child_and_Adolescent_Psychiatry.aspx (accessed July 18, 2023).

AAHPM (American Academy of Hospice and Palliative Medicine). 2023. *ABMS subspecialty certification in hospice and palliative medicine.* https://aahpm.org/certification/subspecialty-certification (accessed May 10, 2023).

AAMC (Association of American Medical Colleges). 2022a. *Table C2. Number of individuals who completed residency and are practicing in federally designated medically underserved areas, by last completed GME specialty: Residents who completed training, 2012–21.* https://www.aamc.org/data-reports/students-residents/data/report-residents/2022/table-c2-number-individuals-who-completed-residency-and-are-practicing (accessed April 23, 2023).

AAMC. 2022b. *Table C4. Physician retention in state of residency training, by last completed GME specialty.* https://www.aamc.org/data-reports/students-residents/data/report-residents/2021/table-c4-physician-retention-state-residency-training-last-completed-gme (accessed April 23, 2023).

AAMC. 2023. *Number of people per active physician by specialty, 2021.* https://www.aamc.org/data-reports/workforce/data/number-people-active-physician-specialty-2021 (accessed April 23, 2023.)

AANP (American Association of Nurse Practitioners). 2022. *NP fact sheet.* https://www.aanp.org/about/all-about-nps/np-fact-sheet (accessed December 29, 2022).

AANP. 2023. *Nurse practitioner (NP) certification.* https://www.aanp.org/student-resources/np-certification (accessed May 6, 2023).

ABFM. (American Board of Family Medicine). 2023a. *Added qualifications: Adolescent Medicine.* https://www.theabfm.org/added-qualifications/adolescent-medicine (accessed May 10, 2023).

ABFM. 2023b. *Fellowship directory.* https://www.aafp.org/medical-education/directory/fellowship/search (accessed May 10, 2023).

ABMS (American Board of Medical Specialties). 2023. *Specialty and subspecialty certificates.* https://www.abms.org/member-boards/specialty-subspecialty-certificates (accessed November 15, 2022).

ABP (American Board of Pediatrics). 2004. *Training requirements for subspecialty certification.* https://www.abp.org/sites/abp/files/trainingrequirements.pdf (accessed May 9, 2023).

ABP. 2022. *Hospice and palliative medicine certification.* https://www.abp.org/content/hospice-and-palliative-medicine-certification (accessed May 10, 2023).

ABP. 2023a. *Entrustable professional activities for subspecialties.* https://www.abp.org/content/entrustable-professional-activities-subspecialties (accessed May 9, 2023).

APB. 2023b. *Pediatricians ever certified since 1934.* https://www.abp.org/dashboards/pediatricians-ever-certified-1934 (accessed July 16, 2023).

ABP. 2023c. *General pediatrician age/gender distribution and summary: Pediatrician counts by continuing certification status.* https://www.abp.org/dashboards/general-pediatrician-agegender-distribution-and-summary (accessed July 16, 2023).

ABP. 2023d. *Latest race and ethnicity data for pediatricians and pediatric trainees: 1) Comparison to AAMC data and US populations.* https://www.abp.org/dashboards/latest-race-and-ethnicity-data-pediatricians-and-pediatric-trainees (accessed July 17, 2023).

ABP. 2023e. *Yearly growth in general pediatrics residents by demographics and program characteristics: Residents by demographics.* https://www.abp.org/dashboards/yearly-growth-general-pediatrics-residents-demographics-and-program-characteristics (accessed July 17, 2023).

ABP. 2023f. *Yearly growth in general pediatrics residents by demographics and program characteristics: Home, key findings, and summary of all residents.* https://www.abp.org/dashboards/yearly-growth-general-pediatrics-residents-demographics-and-program-characteristics (accessed July 17, 2023).

ABP. 2023g. *Yearly growth in general pediatrics residents by demographics and program characteristics: Residents by race and ethnicity.* https://www.abp.org/dashboards/yearly-growth-general-pediatrics-residents-demographics-and-program-characteristics (accessed July 17, 2023).

ABP. 2023h. *Pediatric program map and listing.* https://www.abp.org/dashboards/pediatric-program-map-and-listing (accessed July 17, 2023).
ABP. 2023i. *Comparison of ABP data to the NRMP match data.* https://www.abp.org/content/comparison-abp-data-nrmp-match-data (accessed July 17, 2023).
ABP. 2023j. *Yearly growth in pediatric fellows by demographics and program characteristics: First-year fellows by demographics (combined view).* https://www.abp.org/dashboards/yearly-growth-pediatric-fellows-subspecialty-demographics-and-program-characteristics (accessed July 17, 2023).
ABP. 2023k. *Yearly growth in pediatric fellows by demographics and program characteristics: Home, key findings, and summary of all fellows.* https://www.abp.org/dashboards/yearly-growth-pediatric-fellows-subspecialty-demographics-and-program-characteristics (accessed July 17, 2023).
ABP. 2023l. *Yearly growth in pediatric fellows by demographics and program characteristics: Fellows by race and ethnicity.* https://www.abp.org/dashboards/yearly-growth-pediatric-fellows-subspecialty-demographics-and-program-characteristics (accessed July 17, 2023).
ABP. 2023m. *Pediatric subspecialists ever certified.* https://www.abp.org/dashboards/pediatric-subspecialists-ever-certified (accessed July 17, 2023).
ABP. 2023n. *Survey results: 2018–2022 maintenance of certification enrollment surveys: Hours worked and work profiles.* https://www.abp.org/dashboards/results-continuing-certification-moc-enrollment-surveys-2018-2022 (accessed July 17, 2023).
ABP. 2023o. *Survey results: 2018–2022 maintenance of certification enrollment surveys: Primary work settings.* https://www.abp.org/dashboards/results-continuing-certification-moc-enrollment-surveys-2018–2022 (accessed July 17, 2023).
ABP. 2023p. *Latest race and ethnicity data for pediatricians and pediatric trainees: 4) Estimates by year of initial certification compared to the US population of children over time.* https://www.abp.org/dashboards/latest-race-and-ethnicity-data-pediatricians-and-pediatric-trainees (accessed July 17, 2023).
ABP. 2023q. *Latest race and ethnicity data for pediatricians and pediatric trainees: 5) Estimates by subpopulations as distinct groups.* https://www.abp.org/dashboards/latest-race-and-ethnicity-data-pediatricians-and-pediatric-trainees (accessed July 17, 2023).
ABP. 2023r. *Yearly growth in pediatric fellows by demographics and program characteristics: Fellows by demographics (by subspecialty).* https://www.abp.org/dashboards/yearly-growth-pediatric-fellows-subspecialty-demographics-and-program-characteristics (accessed July 17, 2023).
ABP. 2023s. *Pediatrics-psychiatry/child and adolescent psychiatry.* https://www.abp.org/content/pediatrics-psychiatrychild-and-adolescent-psychiatry (accessed May 10, 2023).
ACGME. 2021. *Data resource book: Academic year 2020-2021.* https://www.acgme.org/globalassets/pfassets/publicationsbooks/2020-2021_acgme_databook_document.pdf (accessed May 11, 2023).
ACGME. 2022a. *ACGME program requirements for graduate medical education in pediatrics.* https://www.acgme.org/globalassets/pfassets/programrequirements/320_pediatrics_2022_tcc.pdf (accessed May 9, 2023).
ACGME. 2022b. *ACGME program requirements for graduate medical education in family medicine.* https://www.acgme.org/globalassets/pfassets/programrequirements/120_familymedicine_2022.pdf (accessed January 3, 2023).
Aiken, L. H., D. M. Sloane, H. M. Brom, B. A. Todd, H. Barnes, J. P. Cimiotti, R. S. Cunningham, and M. D. McHugh. 2021. Value of nurse practitioner inpatient hospital staffing. *Med Care* 59(10):857-863.
Alaish, S. M., and A. V. Garcia. 2019. Who moved my fellow: Changes to Accreditation Council for Graduate Medical Education fellowships in pediatric surgery and what may be yet to come. *Current Opinion in Pediatrics* 31(3):409-413.

Alaish, S. M., D. M. Powell, J. H. T. Waldhausen, and S. P. Dunn. 2020. The Right Child/Right Surgeon initiative: A position statement on pediatric surgical training, sub-specialization, and continuous certification from the American Pediatric Surgical Association. *Journal of Pediatric Surgery* 55(12):2566-2574.

Alberto, C. K., J. Kemmick Pintor, A. Martinez-Donate, L. P. Tabb, B. Langellier, and J. P. Stimpson. 2021. Association of maternal-clinician ethnic concordance with Latinx youth receipt of family-centered care. *JAMA Network Open* 4(11):e2133857.

AMSPDC (Association of Medical School Pediatric Department Chairs). 2020. *Pediatric subspecialty supply model information sheet.* https://media.amspdc.org/wp-content/uploads/2020/10/22134843/BriefStatement_SubModelingProject.pdf (accessed May 6, 2023).

ANA (American Nurses Association). 2023. *Advanced practice registered nurse.* https://www.nursingworld.org/practice-policy/workforce/what-is-nursing/aprn (accessed July 19, 2023).

APA (American Psychological Association). 2023. *What do practicing psychologists do?* https://www.apa.org/topics/psychotherapy/about-psychologists (accessed May 10, 2023).

Apple, R. W., and E. G. Clemente. 2022. Role of psychologists in pediatric subspecialties. *Pediatr Clin North Am* 69(5):xv-xvi.

APRN (Advanced Practice Registered Nurses) Joint Dialogue Group. 2008. *Consensus model for APRN regulation: Licensure, accreditation, certification & education.* https://www.ncsbn.org/public-files/Consensus_Model_for_APRN_Regulation_July_2008.pdf (accessed April 26, 2023).

Auerbach, D. I., P. I. Buerhaus, and D. O. Staiger. 2020. Implications of the rapid growth of the nurse practitioner workforce in the US. *Health Affairs* 39(2):273-279.

Auerbach, D. I., D. O. Staiger, and P. I. Buerhaus. 2018. Growing ranks of advanced practice clinicians—implications for the physician workforce. *New England Journal of Medicine* 378(25):2358-2360.

Barber Doucet, H., Ward, V. L., T. J. Johnson, and L. K. Lee. 2021. Implicit bias and caring for diverse populations: Pediatric trainee attitudes and gaps in training. *Clinical Pediatrics* 60(9-10):408-417.

Bazemore, A. W., L. A. Makaroff, J. C. Puffer, P. Parhat, R. L. Phillips, I. M. Xierali, and J. Rinaldo. 2012. Declining numbers of family physicians are caring for children. *Journal of the American Board of Family Medicine* 25(2):139-140.

Beck, A. J., C. Page, J. Buche, D. Rittman, and M. Gaiser. 2018. *Estimating the distribution of the U.S. psychiatric subspecialist workforce.* https://behavioralhealthworkforce.org/wp-content/uploads/2019/02/Y3-FA2-P2-Psych-Sub_Full-Report-FINAL2.19.2019.pdf (accessed May 10, 2023).

Berry, L. L., B. L. Rock, B. S. Houskamp, J. Brueggeman, and L. Tucker. 2013. Care coordination for patients with complex health profiles in inpatient and outpatient settings. *Mayo Clinic Proceedings* 88(2):184-194.

Boat, T. F., M. L. Land, L. K. Leslie, K. E. Hoagwood, E. Hawkins-Walsh, M. A. McCabe, M. W. Fraser, L. de Saxe Zerden, B. M. Lombardi, G. K. Fritz, B. Kiyoe Frogner, J. D. Hawkins, and M. Sweeney. 2016. Workforce development to enhance the cognitive, affective, and behavioral health of children and youth: Opportunities and barriers in child health care training. *NAM Perspectives.* Discussion Paper, National Academy of Medicine, Washington, DC.

Bogetz, J. F., A. Anderson, M. Holland, and R. Macauley. 2022. Pediatric hospice and palliative care services and needs across the northwest United States. *Journal of Pain and Symptom Management* 64(1):e7-e14.

Brock, K. E., 2021. Urgent appeal from hospice nurses for pediatric palliative care training and community. *JAMA Network Open* 4(10):e2127958.

Buerhaus, P. 2018. Nurse practitioners: A solution to America's primary care crisis. *American Enterprise Institute* 1-30.

Catalani, C. E., S. E. Findley, S. Matos, and R. Rodriguez. 2009. Community health worker insights on their training and certification. *Progress in Community Health Partnerships: Research, Education, and Action* 3(3):227-235.

Children's National. 2023. *Social work services in the Heart Institute.* https://childrensnational.org/departments/childrens-national-heart-institute/resources-for-families/social-work-heart-institute (accessed May 6, 2023).

Centers for Medicare & Medicaid Services (CMS). 2022. *NPI: What you need to know.* https://www.cms.gov/outreach-and-education/medicare-learning-network-mln/mlnproducts/downloads/npi-what-you-need-to-know.pdf (accessed July 20, 2023).

Cohen, D., and A. Coco. 2010. Trends in well-child visits to family physicians by children younger than 2 years of age. *Annals of Family Medicine.* 8(3):245-248.

Colvin, J. D., M. Hall, J. G. Berry, L. M. Gottlieb, J. L. Bettenhausen, S. S. Shah, E. S. Fieldston, P. H. Conway, and P. J. Chung. 2016a. Financial loss for inpatient care of Medicaid-insured children. *JAMA Pediatrics* 170(11):1055-1062.

Colvin, J. D., M. Hall, L. Gottlieb, J. L. Bettenhausen, S. S. Shah, J. G. Berry, and P. J. Chung. 2016b. Hospitalizations of low-income children and children with severe health conditions: Implications of the Patient Protection and Affordable Care Act. *JAMA Pediatrics* 170(2):176-178.

Cornell, P. Y., C. W. Halladay, J. Ader, J. Halaszynski, M. Hogue, C. E. McClain, J. W. Silva, L. D. Taylor, and J. L. Rudolph. 2020. Embedding social workers in Veterans Health Administration primary care teams reduces emergency department visits. *Health Affairs* 39(4):603–612.

Correll, C. K., L. G. Spector, L. Zhang, B. A. Binsdtadt, and R. K. Vehe. 2015. Barriers and alternatives to pediatric rheumatology referrals: Survey of general pediatricians in the United States. *Pediatric Rheumatology* 13:32.

Cosgrove, S., M. Moore-Monroy, C. Jenkins, S. R. Castillo, C. Williams, E. Parris, J. H. Tran, M. D. Rivera, and J. N. Brownstein. 2014. Community health workers as an integral strategy in the reach U.S. program to eliminate health inequities. *Health Promotion Practice* 15(6):795-802.

Coutinho, M. T., S. S. Subzwari, E. L. McQuaid, and D. Koinis-Mitchell. 2020. Community health workers' role in supporting pediatric asthma management: A review. *Clinical Practice in Pediatric Psychology* 8(2):195-210.

Doan, Q., V. Sabhaney, N. Kissoon, D. Johnson, S. Sheps, H. Wong, and J. Singer. 2012. The role of physician assistants in a pediatric emergency department: A center review and survey. *Emergency Care* 28(8):783-788.

Doan, Q., S. Piteau, S. Sheps, J. Singer, H. Wong, D. Johnson, and N. Kissoon. 2015. The role of physician assistants in pediatric emergency medicine: The physician's view. *Canadian Journal of Emergency Medicine* 15(6):321-329.

Drake, F. T., S. Aarabi, B. T., Garland, C. R. Huntington, J. McAteer, M. K. Richards, N. K. Zern, and K. W. Gow. 2017. Accreditation Council for Graduate Medical Education (ACGME) surgery resident operative logs. *Annals of Surgery* 265(5):923-929.

Eden, A. R., Z. J. Morgan, A. Jetty, and L. E. Peterson. 2020. Proportion of family physicians caring for children is declining. *Journal of the American Board of Family Medicine* 33(6):830-831.

Farooqui, Z., A. R. Cortez, J. R. Potts III, G. M. Tiao, D. von Allmen, R. C. Quillin, A. J. Bondoc, and A. P. Garrison. 2023. 10 year analysis of pediatric surgery fellowship match and operative experience: Concerning trends? *Annals of Surgery* 277(2):e475-e482.

FOPO (Federation of Pediatric Organizations). 2001. Federation of Pediatric Organizations subspecialty forum. *The Journal of Pediatrics* 139(4):487-493.

Fox, P., P. G. Porter, S. H. Lob, J. H. Boer, D. A. Rocha, and J. W. Adelson. 2007. Improving asthma-related health outcomes among low-income, multiethnic, school-aged children: Results of a demonstration project that combined continuous quality improvement and community health worker strategies. *Pediatrics* 120(4):e902-e911.

Freed, G. L., T. A. Nahra, and J. R. C. Wheeler. 2004. Which physicians are providing health care to America's children?: Trends and changes during the past 20 years. *Archives of Pediatrics & Adolescent Medicine* 158(1):22-26.

Freed, G. L., K. M. Dunham, C. J. Loveland-Cherry, and K. K. Martyn. 2010a. Pediatric nurse practitioners in the United States: Current distribution and recent trends in training. *Journal of Pediatrics* 157(4):589-593.e581.

Freed, G. L., K. M. Dunham, A. Gebremariam, G. R. C. Wheeler, and the Research Advisory Committee of the American Board of Pediatrics. 2010b. Which pediatricians are providing care to America's children? An update on the trends and changes during the past 26 years. *The Journal of Pediatrics* 157(1):148-152.e1.

Freed, G. L., K. M. Dunham, C. Loveland-Cherry, K. K. Martyn, M. J. Moote, L. Althouse, W. Balistreri, A. Cohen, L. First, M. Land, G. Lister, G. McGuinness, J. McMillan, P. Miles, J. St Geme, and J. Stockman. 2011. Nurse practitioners and physician assistants employed by general and subspecialty pediatricians. *Pediatrics* 128(4):665-672.

Freed, G. L., L. M. Moran, L. A. Althouse, K. D. Van, L. K. Leslie, and Research Advisory Committee of American Board of Pediatrics. 2016. Jobs and career plans of new pediatric subspecialists. *Pediatrics* 137(3).

Freed, G. L., L. M. Moran, K. D. Van, L. K. Leslie, and Research Advisory Committee of American Board of Pediatrics. 2017. Current workforce of pediatric subspecialists in the United States. *Pediatrics* 139(5).

Freed, G. L., and K. L. Wickham. 2023. Assessing the pediatric subspecialty pipeline: It is all about the data source. *Pediatric Research* 93(7):1907-1912.

Gans, D., M. Battistelli, M. Ramirez, L. Cabezas, and N. Pourat. 2013. *Assuring children's access to pediatric subspecialty care in California*. https://www.lpfch.org/sites/default/files/field/publications/ucla_subspecialty_care_issue_brief_4-13.pdf (accessed May 11, 2023).

Gigli, K. H., M. S. Dietrich, P. I. Buerhaus, and A. F. Minnick. 2018. PICU provider supply and demand: A national survey. *Pediatric Critical Care Medicine* 19(8):e378-e386.

Gigli, K. H., B. S. Davis, G. R. Martsolf, and J. M. Kahn. 2021. Advanced practice provider-inclusive staffing models and patient outcomes in pediatric critical care. *Medical Care* 59(7):597-603.

Gigli, K. H., G. R. Martsolf, R. J. Vinci, and P. I. Buerhaus. 2023. A cross-sectional examination of the nurse practitioner workforce caring for children in the United States. *The Journal of Pediatrics* In press: doi.org/10.1016/j.peds.2023.02.020.

Gonçalves, M. I. R., D. A. Mendes, S. Caldeira, E. Jesus, and E. Nunes. 2022. Nurse-led care management models for patients with multimorbidity in hospital settings: A scoping review. *Journal of Nursing Management* 30(6):1960-1973.

Gonzalez, J., and K. Gigli. 2021. Navigating population foci and implications for nurse practitioner scope of practice. *Journal for Nurse Practitioners* 17(7):846-850.

Gorin, S. S., D. Haggstrom, P. K. J. Han, K. M. Fairfield, P. Krebs, and S. B. Clauser. 2017. Cancer care coordination: A systematic review and meta-analysis of over 30 years of empirical studies. *Annals of Behavioral Medicine* 51(4):532-546.

Green, C., R. E. K. Stein, A. Storfer-Isser, A. S. Garner, B. D. Kerker, M. Szilagyi, K. E. Hoagwood, and S. M. Horwitz. 2019. Do subspecialists ask about and refer families with psychosocial concerns? A comparison with general pediatricians. *Maternal and Child Health Journal* 23(1):61-71.

Green, C. M., J. K. Leyenaar, A. Tucker, and L. K. Leslie. 2022. Preparedness of pediatric subspecialty fellows to address emotional and mental health needs among children with chronic medical conditions. *JAMA Pediatrics* 176(12):1266-1268.

Greenwood, B. N., R. R. Hardeman, L. Huang, and A. Sojourner. 2020. Physician-patient racial concordance and disparities in birthing mortality for newborns. *Proceedings of the National Academy of Sciences* 117(35):21194-21200.

Hadland, S. E., E. Wood, and S. Levy. 2016. How the paediatric workforce can address the opioid crisis. *Lancet* 388(10051):1260-1261.

Hilgenberg, S. L., M. P. Frintner, R. L. Blankenberg, H. M. Haftel, and C. E. Gellin. 2021. Categorical pediatric residency program curriculum needs: A study of graduating residents and residency program leadership. *Academic Pediatrics* 21(4):589-593.

Hospital for Special Surgery. 2023. *Lerner Children's Pavilion: Pediatric social work/case management services.* https://www.hss.edu/pediatric-social-work.asp (accessed May 6, 2023).

Hoyt, A., M. O'Reilly-Jacob, and M. Souris-Kraemer. 2022. Certification alignment of nurse practitioners in acute care. *Nursing Outlook* 70(3):417-428.

HRSA (Health Resources & Services Administration). 2019. *2018 National Sample Survey of Registered Nurses: Brief summary of results.* Rockville, MD: U.S. Department of Health and Human Services.

HRSA. 2023. *Allied health workforce projections, 2016–2030: Community health workers.* https://bhw.hrsa.gov/sites/default/files/bureau-health-workforce/data-research/community-health-workers-2016-2030.pdf (accessed May 10, 2023).

ICN (International Council of Nurses). 2022. *Nursing definitions.* https://www.icn.ch/nursing-policy/nursing-definitions (accessed December 29, 2022).

IOM (Institute of Medicine). 2011. *The future of nursing: Leading change, advancing health.* Washington, DC: The National Academies Press.

Jetty, A., M. J. Romano, Y. Jabbarpour, S. Petterson, and A. Bazemore. 2021. A cross-sectional study of factors associated with pediatric scope of care in family medicine. *Journal of the American Board of Family Medicine* 34(1):196-207.

Johns Hopkins Medicine. 2023. *Johns Hopkins Children's Center: Social work.* https://www.hopkinsmedicine.org/johns-hopkins-childrens-center/patients-and-families/our-services/social-work (accessed May 6, 2023).

Johnson, K. A., A. Morvant, K. James, and L. C. Lindley. 2021. Changing pediatric hospice and palliative care through Medicaid partnerships. *Pediatrics* 148(5):e2021049968.

Jones, B., J. Currin-McCulloch, W. Pelletier, V. Sardi-Brown, P. Brown, and L. Wiener. 2018. Psychosocial standards of care for children with cancer and their families: A national survey of pediatric oncology social workers. *Social Work in Health Care* 57(4):221-249.

Joo, J. Y., and D. L. Huber. 2017. Barriers in case managers' roles: A qualitative systematic review. *Western Journal of Nursing Research* 40(10):1522-1542.

Kelly, E., N. Ivers, R. Zawi, L. Barnieh, D. Manns, D. L. Lorenzetti, D. Nicholas, M. Tonelli, B. Hemmelgarn, R. Lewanczuk, A. Edwards, T. Braun, and K. A. McBrien. 2015. Patient navigators for people with chronic disease: Protocol for a systematic review. *Systematic Reviews* 4(28). https://doi.org/10.1186/s13643-015-0019-1.

KidsData. 2018. *Children in rural and urban areas (California and U.S. only).* https://www.kidsdata.org/topic/557/children-rural-urban/pie#fmt=745&loc=1&tf=108&ch=969,968&pdist=150 (accessed May 6, 2023).

Krugman, S., L. N. Hodo, Z. J. Morgan, and A. R. Eden. 2023. Challenges meeting training requirements in the care of children in family medicine residency programs: A CERA study. *Family Medicine* 55(4):238-244.

Laurant, M., M. van der Biezen, N. Wijers, K. Watananirun, E. Kontopantelis, and A. J. van Vught. 2018. Nurses as substitutes for doctors in primary care. *Cochrane Database Syst Rev* 7(7):Cd001271.

Lewandowski, W., and K. Adamle. 2009. Substantive areas of clinical nurse specialist practice: A comprehensive review of the literature. *Clinical Nurse Specialist* 23(2):73-90.

Lewin, S., S. Munabi-Babigumira, C. Glenton, K. Daniels, X. Bosch-Capblanch, B. E. van Wyk, J. Odgaard-Jensen, M. Johansen, G. N. Aja, M. Zwarenstein, and I. B. Scheel. 2010. Lay health workers in primary and community health care for maternal and child health and the management of infectious diseases. *Cochrane Database of Systematic Reviews* 2010(3):Cd004015.

Lin, L., and K. Stamm. 2020. *The child and adolescent behavioral health workforce.* https://www.behavioralhealthworkforce.org/project/supply-of-child-and-adolescent-behavioral-health-providers/ (accessed May 10, 2023).

Lopez, K. N., and E. Fuentes-Afflick. 2022. Engaging pediatric subspecialists in pursuit of health equity—breaking out of the silo. *JAMA Pediatrics* 176(9):841-842.

Mack, J.W., E. R. Currie, V. Martello, J. Gittzus, A. Isack, L. Fisher, L. C. Lindley, S. Gilbertson-White, E. Roeland, and M. Bakitas. 2021. Barriers to optimal end-of-life care for adolescents and young adults with cancer: Bereaved caregiver perspectives. *Journal of the National Comprehensive Cancer Network* 19(5):528-533.

Macy, M. L., L. K. Leslie, A. Turner, and G. L. Freed. 2021. Growth and changes in the pediatric medical subspecialty workforce pipeline. *Pediatric Research* 89(5):1297-1303.

Makaroff, L. A., I. M. Xierali, S. M. Petterson, S. A. Shipman, J. C. Puffer, and A. W. Bazemore. 2014. Factors influencing family physicians' contribution to the child health care workforce. *Annals of Family Medicine* 12(5):427-431.

Mathur, M., A. Rampersad, K. Howard, and G. Goldman. 2005. Physician assistants as physician extenders in the pediatric intensive care unit setting—a 5-year experience. *Pediatric Critical Care Medicine* 6(1):14-19.

Maughan, E. D. 2018. School nurses: An investment in student achievement. *Phi Delta Kappan* 99(7):8-14.

Mehta, L. S., K. Fisher, A. K. Rzeszut, R. Lipner, S. Mitchell, M. Dill, D. Acosta, W. J. Oetgen, and P. S. Douglas. 2019. Current demographic status of cardiologists in the United States. *JAMA Cardiology* 4(10):1029-1033.

Merrit Hawkins Team. 2021. *2020/2021 sees highest demand for nurse practitioners.* https://www.merritthawkins.com/news-and-insights/blog/healthcare-news-and-trends/increasing-demand-for-nps-2021/#:~:text=In%20fact%2C%20nurse%20practitioners%20(NPs,healthcare%20facilities%20around%20the%20country (accessed May 5, 2023).

NACNS (National Association of Clinical Nurse Specialists). 2023. *What is a CNS?* https://nacns.org/about-us/what-is-a-cns (accessed July 19, 2023).

NASEM (National Academies of Sciences, Engineering, and Medicine). 2017. *Communities in action: Pathways to health equity.* Washington, DC: The National Academies Press.

NASEM. 2020. *Addressing sickle cell disease: A strategic plan and blueprint for action.* Washington, DC: The National Academies Press.

NASEM. 2021a. *The future of nursing 2020-2030: Charting a path to achieve health equity.* Washington, DC: The National Academies Press.

NASEM. 2021b. *Implementing high-quality primary care: Rebuilding the foundation of health care.* Edited by L. McCauley, R. L. Phillips, Jr., M. Meisnere and S. K. Robinson. Washington, DC: The National Academies Press.

NASW (National Association of Social Workers). 2023a. *Children, adolescents and young adults (CAYA) Specialty Practice Section.* https://www.socialworkers.org/careers/specialty-practice-sections/Children-adolescents-and-young-adults (accessed May 6, 2023).

NASW. 2023b. *Child welfare Specialty Practice Section.* https://www.socialworkers.org/careers/specialty-practice-sections/child-welfare (accessed May 6, 2023).

NCCPA (National Commission on Certification of Physician Assistants). 2020. *2019 statistical profile of recently certified physician assistants.* https://www.nccpa.net/wp-content/uploads/2020/11/2019-Recently-Certified-Report-final_compressed.pdf (accessed May 6, 2023).

NCCPA. 2023. *Pediatrics CAQ.* https://www.nccpa.net/specialty-certificates/#pediatrics (accessed May 6, 2023).

NEJM Catalyst. 2018. *What is care coordination?* https://catalyst.nejm.org/doi/full/10.1056/CAT.18.0291 (accessed July 20, 2023).

NHPCO (National Hospice and Palliative Care Organization). 2023. *Pediatric palliative and hospice care.* https://www.nhpco.org/pediatrics (accessed May 10, 2023).

NONPF (National Organization of Nurse Practitioner Faculties). 2022. *Nurse practitioner role core competencies.* https://cdn.ymaws.com/www.nonpf.org/resource/resmgr/competencies/nonpf_np_role_core_competenc.pdf (accessed December 29, 2022).

NRMP (National Resident Matching Program). 2022. *Results and data: 2022 main residency match.* https://www.nrmp.org/wp-content/uploads/2022/11/2022-Main-Match-Results-and-Data-Final-Revised.pdf (accessed May 6, 2023).

NRMP. 2023a. *Advance data tables: 2023 main residency match.* https://www.nrmp.org/wp-content/uploads/2023/04/Advance-Data-Tables-2023_FINAL-2.pdf (accessed May 6, 2023).

NRMP. 2023b. *Results and data: Specialties Matching Service: 2023 appointment year.* https://www.nrmp.org/wp-content/uploads/2023/04/2023-SMS-Results-and-Data-Book.pdf (accessed May 4, 2023).

Oluyede, L., A. L. Cochran, L. Prunkl, J. Wang, M. Wolfe, and N. C. McDonald. 2022. Unpacking transportation barriers and facilitators to accessing health care: Interviews with care coordinators. *Transportation Research Interdisciplinary Perspectives* 13. https://doi.org/10.1016/j.trip.2022.100565.

Palermo, T. M., D. M. Janicke, E. L. McQuaid, L. L. Mullins, P. M. Robins, and Y. P. Wu. 2014. Recommendations for training in pediatric psychology: Defining core competencies across training levels. *Journal of Pediatric Psychology* 39(9):965-984.

Paskett, E. D., J. P. Harrop, and K. J. Wells. 2011. Patient navigation: An update on the state of the science. *CA: A Cancer Journal for Clinicians* 61(4):237-249.

Perales-Hull, M., and K. Klein. 2022. Barriers to palliative and hospice care in the seriously ill pediatric population. *Journal of Pain and Symptom Management* 63(6):1147.

Perloff, J., C. M., DesRoches, and P. Buerhaus. 2016. Comparing the cost of care provided to Medicare beneficiaries assigned to primary care nurse practitioners and physicians. *Health Services Research* 51(4):1407-1423.

Phillips, R. L., M. S. Dodoo, J. L. McCann, A. Bazemore, G. E. Fryer, L. S. Klein, M. Weitzman, and L. A. Green. 2005. *Report to the Task Force on the Care of Children by Family Physicians.* https://www.graham-center.org/content/dam/rgc/documents/publications-reports/monographs-books/rgcmo-care-children.pdf (accessed April 26, 2023).

Phillips, R. L., A. W. Bazemore, M. S. Dodoo, S. A. Shipman, and L. A. Green. 2006. Family physicians in the child health care workforce: Opportunities for collaboration in improving the health of children. *Pediatrics* 118(3):1200-1206.

PNCB (Pediatric Nursing Certification Board). 2022. *Who provides nursing care for our kids? Pediatric nursing workforce report 2022.* https://www.pncb.org/sites/default/files/resources/PNCB_2022_Pediatric_Nursing_Workforce_Demographic_Report.pdf (accessed December 29, 2022).

Randolph, C. 2021. Community health workers in home visits and asthma outcomes. *Pediatrics* 148(Supplement 3):S56-S57.

Ray, K. N., J. M. Kahn, E. Miller, and A. Mehrotra. 2016. Use of adult-trained medical subspecialists by children seeking medical subspecialty care. *Journal of Pediatrics* 176:173-181.e1.

Reed, S. M., J. Arbet, and L. Staubli. 2021. Clinical nurse specialists in the United States registered with a national provider identifier. *Clinical Nurse Specialist* 35(3):119-128.

Rehner, T., M. Brazeal, and S. T. Doty. 2017. Embedding a social work-led behavioral health program in a primary care system: A 2012–2018 case study. *Journal of Public Health Management and Practice* 23:S40–S46.

Rimsza, M. E., H. S. Ruch-Ross, C. J. Clemens, W. B. Moskowitz, and H. J. Mulvey. 2018. Workforce trends and analysis of selected pediatric subspecialties in the United States. *Academic Pediatrics* 18(7):805-812.

Roberts, M. C., and R. G. Steele. 2017. *Handbook of pediatric psychology: Fifth Edition*: Guilford Press.
Rosenthal, E. L. 1998. A summary of the national community health advisor study. Baltimore, MD: Annie E. Casey Foundation.
Rosenthal, E. L., J. N. Brownstein, C. H. Rush, G. R. Hirsch, A. M. Willaert, J. R. Scott, L. R. Holderby, and D. J. Fox. 2010. Community health workers: Part of the solution. *Health Affairs* 29(7):1338-1342.
Ross, A., J. Arnold, A. Gormley, S. Locke, S. Shanske, and C. Tardiff. 2018. Care coordination in pediatric health care settings: The critical role of social work. *Social Work in Health Care* 58(1):1-13.
Ruggiero, K., P. Pratt, and R. Antonelli. 2019. Improving outcomes through care coordination: Measuring care coordination of nurse practitioners. *Journal of the American Association of Nurse Practitioners* 31(8):476-481.
Rule, A. R. L., K. Reynolds, H. Sucharew, and B. Volck. 2018. Perceived cultural competency skills and deficiencies among pediatric residents and faculty at a large teaching hospital. *Hospital Pediatrics* 8(9):554-569.
Russell, A., J. Fromewick, B. Macdonald, S. Kimmel, K. Franke, K. Leach, and K. Foley. 2021. Drivers of scope of practice in family medicine: A conceptual model. *Annals of Family Medicine* 19(3):217-223.
Saunders, M. M. 2015. Clinical nurse specialists' perceptions of work patterns, outcomes, desires, and emerging trends. *The Journal of Nursing Administration* 45(4):212-217.
Schumacher, D. J., D. C. West, A. Schwartz, S. T. Li, L. Millstein, E. C. Griego, T. Turner, B. E. Herman, R. Englander, J. Hemond, V. Hudson, L. Newhall, K. McNeal Trice, J. Baughn, E. Giudice, H. Famiglietti, J. Tolentino, K. Gifford, and C. Carraccio. 2020. Longitudinal assessment of resident performance using entrustable professional activities. *JAMA Network Open* 3(1):e1919316.
Semanco, M., S. Wright, and R. L. Rich. 2022. Improving initial sepsis management through a nurse-driven rapid response team protocol. *Critical Care Nursing* 42(5):51-57.
Silver, H. K., L. C. Ford, and L. R. Day. 1968. The pediatric nurse-practitioner program: Expanding the role of the nurse to provide increased health care for children. *JAMA* 204(4):298-302.
SPP (Society of Pediatric Psychology). 2023. *Who we are.* https://pedpsych.org/about-us/ (accessed May 10, 2023).
Stevenson, D. K., G. A. McGuinness, J. D. Bancroft, D. M. Boyer, A. R. Cohen, J. T. Gilhooly, M. F. Hazinski, E. S. Holmboe, M. D. Jones, Jr, M. L. Land, Jr, S. S. Long, V. F. Norwood, D. J. Schumacher, T. C. Sectish, J. W. St. Geme, III, and D. C. West. 2014. The initiative on subspecialty clinical training and certification (SCTC): Background and recommendations. *Pediatrics* 133(Supplement_2):S53-S57.
Surgical Advisory Panel, M. D. Klein, C. F. Bannister, C. S. Houck, J. S. Tweddell, M. S. Dias, A. Segura, J. B. Ruben, W. L. Hennrikus, and R. M. Schwend. 2014. Referral to pediatric surgical specialists. *Pediatrics* 133(2):350-356.
Takeshita, J., S. Wang, A. W. Loren, N. Mitra, J. Shults, D. B. Sin, and D. L. Sawinski. 2020. Association of racial/ethnic and gender concordance between patients and physicians with patient experience ratings. *JAMA Open Network* 3(11):2024583.
U.S. Bureau of Labor Statistics (BLS). 2023. *Occupational employment and wages, May 2022: 21-1094 community health workers.* https://www.bls.gov/oes/current/oes211094.htm (accessed May 10, 2023).
Valdivia, H. R. 2022. The pediatric clinical nurse specialist: A children's hospital journey. *Journal of Pediatric Nursing* 66:213-215.

Vasan, A., J. W. Morgan, N. Mitra, C. Xu, J. A. Long, D. A. Asch, and S. Kangovi. 2020. Effects of a standardized community health worker intervention on hospitalization among disadvantaged patients with multiple chronic conditions: A pooled analysis of three clinical trials. *Health Services Research* 55 Suppl 2(Suppl 2):894-901.

Viswanathan, M., J. L. Kraschnewski, B. Nishikawa, L. C. Morgan, A. A. Honeycutt, P. Thieda, K. N. Lohr, and D. E. Jonas. 2010. Outcomes and costs of community health worker interventions: A systematic review. *Medical Care* 48(9):792-808.

Walker, K. O., G. Moreno, and K. Grumbach. 2012. The association among specialty, race, ethnicity, and practice location among California physicians in diverse specialties. *Journal of the National Medical Association* 104(1-2):46-52.

Wasserman, R. C., S. E. Varni, M. C. Hollander, and V. S. Harder. 2019. Change in site of children's primary care: A longitudinal population-based analysis. *Annals of Family Medicine* 17(5):390-395.

White, K., and B. Belachew. 2022. Role of psychologists in pediatric subspecialties: Integrated psychological services overarching concepts across pediatric subspecialties. *Pediatric Clinics of North America* 69(5):825-837.

Wieting, J. M., D. G. Williams, K. A. Kelly, and L. Morales-Egizi. 2018. Appendix 2: American Osteopathic Association specialty board certification. *Journal of Osteopathic Medicine* 118(4):275-279.

Willgerodt, M. A., D. M. Brock, and E. D. Maughan. 2018. Public school nursing practice in the United States. *The Journal of School Nursing* 34(3):232-244.

Woodward, J., and E. Rice. 2015. Case management. *Nursing Clinics of North America* 50(1):109-121.

Xierali, I., L. Castillo-Page, S. Conrad, and M. Nivet. 2014. *Analysis in brief: Analyzing physician workforce racial and ethnic composition associations: Geographic distribution (part II).* https://www.aamc.org/data-reports/analysis-brief/report/analyzing-physician-workforce-racial-and-ethnic-composition-associations (accessed April 20, 2023).

Yheulon, C. G., W. C. Cole, J. J. Ernat, and S. S. Davis, Jr. 2019. Normalized competitive index: Analyzing trends in surgical fellowship training over the past decade (2009–2018). *Journal of Surgical Education* 77(1):74-81.

5

Influences on the Career Path of a Pediatric Subspecialty Physician

The majority of pediatric medical subspecialty physicians in the United States follow the typical career path of 4 years of medical school, followed by 3 years of pediatric residency and then 3 years of subspecialty fellowship training (ABP, 2022a,b).[1] Major decisions along their career paths include: deciding to entering pediatrics in general, choosing to pursue subspecialty training, selecting a specific subspecialty, and choosing where and what type of practice. At each of those decision points, many factors may influence the outcome of that decision, including mentorship, personal interest, financial considerations, and lifestyle preferences. In choosing specialty training, medical students (in general) place the highest value on the content of the specialty and their personal interests, influential role models, and work–life balance (Youngclaus and Fresne, 2020). The decision to pursue a pediatric subspecialty is also affected by many of the same factors. Frintner and colleagues (2021a) used the 2019 American Academy of Pediatrics (AAP) Annual Survey of Graduating Residents to assess what factors influenced decisions to pursue pediatric subspecialty training. Among those who were planning to pursue such training, the highest rated factors were future job opportunities and interest in a specific disease/organ system, with most reporting these factors as essential or very important (90 percent and 88 percent, respectively). See Figure 5-1 for other factors identified as important in the decision to pursue fellowship training in a pediatric subspecialty.

---

[1] One notable exception is that fellowship training for pediatric hospital medicine is 2 years (ABP, 2020). Non-standard pathways to certification may also apply in certain situations (ABP, 2022d).

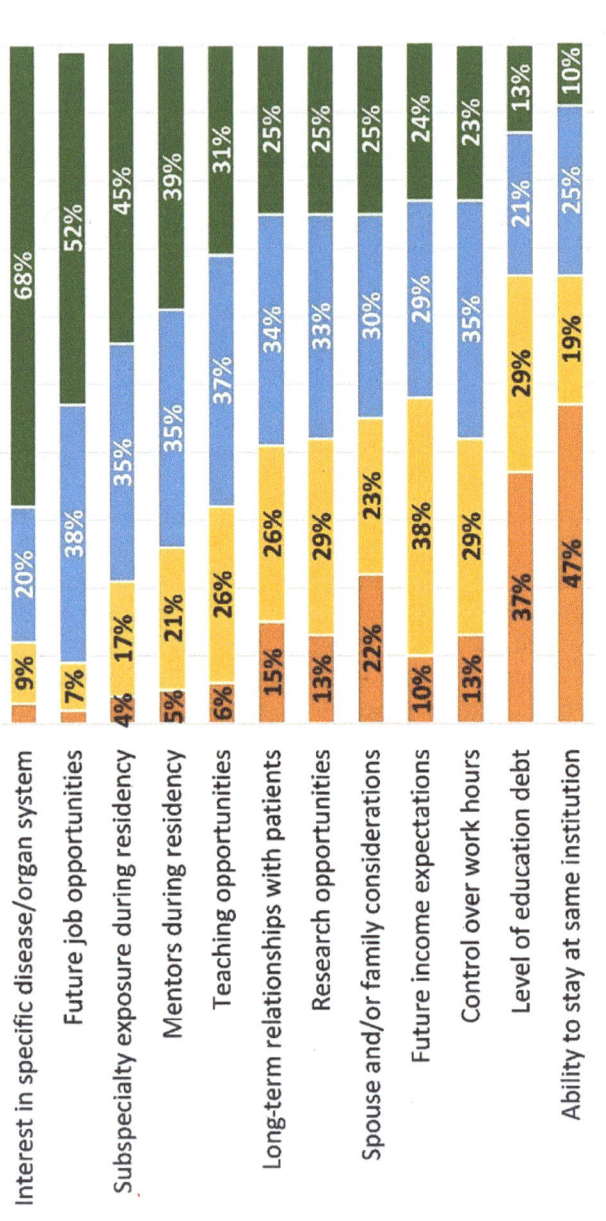

FIGURE 5-1 Factors identified as important in decision to pursue pediatric subspecialty fellowship training.
SOURCE: Frintner et al., 2021a.

This chapter explores the influences—timing of exposure to pediatrics; education and training; coaching, mentoring, and role modeling; financing of graduate education; educational debt and earning potential; lifestyle preferences; and efforts in workforce planning, recruitment, and retention—that can encourage or discourage an individual from pursuing a career as a pediatric subspecialty physician. Many factors that can influence the choice to pursue a career in pediatrics can also influence the retention of clinicians in their chosen fields. Given limited evidence on some of these factors specific to pediatric subspecialists, drivers of career choices in medicine in general are also discussed, but the primary focus of this chapter is on the influences for a career as a pediatric subspecialty physician.

EXPOSURE TO PEDIATRICS

Early exposure to the medical specialty of pediatrics at various critical touch points, including high school and college, medical school, and early residency training, has been hypothesized to be critical in the decision to pursue a career in pediatrics and the pediatric subspecialties (Donnelly et al., 2007; Lindgren and Shah, 2023; Nelson et al., 2020; Vinci et al., 2021).

Before Medical School

An individual's drive to pursue a career in pediatrics may be profoundly shaped by experiences that occur before entering medical school. The Association of American Medical Colleges (AAMC) compared students' answers regarding a specialty preference on the 2022 Medical School Graduation Questionnaire to their previous answers on the Matriculating Student Questionnaire (administered during the summer before the first year of medical school) (AAMC, 2022a). Among all medical students, only 28 percent of students indicated the same preferred specialty upon graduation as they had intended upon matriculation. However, among students who indicated a preference for pediatrics upon graduation, nearly 45 percent had selected pediatrics at the beginning of medical school, suggesting that earlier life experiences may have had a significant impact on deciding to pursue a career in pediatrics. See Box 5-1 for clinician perspectives on the influence of their early exposure (before medical school) to pediatrics.

During Medical School and Residency

Experiences during medical school and residency also influence a student's choice of specialty or subspecialty (Hauer et al., 2008; Pfarrwaller et al., 2015, 2017; Sozio et al., 2019; Tsai et al., 2022). The faculty of each medical school design the medical education curriculum, and there are no

> **BOX 5-1**
> **Clinician Perspectives—Exposure Before Medical School**
>
> "I opted for pediatrics, and adolescent medicine specifically, due to the joys of working with teens as a prior high school teacher."
> **– Chair and Chief of Pediatrics, New Hampshire**
>
> "I knew I wanted to be a [developmental and behavioral pediatrician] since high school when I worked at a county-run summer camp for kids with developmental disabilities."
> **– Attending Physician, Developmental and Behavioral Pediatrics, Philadelphia, PA**
>
> "I knew I wanted to go into pediatrics since the ninth grade."
> **– Attending Neonatologist, Chicago, IL**
>
> *These quotes were collected from the committee's online call for trainee, clinician, and family perspectives.*

specific requirements from the Liaison Committee on Medical Education (LCME) for exposure to topics such as pediatrics (LCME, 2023). Thus, medical students have variable exposure to pediatrics, and opportunities to enhance that exposure may be limited or occur late in the educational curriculum (Guiot et al., 2013; Laitman et al., 2019). Several institutions have offered preclinical electives in pediatrics in an effort to increase students' confidence in caring for pediatric populations as well as to increase their interest in pediatrics as a career, but evidence of their impact is extremely limited (Keating et al., 2013; Laitman et al., 2019; Saba et al., 2015). See Box 5-2 for trainee and clinician perspectives on exposure to pediatrics during training.

Timing of Fellowship Decisions

Macy et al. (2018) found that 68 percent of individuals who entered pediatric subspecialty fellowship training first reported plans to do so at the start of their internship, and few changed plans to pursue such training. However, their selection of a specific subspecialty occurred across all 3 years of residency training, with the most common time being July of their second year of residency; nearly one-fifth of residents who entered fellowship training changed their choice of a specific subspecialty during

> **BOX 5-2**
> **Trainee and Clinician Perspectives—**
> **Exposure During Medical School and Residency**
>
> "I discovered my interest in rheumatology during a fourth year elective in orthopedics where one week was spent with adult rheumatology. I then attended a residency where early electives were offered and I took pediatric rheumatology, which cemented my interest."
> **– Attending Physician, Pediatric Rheumatology, Fargo, ND**
>
> "I am planning to go into pediatric rheumatology. I became interested by seeing young adult patients with pediatric-onset rheumatic disease during an adult rheumatology rotation."
> **– Fourth Year Medical Student, Madison, WI**
>
> "Medical training at many larger programs in residency tends to be very hospital inpatient-heavy as residents are seen as the primary workforce, and it results in fewer opportunities for outpatient exposure and procedures."
> **– Second Year Pediatric Pulmonology Fellow from Birmingham, AL**
>
> *These quotes were collected from the committee's online call for trainee, clinician, and family perspectives.*

residency (Macy et al., 2018). In addition, international medical graduates were more likely than American medical graduates to decide on a specific pediatric subspecialty earlier in training.

Interest in the Specific Area of Specialization

One influence that may be intangible in influencing an individual's choice of specialty or subspecialty is an academic or personal interest—something that potentially may be influenced by early exposure to that specialty or subspecialty. As noted earlier, simply being interested in the specific topic has been shown to be influential on medical students' choice of specialty in general (Levaillant et al., 2020; Rao et al., 2017; Yang et al., 2019). In pediatrics, one survey of pediatrics residents found that "interest in a specific disease/patient population" was the highest ranked career factor in pursuing a pediatrics career (Orr et al., 2023), and a survey of graduating pediatric residents found that "interest in the specific disease/organ" was one of the most highly rated factors as influencing their decision to pursue a specific fellowship (Haftel et al., 2020). The importance of interest in the specific area or the intellectual stimulation of the field has been documented for new pediatric subspecialists in general (Freed et al., 2016) as well as specifically in several pediatric subspecialties, including pediatric nephrology (Weinstein et al., 2010), pediatric endocrinology (Kumar et al., 2021), and pediatric pulmonology (Nelson et al., 2020). See Box 5-3 for trainee and clinician perspectives on how personal interest influenced their career choices.

EDUCATION AND TRAINING MODEL

While Chapter 1 presented a history of the development of subspecialty training and Chapter 4 provided the landscape of the current pediatric workforce, including an overview of the basic requirements of pediatric residency and fellowship training, the following sections emphasize some specific aspects of formal medical education and training that may directly influence an individual's decision to pursue subspecialty training.

BOX 5-3
Trainee and Clinician Perspectives—Personal Interest

"I chose pediatric nephrology because of my interest and awe of the kidneys and their varied functions…I also just loved the mix of conditions seen by nephrologists."
– Pediatric Nephrologist, Seattle, WA

"I chose pediatric infectious diseases because I had an interest in vaccine research and I enjoy the broad differential diagnoses encountered in my specialty."
– Pediatric Infectious Disease Attending, Baltimore, MD

"I went into pediatric endocrinology because hormones are a fascinating puzzle and I can generally provide interventions that improve quality of life for patients."
– Second Year Pediatric Endocrinologist, Denver, CO

These quotes were collected from the committee's online call for trainee, clinician, and family perspectives.

Requirements for Scholarly Activity in Fellowship

Currently, all pediatric subspecialty fellowships have a requirement for a core curriculum in scholarly activity (ABP, 2004, 2022b). The curricula for these activities are intended to develop an understanding of research-related skills such as biostatistics, research methodology, study design, and preparation of applications for research funding. Scholarly activity can be pursued in areas such as basic, clinical, and translational research; health services research; quality improvement; bioethics; education; and public policy. Scholarly projects are overseen by local scholarship oversight committees. Examples of appropriate scholarly activities include bench or clinical research, rigorous meta-analyses or systematic reviews, a critical analysis of a relevant public policy, or a curriculum development project (with an assessment component). Most fellows complete bench or clinical research (84 percent) and/or quality improvement activities or clinical care guideline development (50 percent) to meet these requirements (Freed et al., 2014a). At the end of the fellowship program, the fellow must finalize and submit a specific written product (e.g., peer-reviewed publication, successful grant application) (ABP, 2022c). However, the outcomes of pediatric subspecialty fellowship activities have not been fully assessed for either their contribution to the larger research enterprise or their impact on career trajectories.

The value of requiring all fellows to participate in scholarly activity as currently required, particularly for those individuals who do not plan to pursue a career that includes research, is an ongoing debate. Several justifications for this requirement have been proposed, including a need for subspecialists to have more a detailed understanding of the scientific process and the ability to critically assess new literature in order to safely bring new diagnostics and treatments to the children they care for, ones who are likely to have the most complex care needs; to provide exposure to career opportunities in research; and a maturation effect in which a trainee more fully develops and practices the total skill set of the subspecialist (e.g., teaching skills). Others have noted that this approach costs significant money and time (which may be a negative influence on the choice to pursue subspecialty training), and may be suboptimally executed because of lack of resources, mentorship, and in-depth education in research. See Box 5-4 for clinician perspectives on the requirement for scholarly activity. See Chapter 6 for more on the physician–scientist pipeline. The impact of research training requirements on the overall length of training is discussed later in this chapter.

> **BOX 5-4**
> **Clinician Perspectives—Requirement for Scholarly Activity**
>
> "We need to enforce more scholarship in our trainees to better society."
> **– Practicing Physician–Scientist for over 10 Years, Houston, TX**
>
> "The research year in pediatric specialty fellowships needs to be OPTIONAL. This does not create more scientists and pushes people away from training when they don't want to do that."
> **– Pediatric Emergency Medicine Attending for 11 Years, Des Moines, IA**
>
> "Barriers included a strong focus on lab research, which is less relevant to clinicians."
> **– First Year Pediatric Oncology Attending, Dallas, TX**
>
> *These quotes were collected from the committee's online call for trainee, clinician, and family perspectives.*

Comparison with Internal Medicine Fellowships

The internal medicine model of fellowship training may provide insights on how to address issues of low enrollment into some pediatric subspecialties. Specifically, many internal medicine fellowships with similar clinical concentrations to pediatric fellowships (e.g., adolescent medicine, critical care, endocrinology, infectious disease, nephrology, pulmonary disease, rheumatology) only require 2 years of training (ABIM, 2023a). The American Board of Internal Medicine (ABIM) outlines specific clinical competence requirements for these fellowships, but does not have specific research requirements. ABIM does provide a research pathway for trainees who plan to pursue research careers; planning for this track is encouraged to occur during the first year of residency, and there are specific requirements for clinical training to accompany the research program (ABIM, 2023b). Internal medicine, however, also struggles with enrollment into some subspecialties. As shown in Table 5-1, the fill rates for ABIM-certified subspecialties with similar clinical concentrations for American Board of Pediatrics (ABP)-certified subspecialties tend to have higher fill rates overall. These data are for 2022 and show a point in time example that compares fellowship fill rates for pediatric versus adult subspecialties. (See Table 4-2 in Chapter 4 for data on average pediatric subspecialty fill rates over time.) Although there may be many reasons for these higher fill rates, including higher levels of compensation for adult subspecialists, training requirements

TABLE 5-1 Selected ABP-Certified and ABIM-Certified Subspecialties by Fellowship Fill Rate, 2022

Subspecialty Area	Pediatrics		Internal Medicine
	NRMP-Reported Fill Rate	ABP-Calculated Final Fill Rate	NRMP-Reported Fill Rate
Endocrinology	59.1%	75.5%	98.3%
Infectious Diseases	52.4%	69.7%	82.1%
Nephrology	55.0%	70.0%	69.2%
Pulmonology	73.5%	85.5%	92.0%
Rheumatology	69.2%	97.4%	97.8%

NOTES: Data reported from the NRMP do not necessarily reflect the final fill rate of training programs as some residents will be accepted outside of the NRMP process. Final fill rates for internal medicine subspecialties are unavailable, and so may also be higher than the NRMP-reported fill rates. See Chapter 4 for more information on ABP-calculated final fill rates for pediatric subspecialties.
SOURCES: ABP, 2023a; NRMP, 2022.

might be one factor that contributes to the decisions of trainees to pursue subspecialty training.

Overall Length of Education and Training

The length and structure of education and training to become a pediatric subspecialist may influence the choice of pursuing a subspecialty.

Initiatives to Accelerate Medical School Training

Several initiatives have explored opportunities to shorten the overall length of time required to become a physician. These initiatives provide examples of how education and training may be accelerated without compromising quality. The first modern-day accelerated baccalaureate medical programs opened in the early 1960s (Drees and Omurtag, 2012). The initial goal of these programs was to lessen the financial burden of medical education by allowing for the completion of a combined undergraduate and graduate medical education in 6 to 7 years rather than the typical 8 years; however, they soon became recognized as a viable way to quickly generate well-trained physicians (CAMPP, 2023; Drees and Omurtag, 2012; Kistemaker and Montez, 2022).

The Consortium of Accelerated Medical Pathway Programs was established in 2015 to develop 3-year M.D. programs to expedite medical education and offer guidance to schools seeking to develop similar programs (CAMPP, 2023). Their primary goal is to make medical education more efficient and less expensive while maintaining student performance and competency. In 2012, there were only two accelerated M.D. programs in the country; by 2014 the number had grown to eight (Cangiarella, 2021). Today the Consortium includes more than 30 members who either offer or are planning to offer such programs. Graduates of accelerated programs perceive being prepared for residency and graduate with less debt as compared to 4-year M.D. students (Cangiarella et al., 2022; Leong et al., 2022).

Length of Residency and Fellowship Training

Overall length of training may influence the career path of a pediatric subspecialist; the appropriate length of training, particularly subspecialty fellowship training, is intertwined with the requirement for research during fellowship. In 2010, ABP hosted an Invitational Conference on Subspecialty Clinical Training and Certification (SCTC), with a task force subsequently charged with "examining the current model of pediatrics subspecialty fellowship training and certification with an emphasis on competency-based clinical training and recommending changes in the current requirements, if warranted" (Stevenson et al., 2014, pg.1). While the task force originally intended to focus on clinical training, its charge expanded to include the scholarly activity requirements of training, as those topics are intertwined. As part of the SCTC initiative, researchers surveyed current fellows (Freed et al., 2014a), program directors (Freed et al., 2014b), and recent graduates and mid-career professionals (Freed et al., 2014c) for each subspecialty (ABP, 2014; Freed et al., 2014d). These surveys revealed a wide range of opinions on the length of training and the clinical and research requirements by career stage.

While 87 percent of recent graduates and mid-career professionals agreed that the 12-month requirement for clinical training was appropriate, only 58 percent thought that the 12-month requirement for scholarly activity was appropriate (Freed et al., 2014c). Among those who did not agree with the 12-month requirement for scholarly activity, there were a range of opinions on whether that time should be increased, decreased, or eliminated. Although 76 percent of recent graduates and mid-career professionals thought that clinical training time should be equivalent for all fellows regardless of career path, only 46 percent thought the duration of scholarly activity should be equivalent; 31 percent of recent graduates and 26 percent of mid-career professionals thought there should be different tracks for clinical and research careers (Freed et al., 2014c). Furthermore, 43 percent of current fellows and 48 percent of recent graduates and mid-career professionals stated that their experience with scholarly activity did not affect their choice of a career path (Freed et al., 2014a,c). While 12 percent of current fellows and 22 percent of recent graduates and mid-career professionals said the scholarly activity experience influenced them to work primarily in research, 13 percent of current fellows and 12 percent of recent graduates and mid-career professionals said the experience led them to change their career path to work primarily as a clinician (Freed et al., 2014a,c). The task force concluded that the joint ABP–Accreditation Council for Graduate Medical Education (ACGME) requirements were sufficiently flexible for all subspecialties and trainees to achieve their goals (Stevenson et al., 2014). The task force also concluded that "although the current requirement for 3 years of subspecialty training will remain for now, as the ability to measure subspecialty training outcomes improves, the ABP may, in a staged and deliberate fashion, consider allowing fellowship training of shorter, longer, or variable lengths" (Stevenson et al., 2014, pg. S55). For example, the addition of pediatric hospital medicine as a certified subspecialty was approved as a predesigned 2-year fellowship (ABP, 2020). Importantly, the SCTC surveys were conducted more than 10 years ago, and it is unclear if the results would be the same today. See Box 5-5 for trainee and clinician perspectives on the length of fellowship training.

Alternative Pathways

While the standard model of research training in pediatric fellowship has routinely been implemented by programs as 12 to 24 months within the 3 years, ABP has alternate pathways available (see Box 5-6) (ABP, 2022d). Notably, these pathways have been specifically designed to provide options for future research-oriented trainees. Alternate pathways do not exist for trainees who want to focus their careers on clinical care. During one of the committee's public webinars, Joanna Lewis, pediatric residency program director and director for mobile health services at Advocate Children's Hospital in Park Ridge, IL, stated:

> [Residents] see these physicians with very robust, fulfilling, satisfying clinical careers that do not involve research and they don't find that fellowships seem to offer them the path to get to that spot. I think that becomes challenging for some of our residents when they're making the decision about what fellowship to head into … I think a two-year fellowship with some experience with research—they all know that within subspecialty care and within all of us, our work is made better by there being research done and having evidence-based practice, and that doesn't come out of thin air. I do think the three-year seems particularly daunting, especially to our residents that have a lot of debt and know that in some of these subspecialties they will put three more years into not making more money than if they went into general pediatrics right away. Also, many of our residents are helping to support their family members, so it is even more of a strain to continue to take on additional training.[2]

---

[2] The webinar recording can be accessed at https://www.nationalacademies.org/event/09-06-2022/the-pediatric-subspecialty-workforce-and-its-impact-on-child-health-and-well-being-webinar-2.

BOX 5-5
Resident, Fellow, and Clinician Perspectives—
Length of Fellowship Training

"AAP needs to consider making fellowships 2 years so that more people will consider applying. We are already incredibly underpaid and lose out on lifetime earnings by going into fellowship."
– **Pediatric PGY-3, DBP Applicant, Babylon, NY**

"I think one barrier is that the [American Board of Pediatrics] requires 3 years for [fellowship training]. I wish there were two tracks, one clinical that was 2 years and one for research that would be a 3-year fellowship. I think there would be more people going into this field."
– **Pediatric Pulmonologist, Grand Rapids, MI**

"With 3 years of subspecialty training required and with only one year of that clinical (the rest of the time is research), I think this is a barrier for clinicians who might want to go into [pediatric infectious diseases] but are not interested in spending 2 years doing research. Plus, there is a further financial cost due to prolonging training unnecessarily for those not interested in research."
– **Clinician and Assistant Professor in Pediatric Infectious Diseases**

"Barriers included longer fellowship with research requirements that are not found on the adult side, which coupled with diminished earning potential sets us back financially for several more years and makes it more difficult not only to pay off loans but also to adequately start saving for and starting a family."
– **Second Year Pediatric Pulmonology Fellow, Birmingham, AL**

"Fellowship means 3 years of delaying the start of independent practice, which means continuing to survive on meager training salaries, working long hours, delaying paying off student loans, potentially delaying having children, or expanding one's family."
– **Third Year Pediatric Critical Care Fellow**

These quotes were collected from the committee's online call for trainee, clinician, and family perspectives.

> **BOX 5-6**
> **Alternate ABP Pathways**
>
> 1. The **Accelerated Research Pathway (ARP)** supports "candidates who are committed to an academic career as physician–scientists with a strong research emphasis in a pediatric subspecialty." Candidates may begin fellowship after completion of 2 years of general pediatric residency training, then complete 4 years of fellowship training with expectations of a more robust experience in research than standard trainees. This pathway is used most commonly by those who have had prior experience in a clinical or research field and does not shorten overall training, but shifts time away from the broader experiences in general pediatric training (ABP, 2022e).
>
> 2. **The Integrated Research Pathway** is designed to support trainees with significant prior experience in research and allow them to maintain and grow that trajectory while training in pediatrics and a subspecialty. This pathway is open to individuals with M.D./Ph.D. degrees or others who can demonstrate equivalent experience. This pathway uses the streamlined clinical curriculum of the ARP and integrates 12 months of ongoing research within the 3 years of general pediatrics residency. This pathway may interface with fast tracking in a subspecialty to allow for shortened overall training given the prior attainment of scholarly goals (ABP, 2022f).
>
> 3. **Subspecialty Fast Tracking** recognizes the research accomplishments of fellows that occurred before or during residency. In this situation, the requirement for scholarly activity may be waived. However, individuals who entered training through the Accelerated Research Pathway would not be eligible for fast tracking (ABP, 2022g).
>
> 4. **Dual Subspecialty Training** allows for dual certification in pediatric subspecialties in a reduced amount of time. Fellowship programs must be at the same institution (ABP, 2022h).

Training Locations

The location of residency and fellowship programs may impact both an individual's choice of a residency or fellowship, choice of subspecialty, and subsequent choice of practice location upon graduation. In general, physicians have a high likelihood of practicing in the state in which they completed graduate medical education (GME) (Fagan et al., 2015; Seifer et al., 1995) and training in rural and underserved settings increases future practice in these settings (Goodfellow et al., 2016; Morris et al., 2008; Phillips et al., 2013; Russell et al., 2022).

The 2022 AAMC Report on Residents reveals that 60 percent of the individuals who completed pediatric residency training from 2012 through 2021 and did not pursue subspecialty training are practicing in the state where they did their residency training (AAMC, 2022b). Similarly, as shown in Table 5-2, on average, more than half of pediatric subspecialists ultimately practice in the states where they complete their residency training. This may be due to a tendency for subspecialists to pursue fellowship training at the same institution as their residency, or lifestyle factors that influence an individual's choice of training location. Women are more likely than men to remain in the state where they completed their residency training.

COACHING, MENTORSHIP, AND ROLE MODELING

Early and consistent presence of coaches, mentors, and role models can be important influences on an individual's choice to both specialize in pediatrics as well as pursue training in a pediatric subspecialty. A definition of mentorship put forth in the National Academies report *The Science of Effective Mentorship in STEMM* (Science, Technology, Engineering, Mathematics, and Medicine) is "a professional, working alliance in which individuals work together over time to support the personal and professional growth, development, and success of the relational partners through the provision of career and psychosocial support" (NASEM, 2019a, pg 2). That report highlighted the multiple forms that mentorship can take, ranging from the typical/standard dyadic relationship, peer and near-peer interactions, and experience, to national workshops, seminars, and programs. The emphasis on psychosocial as well as career support highlights the important roles of emotional support and role modeling, which can be particularly impactful for mentees from backgrounds underrepresented in medicine (URiM). These supports can potentially mitigate unsupportive or hostile environments while reforms or strategies are implemented at institutional or societal levels to combat/dismantle structural racism and other barriers to the inclusion, retention, and advancement of pediatric subspecialists from

TABLE 5-2 Pediatric Subspecialist Retention in State of Residency Training by Gender, 2012–2021

Subspecialty	Percentage Remaining in State (Overall)	Percentage Remaining in State (Men)	Percentage Remaining in State (Women)
Adolescent Medicine	60.2	56.1	61.4
Child Abuse Pediatrics	54.4	33.3	57.7
Developmental-Behavioral Pediatrics	60.7	43.5	64.2
Neonatal-Perinatal Medicine	59.5	52.6	62.6
Pediatric Cardiology	45.0	42.0	48.5
Pediatric Critical Care Medicine	56.0	53.2	58.0
Pediatric Emergency Medicine	61.5	56.9	64.0
Pediatric Endocrinology	60.5	57.2	61.4
Pediatric Gastroenterology	57.9	51.9	61.7
Pediatric Hematology/Oncology	60.5	59.5	61.2
Pediatric Hospital Medicine[a]	78.9	100.0	66.7
Pediatric Infectious Diseases	58.7	62.4	56.6
Pediatric Nephrology	57.1	61.1	55.5
Pediatric Pulmonology	63.8	60.3	65.7
Pediatric Rheumatology	59.3	48.3	63.4

NOTE: [a]The percentage for pediatric hospital medicine reflects only a very small number of residents given that the first examination for certification was administered in 2020.
SOURCES: AAMC, 2022b,c.

URiM backgrounds. Early exposure to mentors and role models may be particularly important for students from URiM backgrounds. For example, one small study of 20 medical students from URiM backgrounds showed that mentorship and having role models from URiM backgrounds influenced their decisions to pursue academic pediatrics (Dixon et al., 2021).

In academic medicine, mentored experiences have been associated with a number of positive benefits, including job satisfaction and higher academic self-efficacy, although there are reports of less-than-optimal mentoring during fellowship training (Diekroger et al., 2017; Feldman et al., 2010). Mentors can serve as role models and advisors for future subspecialists, and their presence can enhance mentees' learning experiences (Nelson et al., 2020). One study of graduating pediatrics residents showed that most (87 percent) had a mentor who provided career advice; of those, nearly half (45 percent) had mentors who were subspecialists (Umoren and Frintner,

2014). The study further found that residents with subspecialist mentors were more likely to seek subspecialty training. A survey of 12 pediatric hospitalist fellows showed that most reported subspecialty-specific mentorship as being important during residency in supplementing the development of clinical skills (Patel et al., 2021). Within the subspecialty of pediatric infectious disease, faculty and fellows have encouraged students to join the subspecialty by inviting them to shadow their clinical practice and connecting them with minority prehealth professional organizations (Rogo et al., 2022).

FINANCING OF GRADUATE MEDICAL EDUCATION

GME, which includes initial residency and subsequent fellowship training, is a critical step in the physician pipeline. It is through GME that physicians specialize and subspecialize. In addition, to be independently licensed in any state, physicians must complete at least one year of GME in a U.S. program (FSMB, 2018).[3] Therefore, the availability of GME positions determines both the overall number and the specialty distribution of the physician workforce.

GME also represents the largest public investment in the health workforce. Funding for pediatric residency programs can come from Medicare, Medicaid, the Children's Hospital Graduate Medical Education (CHGME) program, and the Teaching Health Center Graduate Medical Education (THCGME)[4] program. In FY2020, Medicare GME provided the largest share of GME funding estimated at $16.2 billion (CRS, 2022); in FY2022, Medicaid GME provided $7.4 billion of federal and state funding (AAMC, 2023). In 2018, THCGME obligated $119 million to increase the number of primary care residents and dentists training in community-based, ambulatory patient care centers (GAO, 2021a). (Financing levels of CHGME are discussed later in this section.)

According to AAMC, in academic year 2021–2022, there were 9,219 pediatric residents, 1,519 residents in the combined program of internal medicine/pediatrics, and 4,417 pediatric medical subspecialty fellows[5]

---

[3] In most states, additional years of GME are required for international medical graduates. Some states accept GME completed in Canada to meet licensing requirements (FSMB, 2018).

[4] The THCGME program was established in the *Patient Protection and Affordable Care Act of 2010*. The program provides GME payments to new or expanded primary care residency programs located in community-based settings. In academic year 2022–2023, 4 out of 102 awardees were in pediatrics (HRSA, 2022c).

[5] The count of pediatric medical subspecialty fellows includes fellows from the 15 ABP-certified subspecialties plus fellows in clinical informatics (30 total), pediatric sports medicine (25 total), and pediatric transplant hepatology (16 total) (AAMC, 2022d).

(AAMC, 2022d). The CHGME program supported the training of 6,124 pediatrics residents[6] and 3,201 pediatric medical subspecialty fellows (including 206 child and adolescent psychiatry fellows) in 2021–2022 (HRSA, 2023a). While some pediatricians are trained in Medicare GME hospitals, the majority of pediatric medical subspecialty fellows were trained in freestanding children's hospitals supported by the CHGME program.

Role of Medicare in Graduate Medical Education

Medicare GME payments make up the largest portion of public funding for residency training programs. Medicare GME is mandatory funding with payments, based on the statutory formulas, guaranteed annually. In 2018, Medicare provided GME payments to 1,319 hospitals, and 70 percent of training hospitals were training at least one more resident than was covered by the Medicare-funded cap (GAO, 2021b). A 2008 study found that much of the growth in residency positions after the *Balanced Budget Act of 1997* established hospital resident caps was in non-primary care specialty and subspecialty fields (Salsberg et al., 2008). Medicare GME has been criticized for concerns of overpayment, geographic maldistribution, and lack of transparency and accountability. The Medicare Payment Advisory Commission (MedPAC) and the Institute of Medicine (IOM)[7] have both recommended major GME reforms. In their June 2010 *Report to Congress*, MedPAC identified two major areas of concern for GME—workforce mix and education and training in the skills needed to improve the value of health care delivery systems—and included among their recommendations:

1. Congress should authorize the Secretary of the U.S. Department of Health and Human Services (Secretary) to change Medicare's GME funding, establishing new standards for distributing funds, goals for learning, and performance-based funding;
2. The Secretary should conduct workforce analysis to determine the number of residency positions, in total and by specialty, needed in the United States, and annually publish a report on GME payments and associated costs to hospitals; and

---

[6] The pediatric residents included general pediatrics residents as well as residents from eight types of combined pediatrics programs (HRSA, 2023a).

[7] As of March 2016, the Health and Medicine Division of the National Academies of Sciences, Engineering, and Medicine (National Academies) continues the consensus studies and convening activities previously carried out by the Institute of Medicine (IOM). The IOM name is used to refer to reports issued prior to July 2015.

3. The Secretary should study strategies for increasing workforce diversity (MedPAC, 2010).

In 2014, the IOM found GME financing to be outdated and in need of significant reform (IOM, 2014). The IOM recommended maintaining the current level of Medicare GME funding, but replacing the direct and indirect payments with a single, streamlined, performance-based payment within existing funds, establishing a GME Transformation Fund to "develop and evaluate innovative GME programs, to determine and validate appropriate GME performance measures, to pilot alternative GME payment methods, and to award new Medicare-funded GME training positions in priority disciplines and geographic areas" (IOM, 2014, p.133). The IOM also recommended the creation of a GME Policy Council at the level of the Secretary of the U.S. Department of Health and Human Services and a GME Center in the Centers for Medicare & Medicaid Services to administer reforms, manage demonstrations of new payment models, and ensure strategic investments. To date, these recommendations have not been implemented.

Role of the Children's Hospital Graduate Medical Education Program

The CHGME program was established in the *Healthcare Research and Quality Act of 1999* to provide GME payments to freestanding children's hospitals. Prior to the CHGME program, the Medicare program provided payments based on the Medicare share of total inpatient days for direct GME payments and as an add-on to the Medicare inpatient prospective payment system for indirect GME payments. Therefore, freestanding children's hospitals qualified for minimal Medicare GME payments because so few children are on Medicare. The CHGME program filled a gap in federal GME support.

Since its inception in 2000, the CHGME program has been authorized for annual appropriations of $280–$330 million, and briefly from 2002 to 2005, to "such sums as may be necessary" (CRS, 2021). Program funding has had significant year-to-year variation (see Figure 5-2), but since FY2014, there has been a steady increase in appropriations. The program was funded at $375 million for FY2022 and 385 million[8] for FY2023, which is historically the highest level of funding for the program and above the currently authorized level of $325 million (CRS, 2023). The number of CHGME hospitals has ranged from 54 to 61 (CRS, 2023). In FY2022, there were 59 CHGME hospitals across 29 states, the District of Columbia, and

---

[8] The CHGME funding level for FY2023 was corrected after release of the report to the sponsors.

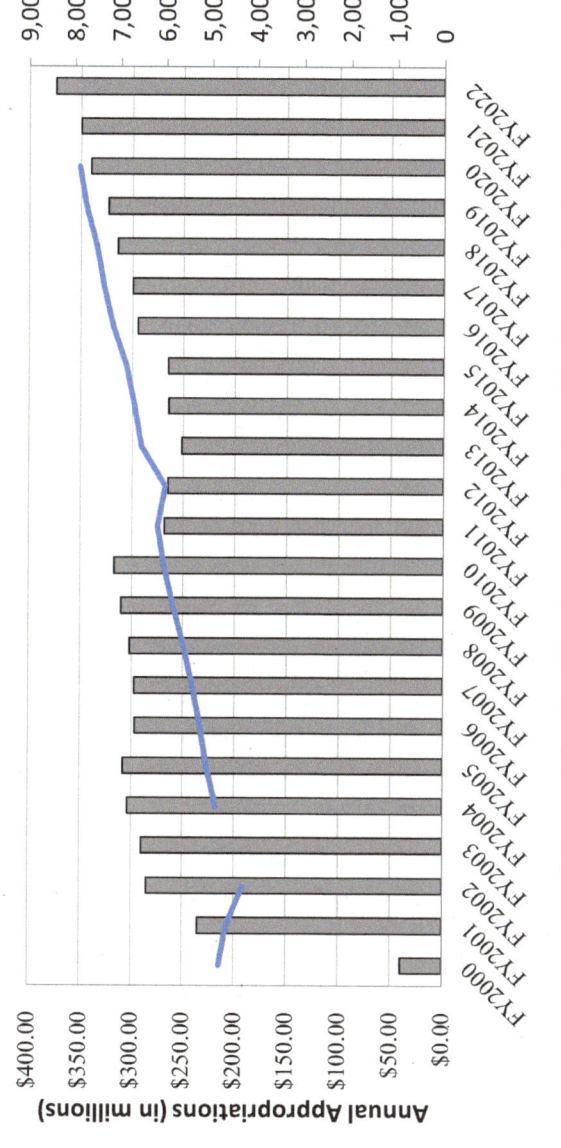

FIGURE 5-2 CHGME annual appropriations and residents supported.
NOTE: *Data for FY2003 residents are missing.
SOURCES: CRS, 2021; HRSA, 2022a.

Puerto Rico. Annual award amounts ranged from $30,273 to $26.2 million (median award $4.1 million).[9]

Although CHGME payments are similar to Medicare GME in structure, there are key differences. Similar to Medicare, direct and indirect payments are calculated based on formulas, and a cap on the number of residents is applied to each hospital. The resident cap limits the number of resident positions eligible for payment, although hospitals can train above the cap if they are able to fund the extra positions. During one of the committee's public webinars, Mary Leonard, Arline and Pete Harman Professor and Chair of the Department of Pediatrics at Stanford University, director of the Stanford Maternal and Child Health Research Institute, and physician-in-chief of Lucile Packard Children's Hospital, described difficulties related to the small clinical margin in pediatric departments:

> Our children's hospital has a very small margin compared to the adult hospital….It has huge implications for funding the education programs… my single biggest line item, just the discretionary funding and how I use my clinical profit, is fellowships…it's increasingly becoming a challenge for my department. We're very, very fortunate…the Lucile Packard Children's Hospital spends $40 million on GME. And so, they fund all my first year fellows and for some they fund the second and third year. It's the obvious ones. It's [neonatal-perinatal] and critical care. But I have 54 second and third year fellows who I am responsible for covering their salary…We were so fortunate about 20 years ago to get an endowment to support some of our second and third year fellows, but that is completely flat, whereas my number of fellows has increased very, very dramatically. So, this year it was a tipping point in terms of the challenges that I'm having because I'm thrilled when we get ACGME approval and hospital support to expand my nephrology fellowship or my ID fellowship, and then I go…I have four more mouths to feed.[10]

In contrast to Medicare, CHGME is a discretionary program and payments are ultimately limited by the amount of annual appropriations. Hospitals receive a portion of their payments based on the annual appropriation level and new CHGME hospitals can mean decreased payments across existing hospitals. In 2018, the GAO estimated that the average unadjusted Medicare GME payment per full-time resident in 2015 was $117,674 while CHGME paid $51,778 per resident and Medicaid GME paid $36,540 per resident (GAO, 2018). Under the CHGME program,

---

[9] These data were generated using the "Find Grants" dashboard at https://data.hrsa.gov/tools/find-grants (accessed May 7, 2023).

[10] The webinar recording can be accessed at https://www.nationalacademies.org/event/07-19-2022/the-pediatric-subspecialty-workforce-and-its-impact-on-child-health-and-well-being-webinar-1.

hospitals must report on the number of residents trained in each specialty, the types of training provided related to the health care needs of different populations (e.g., children who are underserved due to family income or rural/urban location), changes in curriculum and training experiences, and the number of residents who graduate and practice within the same state. In her presentation to this committee, Dr. Leonard discussed the impact of CHGME funding on fellowships:

> [CHGME] supports the training of most of the country's subspecialists, but the funding per training is less than half of that for Medicare GME. Medicare GME is growing reliably annually, but the CHGME is not. So, that's been a big issue. And there's a really nice body of literature around fellowship funding insecurity. Not surprisingly, the disciplines that earn money for the hospital, the NICU [Neonatal Intensive Care Unit], the PICU [Pediatric Intensive Care Unit], emergency medicine, some of the big fellowships are really getting the preponderance of the funding from the hospitals...there is no financial support through CHGME for the research training that's necessary to facilitate the career development of physician scientists and to meet the ABP [American Board of Pediatrics] requirement for scholarly activity.[11]

The CHGME program is unique in that the 2013 reauthorization of the program established a Quality Bonus System (QBS) to link payment to program quality measures. The FY2023 CHGME funding opportunity states that the goal of QBS is "to recognize CHGME Payment Program awardees that provide high-quality training and to incentivize the participating children's hospitals to meet the pediatric workforce needs of the nation" (HRSA, 2022b). In FY2023, hospitals must meet a pay-for-reporting requirement to qualify for the quality bonus payment (i.e., hospitals must complete individual-level documentation for all residents supported by the CHGME program). In FY2019, the Health Resources and Services Administration (HRSA) awarded a QBS evaluation contract to develop quality measures for GME programs. However, quality measures have not been released beyond the pay-for-reporting requirement. The available funds for QBS are limited in statute to any amount remaining after payments are made to a set of hospitals deemed newly qualified for the CHGME program in the 2013 reauthorization. The total amount for the newly qualified hospitals and the Quality Bonus Systems cannot exceed $7 million. In FY2021, the CHGME program provided $1.8 million in QBS payments to 32 of the 59 awardees (HRSA, 2022a). While the QBS is an important policy mechanism to link

---

[11] The webinar recording can be accessed at https://www.nationalacademies.org/event/07-19-2022/the-pediatric-subspecialty-workforce-and-its-impact-on-child-health-and-well-being-webinar-1.

GME funds to priority pediatric workforce needs, the available amount spread across up to 59 hospitals is unlikely to be sufficient to incentivize meaningful change.

Role of Medicaid in Graduate Medical Education

State Medicaid programs can also support GME. As noted earlier, federal and state payments for Medicaid GME (including 44 states and DC) reached an estimated $7.4 billion in 2022 (AAMC, 2023). While many states mirror the Medicare direct and indirect payment method, some states have used their Medicaid programs to innovate, including consolidating to a single GME payment, providing payments directly to medical schools or ambulatory care centers, and other health profession trainees, most often graduate nurses. Additional state innovations include creating GME innovation pools, funding rural rotations and/or providing funding to start new residency programs or expand existing programs, and establishing oversight bodies to bring interested parties together and decide how funds could be targeted to meet specialty, geographic, or other workforce needs (Fraher et al., 2017).

EDUCATIONAL DEBT AND EARNING POTENTIAL

Financial disincentives such as educational debt and earning potential may influence an individual's choice to pursue training in pediatrics in general, as well as the choice to pursue additional training in a specific subspecialty. As discussed previously, debt burden and income do not typically rank among the highest factors in surveys of influences on career decisions; however, such disincentives may weigh more heavily on the decisions for certain groups.

Educational Debt

Data from AAMC show the median educational debt for medical students in general (including both medical school debt and educational debt incurred before medical school) in 2019 was $200,000 (Youngclaus and Fresne, 2020). Debt ranked lower in importance as an influence on specialty choice for medical students than other factors such as the content of the specialty area, role models, and work–life balance. However, educational debt may more strongly influence the choice of a career in primary care for medical students from economically disadvantaged backgrounds (Phillips et al., 2014).

In pediatrics, roughly 75 percent of graduating residents report having educational debt; that percentage has remained consistent over the past decade, while the average amount of debt has steadily increased (Cull et al., 2017). A large amount of educational debt combined with typically lower earning potential for pediatrics and the pediatric subspecialties (as compared with their adult internal medicine counterparts) may hinder recruitment (Catenaccio et al., 2021a; Catenaccio et al., 2021b; Rochlin and Simon, 2011). Using 2013 survey data from the AAP Pediatrician Life and Career Experience Study, Cull et al. (2017) found that pediatric subspecialists were more likely than other pediatricians to be concerned about their debt, even up to 10 years after completing training.

Furthermore, there are disparities in the level of debt burden. For example, medical students from URiM backgrounds have more educational debt, which may further complicate recruitment of URiM candidates to subspecialty careers (Dugger et al., 2013; Orr et al., 2023; Toretsky et al., 2018, 2019; Youngclaus and Fresne, 2020). In 2019, medical school graduates (in general) who identify as Black, not Hispanic had a median education debt of $230,000, in comparison with a median debt of $200,000 for all students, $200,000 for White, not Hispanic students, and $190,000 for Hispanic students (Youngclaus and Fresne, 2020). Orr et al. (2023) found that self-reported educational debt was associated with a trainee's self-reported race/ethnicity, with one-third of individuals who identify as Black/African American having more than $300,000 in educational debt. See Box 5-7 for clinician perspectives on their debt burden.

Earning Potential

In the broader literature on earnings, female-dominated professions tend to have lower earnings than male-dominated ones, including medicine (IWPR, 2021; Levanon et al., 2009; Pelley, 2020). For example, a cross-sectional study of more than 54,000 academic physicians found that women had lower starting salaries than men in 42 of 45 subspecialties and lower earning potential in 43 of the 45 subspecialties (Catenaccio et al., 2022). Regarding pediatrics specifically, Frintner et al. (2019) concluded that "early- to mid-career female pediatricians earned less than male pediatricians" and added that "this difference persisted after adjustment for important labor force, physician-specific job, and work–family characteristics." They initially found that women earn 76 percent of what men earn, or approximately $51,000 less. Adjusting for a variety of workforce, job, and work–family characteristics, they found that women earned approximately 94 percent of men's earnings, or roughly $8,000 less annually (Frintner et al., 2019). These findings are particularly important for pediatrics and the pediatric subspecialties given the increasing percentage of women pursuing careers in pediatrics and the pediatric subspecialties (see Chapter 4).

> **BOX 5-7**
> **Clinician Perspectives—Debt Burden**
>
> "I do not necessarily regret the decision, but the opportunity cost has been MASSIVE in terms of lost salary."
> **– Physician-Investigator, Boston, MA**
>
> "Financial concerns are the most significant barrier—the only reason I felt able to go into such a low-paying specialty was because I did not have any debt from medical school."
> **– Clinician and Professor in Pediatric Infectious Diseases**
>
> "The biggest barrier to consider was impact on my ability to start repaying loans."
> **– Professor of Pediatrics, Atlanta, GA**
>
> "We make less money after 3 additional years of postgraduate fellowship training than we would working as primary care pediatricians right out of residency. I carry enormous student loans and have made financial sacrifices to remain in this field to help meet the immense needs of children and families."
> **– Attending Physician, Developmental and Behavioral Pediatrics, Philadelphia, PA**
>
> *These quotes were collected from the committee's online call for trainee, clinician, and family perspectives.*

Pediatricians are among the lowest paid specialists, even among primary care specialties (Doximity and Curative, 2023; Kane, 2022). Frintner et al. (2019) found that pediatricians in the larger subspecialties (e.g., neonatology, cardiology, critical care, emergency medicine, gastroenterology, and hematology/oncology) reported overall mean earnings of $231,930, while pediatricians in the smaller subspecialties (all other pediatric medical subspecialties) reported overall mean earnings of $168,245, and general pediatricians reported overall mean earnings of $180,250. A more recent survey (in 2022) on payment for physician specialties revealed that pediatrics overall and pediatric subspecialties tended to have the lowest compensation, and surgical specialties received the highest compensation; in fact, ABP-certified pediatric subspecialties represented 8 of the 20 lowest paying specialties, and the 5 specialties with the lowest compensation were all ABP-certified subspecialties (i.e., pediatric endocrinology, pediatric infectious disease, pediatric rheumatology, pediatric hematology and oncology, and pediatric nephrology) (Doximity and Curative, 2023). Among these five subspecialties, total average compensation ranged from $218,266 for pediatric endocrinology to $238,208 for pediatric nephrology.

Lakshminrusimha and colleagues (2023) found that the benchmark compensation for most academic pediatric medical subspecialties was lower than the benchmark compensation for their adult counterparts. For example, the compensation for pediatric gastroenterology was 70 percent of the compensation for adult gastroenterology; pediatric infectious disease, pediatric rheumatology, and pediatric endocrinology academics were compensated at 90 percent of the compensation of their adult counterparts. On the other hand, they showed that pediatric surgeons earned 134 percent of the compensation for adult surgeons (Lakshminrusimha et al., 2023).

A 2021 study showed that the lifetime financial return on investment for pediatric subspecialty training, compared with general pediatrics, was negative for 12 of the 15 subspecialties examined (Catenaccio et al., 2021b). Only subspecialty training in cardiology, critical care, and neonatology resulted in a positive lifetime financial return (Figure 5-3). Furthermore, the relative difference in financial returns among subspecialties is increasing. Over a 10-year period, the difference between subspecialties with positive financial returns (as compared with general pediatrics) and subspecialties

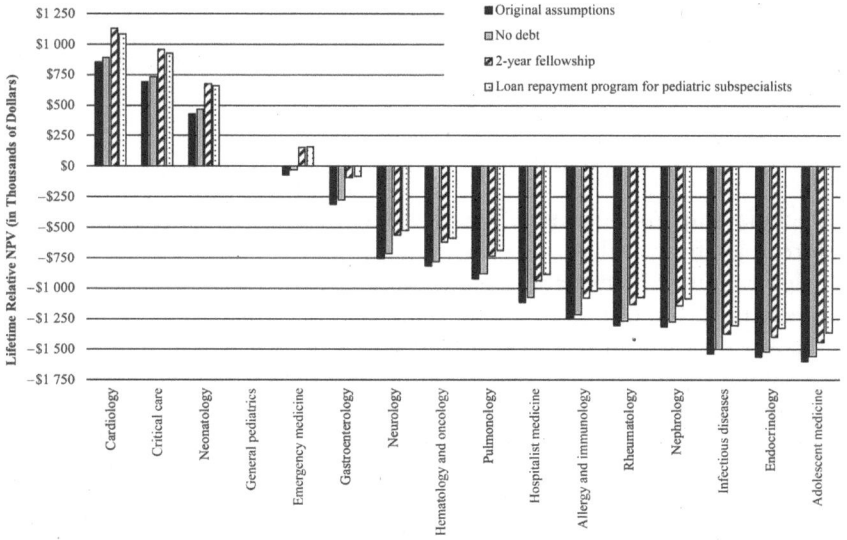

FIGURE 5-3 Lifetime financial returns for subspecialty pediatric training, 2018.
SOURCE: Adapted from Catenaccio et al., 2021b. Reproduced with permission from Pediatrics, Copyright ©2021 by the AAP.

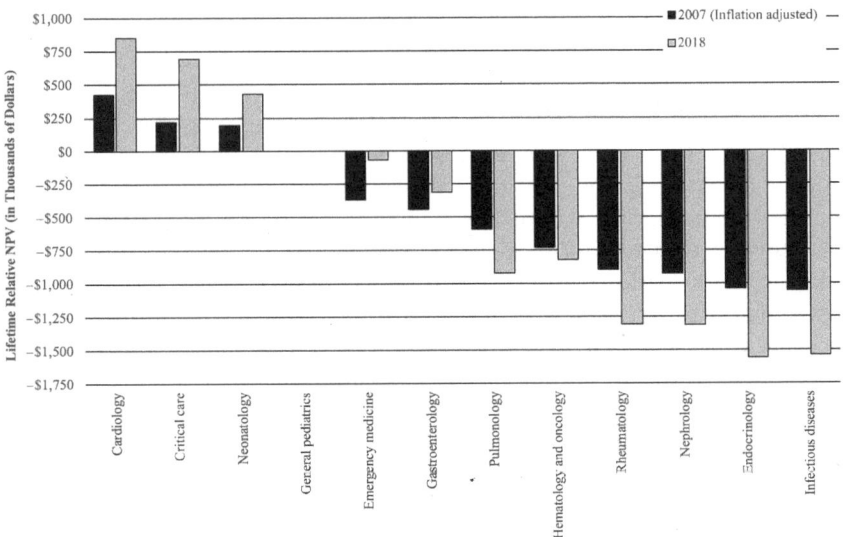

FIGURE 5-4 Lifetime financial returns for subspecialty pediatric training, 2007 versus 2018.
SOURCES: Adapted from Catenaccio et al., 2021b. Reproduced with permission from Pediatrics, Copyright ©2021 by the AAP.

with negative financial returns is even greater. (See Figure 5-4.) See Chapter 8 for more on physician payment.

Scholarship and Loan Repayment Programs

Scholarship and loan repayment programs aim to reduce financial barriers to entry for health professions careers and/or provide a financial incentive, leveraging student debt, for a desired health workforce outcome such as specialty choice or practice in an underserved setting. In 2019, among all medical students with the highest levels of debt, nearly half reported plans to seek loan forgiveness through a public service program (Youngclaus and Fresne, 2020).

National Health Service Corps

HRSA's National Health Service Corps (NHSC) is one of the best known programs providing scholarships or loan repayment in exchange for a minimum of 2 years of clinical services provided in an area with a shortage of health professionals. NHSC supports primary care physicians, nurse practitioners, physician assistants, dentists, pharmacists, and mental health professionals (HRSA, 2021). Pediatric behavioral and mental health subspecialists qualify for NHSC, but other types of pediatric subspecialists are not eligible. In 2022, NHSC supported 2,587 primary care physicians as well as 4,031 nurse practitioners and 1,558 physician assistants providing primary care (HRSA, 2023b). Nearly 70 percent of NHSC primary care practitioners are retained in a health professional shortage area over the 10 years after service (The Lewin Group, Inc., 2016).

Pediatric Specialty Loan Repayment Program

The Pediatric Specialty Loan Repayment Program, administered by HRSA, was established in the *Patient Protection and Affordable Care Act*, offering up to a $35,000 loan repayment a year for each year of full-time services providing pediatric medical subspecialty, pediatric surgical specialty, or child and adolescent mental and behavioral health care, including substance abuse prevention and treatment services for up to 3 years. The qualifying time of service can be during residency or fellowship training. The program was originally authorized at $30 million annually for pediatric medical and surgical specialists and $20 million for child and adolescent behavioral health specialists. However, the program was funded for the first time in FY2022 at only $5 million as part of the *Consolidated Appropriations Act*[12] and again in FY2023 at $10 million (HRSA, 2023c). In June 2023, HRSA opened the first application cycle for this program, expecting to make up to 150 awards with the initial $15 million appropriated by Congress (HRSA, 2023d). Similar to the NHSC, the program has a full-time service commitment; this requires that the specialist provide clinical care for at least 36 hours per week and for at least 45 weeks per year. The clinical care requirement applies for those in practice and in residency or fellowship training. This requirement may preclude pediatric subspecialty researchers from applying for this program.

National Institutes of Health (NIH) Loan Repayment Programs

Loan repayment for pediatric research is another potentially important program for pediatric subspecialty careers. "Since 1988, the NIH Loan Repayment Programs have been successful in recruiting and retaining early-stage investigators into promising biomedical and behavioral research careers" (Lauer, 2019). One of the programs focuses specifically on pediatric research. In this program, NIH can repay up to $50,000 in educational

---

[12] *The Consolidated Appropriations Act of 2022*, Public Law 117-103, 117th Cong., 2d sess. (March 15, 2022).

loans per year in exchange for a commitment to research for at least 20 hours per week for at least 2 years (with possibility for renewal) (NIH, 2022a). In FY 2022, the mean award for new applications was $88,669 while the mean for renewals was $47,720; the mean age of new awardees was 36 years (NIH, 2023). (See Chapter 6 for more on NIH Loan Repayment Programs.)

J-1 Visa Waiver Program

The J-1 Visa Waiver program is one policy mechanism used to recruit and retain non-U.S. citizen international medical graduates. International medical graduates are an important part of the physician workforce. As noted in Chapter 4, nearly 21 percent of general pediatrics residents (not in combined programs or alternate pathways) and 27 percent of first-year ABP-certified subspecialty fellows are international medical graduates (ABP, 2023b,c). The J-1 is an exchange visitor visa that allows individuals to receive graduate medical education or other training. A J-1 visa holder would normally be required to physically reside in their country of nationality (or last residence) for at least 2 years upon completion of their exchange program. The J-1 Visa Waiver program waives the 2-year foreign residence requirement. Also known as the Conrad 30 Waiver Program, named after Sen. Kent Conrad from North Dakota who originally sponsored the legislation in 1994, the program provides each state with up to 30 J-1 visa waivers per year. A 2022 study of Maryland's J-1 Visa Waiver program suggests the program has been effective in attracting physicians to work in primary care and with high-need, low-income patients (Quigley, 2022). However, any policies to increase international recruitment of health professionals should consider global health workforce impacts. While global mobility and opportunity are worthy societal goals, U.S policies to address national physician workforce shortages can negatively impact global health systems, particularly in low- and middle-income countries (Mullan, 2005; Tankwanchi et al., 2013).

INFLUENCES ON LIFESTYLE

In general, lifestyle, work–life balance, and spousal considerations are among the factors that have the most influence on medical students and residents' choice of specialty and career path (Levaillant et al., 2020; Newton et al., 2005; Rao et al., 2017; Yang et al., 2019). A factor that has become increasingly important for clinicians in their choice of specialty or subspecialty is the perceived control over work-related lifestyle (Dorsey et al., 2003; Enoch et al., 2013; Haftel et al., 2020). General pediatrics residents as well as pediatric subspecialists have also specifically expressed the importance of lifestyle on their career paths (Amoli et al., 2016; Freed et al., 2009; Freed et al., 2016). One study of pediatric hematologist/oncologists showed that they preferred a balance of direct patient care, inpatient service and office-based outpatient care, and non-clinical time, and that they specifically sought jobs in settings that supported that balance, which were more likely to be larger medical centers with greater concentrations of subspecialists who could share the on-call burden (Frugé et al., 2010).

Gender may also play a role in prioritizing work–life balance and flexibility (e.g., through part-time work) (Enoch et al., 2013; Freed et al., 2017; Wiley et al., 2002; Women Chairs of the Association of Medical School Pediatric Department Chairs, 2007). Women prioritize lifestyle factors and interest in flexible work hours as compared to men (Freed et al., 2009; Harris et al., 2005). Female early-career pediatricians typically spend more time on household responsibilities and the care of their own children than male pediatricians (Starmer et al., 2016, 2019). In addition, one survey of new pediatric subspecialists showed that women were more likely than men to be employed part time and were more likely to foresee part-time work within the coming 5 years (Freed et al., 2016). However, the study also showed that about one-third of the respondents who reported working part time were still working more than 40 hours per week. Powell et al. (2021) found that graduating female pediatric residents were more likely to prioritize factors such as number of overnight calls per month, option to work part time, length of parental leave, and availability of onsite childcare in positions after residency as compared with male residents. See Box 5-8 for trainee and clinician perspectives on the influence of lifestyle factors. See later in this chapter for discussions of job satisfaction and burnout.

WORKFORCE PLANNING AND RECRUITMENT EFFORTS

Federal and state governments along with the private sector invest in a number of programs designed to support and develop the health care workforce, either overall or specifically for pediatric subspecialties. Aside from its role in loan repayment, NHSC, discussed earlier, is one program that seeks to get more clinicians into geographic areas that have shortages of health professionals.

Pediatrics 2025: AMSPDC Workforce Initiative

The Association of Medical School Pediatric Department Chairs (AMSPDC) workforce initiative was created in 2020 to meet the health and wellness needs of children by increasing the number and diversity of students entering pediatrics and improving the supply of pediatric subspecialists (AMSPDC, 2023). The initiative includes four areas of focus, or

> **BOX 5-8**
> **Trainee and Clinician Perspectives on Lifestyle Factors**
>
> "The very small division size (very few faculty members) makes for a crushing lifestyle."
> **– Pediatric Nephrologist, Bethesda, MD**
>
> "I chose pediatric emergency medicine because of the nature of the work and the schedule. Barriers were training time and training location versus where I wanted to settle with my family."
> **– Pediatric Emergency Medicine Attending Physician, Des Moines, IA**
>
> "I love the acuity, challenge, and patient relationships that are formed in a PICU. I practiced general pediatrics for 5 years before returning to fellowship. I've always loved intensive care, but I was also looking for a more standardized schedule and shift work."
> **– Post-PICU Fellow, Reno, NV**
>
> "Only barrier is that I am in academics, and it is hard to fulfill the expectations of my job while still giving time to my family."
> **– Faculty Neonatology, Indianapolis, IN**
>
> "As a practicing nephrologist, I left the field once for general pediatrics practice as my family relocated to [a] city without an opportunity to practice nephrology. Unfortunately, I had few regrets leaving behind an incredibly taxing service regularly warranting work in excess of 80 hours

domains. The first domain, "Changing the Educational Paradigm," focuses primarily on influencing and attracting students into pediatrics and high-priority subspecialties by advocating for educational change to regulatory agencies, exploring ways to redesign educational curricula (including more flexible training pathways), increasing early exposure to subspecialties, and enhancing positive role modeling. The second domain, "Workforce Data/Needs and Access," focuses primarily on understanding the needs and trends within the pediatric workforce, including gathering data on the diversity of pediatric clinicians, models of care, and referral patterns. The third domain, "Economic Strategy," focuses on ways to minimize educational debt and strategies to achieve parity with other providers. The final domain, "Recruitment/Outreach and Early Integration," primarily examines other avenues to attract medical students to pediatrics, including early

> a week [and] on inpatient call as an attending, with little to no sleep and no protections for my health and well-being."
> **– Mid-Career Pediatric Nephrologist**
>
> "I did know that choosing this additional training, known for being extremely demanding of time and emotional energy, would delay my wife's and my desire to start a family. It meant saving money wherever we could to be able to start that family as soon as possible toward the end of fellowship. It meant moving yet again and limiting where we could ever move to where I can do my job."
> **– Third Year Pediatric Critical Care Fellow**
>
> "I chose pediatric emergency medicine because I liked that the workflow of the specialty allows me to focus on clinical care when I am on a shift, but also provides the ability to hand off to a colleague when I go home. The barriers we face in our specialty are the negative impact that variable schedules have on one's health and overall well-being, including switching from days to evenings to overnights. We also experience the barrier of significant variability in what is considered full time in terms of hours per week, given that we routinely work hazard hours without any adjustment in how those hours are accounted for [during] evenings, overnights, weekends, and holidays."
> **– Pediatric Emergency Medicine Faculty, Houston, TX**
>
> *These quotes were collected from the committee's online call for trainee, clinician, and family perspectives.*

exposure at high school and college levels, marketing strategies, increased shadowing opportunities for preclinical medical students, and incorporating pediatrics into preclinical curricula.

Underrepresented Populations

Evidence increasingly supports the importance of a diverse health workforce. In general, physicians from URiM backgrounds or who grew up in rural or urban underserved areas are more likely to serve underserved populations (Goodfellow et al., 2016; Marrast et al., 2014). Patient–provider demographic concordance may be associated with improved patient outcomes (Alsan et al., 2019; Shen et al., 2018; Zhao et al., 2019) and diversity in medical schools produces educational benefits such as cultural awareness and decreased bias (Saha et al., 2008; van Ryn et al., 2015). A recent scoping review of 27 articles across various medical and surgical specialties found that combinations of interventions, including holistic review, lower emphasis on examination scores, and explicit messaging about the importance of diversity, led to increases in URiM applications, interviews, and matriculation into residency and fellowship (Mabeza et al., 2021). However, recruitment to increase representation in the health care workforce continues to be a challenge for the medical field in general. Additionally, recent state-based initiatives to prohibit programs and training aimed at diversity, equity, and inclusion at public colleges and universities may serve as significant barriers to increasing representation or may even influence a prospective fellow's choice of training location (Acevedo, 2023; Curran, 2023; Reddy and Olivares, 2023). Intentional initiatives will be needed to effectively increase representation of URiM physicians. During one of the committee's public webinars, Denise Cora-Bramble, inaugural chief diversity officer at Children's National Medical Center, stated:

> At the national level, what we see is if we look at those numbers of the percentage of those that are [URiM], for residents, there isn't much change if you look at the last 10 years or so. And for fellows, it's actually decreased. I would say that from my perspective, unless we in the institutional level have some very intentional and direct strategies to address this, the numbers are just not going to change by themselves.[13]

General Efforts to Increase Representation in Medicine

HRSA's Health Careers Opportunity Program (HCOP), Centers of Excellence (COE), and Area Health Education Centers (AHEC) focus on enhancing opportunities for medical students from racial/ethnic minority and disadvantaged backgrounds. The goal of HCOP is to identify, recruit, and support students from disadvantaged backgrounds for education and training for a career in health care professions. COE supports health professions schools that have higher enrollments of students from underrepresented racial/ethnic backgrounds. AHEC supports education and training networks between communities and academic organizations with the goal of increasing diversity of health professionals, improving their distribution, and enhancing quality of care.

NIH maintains the Science Education Partnership Award programs, which support educational projects in science, technology, engineering, and mathematics for prekindergarten through grade 12, and summer internship

---

[13] The webinar recording can be accessed at https://www.nationalacademies.org/event/07-19-2022/the-pediatric-subspecialty-workforce-and-its-impact-on-child-health-and-well-being-webinar-1.

programs for high school students, including the High School Scientific Training and Enrichment Program (HiSTEP) and HiSTEP 2.0, which focus on students from high schools in the Washington, DC metropolitan area with a high percentage of financially disadvantaged students (NIH, 2022b). The Indian Health Service supports the Health Professions Recruitment Program for Indians which, in part, helps American Indians and Alaska Natives to pursue careers in health professions (TAGGS, 2022). Older studies examining the impact of these programs demonstrate that interventions at the high school-and college-level programs had positive effects, including matriculation to medical school and employment in health professions (HHS, 2009). Funding levels for these programs are modest. In FY2023, HCOP was funded at $16.0 million, COE at $28.42 million, AHEC at $47.0 million and Indian Health Service Programs at 3.9 million (HRSA, 2023e; TAGGS, 2022).

Efforts to Increase Representation in Pediatrics

Within pediatrics specifically, several programs and practices have been developed to recruit URiM students. Recruitment initiatives implemented by medical schools include increasing the representation of URiM students on admission committees, adopting a more holistic process to review applicants that considers experiences and attributes in addition to academic performance, and eliminating implicit biases (Weyand et al., 2020). Residency programs have made efforts to focus on URiM applicants through outreach via conferences and second-look programs, and institutions have provided fellows with travel rewards for interviews and conducted targeted improvement. However, few data are available on whether these efforts have improved representation among pediatric subspecialty fellows (Weyand et al., 2020).

There is also little evidence on individual institution or organization efforts on specific URiM recruitment in pediatrics. The Nationwide Children's Hospital in Columbus, OH, increased the visibility of URiM faculty during recruitment and outside of the traditional interview process through outreach and social engagements with candidates. As a result of these efforts, the percentage of URiM residents in the program increased from a baseline of 5 percent in 2015 to 21 percent in the 2021 match (Hoff et al., 2021). As one of the newest subspecialties, pediatric hospital medicine has made concerted efforts to increase representation in their applicants by instituting a diversity and inclusion task force to review past recruitment practices for implicit bias or racism, conducting pre-interview events, highlighting opportunities for mentorship during the recruitment process, developing evidence-based best practice recommendations, and surveying matched and unmatched fellowship applicants to analyze effective URiM recruitment strategies (Lopez and Raphael, 2021). The COVID-19 pandemic demonstrated that virtual recruitment for pediatric subspecialty fellowships resulted in improvements in the diversity of application pools in part due to cost savings and less time lost from residency associated with not needing to travel to the fellowship site (Petersen et al., 2022).

Lopez and Fuentes-Afflick (2022) suggested the following workforce interventions to mitigate health inequities across pediatric subspecialty care, specifically by doing the following:

- Explore the obstacles that may pose unique challenges for individuals from URiM when considering a career in pediatric subspecialties, create programs to increase awareness of subspecialty careers, and promote policies to encourage entrance into these fields, such as loan forgiveness.
- Create, develop, and evaluate policies and programs to diversify the pediatric subspecialty workforce, including faculty recruitment of individuals from URiM groups and retention and leadership training.
- Expand and support career advancement through scholarship focused on reducing health inequities in all pediatric subspecialties.
- Implement strategies to diversify applicants to pediatric fellowship programs.

An important factor to recognize is that the pipeline for recruitment into pediatric subspecialties is the cohort of existing pediatrics residents who, in turn, draw from the existing cohort of medical students (Weyand et al., 2020). Therefore, a focus on efforts to increase diversity among pediatric subspecialists alone will not likely be able to increase representation broadly among the subspecialties; rather, more effort is likely needed to increase representation along the entire pipeline, especially at the earliest stages of career development. As noted by Fuentes-Afflick et al. (2022):

Although all specialties compete in a current zero-sum game to recruit [URiM] medical students into their specialty, we anticipate that efforts to enhance the diversity of medical students will have a positive impact on all specialties.

National Health Care Workforce Commission

There has been a long-standing awareness of the need to assess the supply of and demand for the health care workforce at the national level, but to date, little has been done. For example, the National Health Care Workforce Commission was established by the *Patient Protection and Affordable*

Care Act of 2010,[14] with a structure similar to MedPAC and the Medicaid and CHIP Payment and Access Commission. The purpose of the Commission was to advise Congress, the President, states, and localities on health care workforce supply and demand, and the related health workforce priorities, goals, and policies. However, Congress has not appropriated funds for the National Health Care Workforce Commission, preventing it from even meeting to discuss these issues (McDonough, 2021).

RETENTION

Although this chapter focused primarily on the factors that influence an individual to consider pursuing a career in a pediatric subspecialty, the retention of pediatric subspecialists is also important (the retention of pediatric physician–scientists is discussed in more detail in Chapter 6). Longevity as a pediatric subspecialist may be predicted by the personal or professional factors such as concerns surrounding financial considerations (e.g., educational debt and compensation) and clinician burnout, well-being, and job satisfaction. As discussed in Chapter 4, the number of first-year pediatric medical subspecialty fellows has been increasing over the past few decades (Macy et al., 2021). It is critical to support the current pediatric subspecialty workforce, while also considering ways to expand the pipeline and encourage future medical students to consider a pediatric subspecialty career.

Job Satisfaction

In a systematic review of physician satisfaction studies, Scheurer et al. (2009) found that pediatricians generally report higher satisfaction than other specialties. Studies of early and mid-career pediatricians found that more than 80 percent reported being satisfied with their career as a physician (Frintner et al., 2021b; Starmer et al., 2016). In addition, 95 percent of graduating pediatric residents surveyed in 2020 reported they would choose pediatrics again, a trend that has been consistent over the past 20 years (AAP, 2022). In a national longitudinal study of early to mid-career pediatricians, work satisfaction scale scores in 2012–2020 decreased slightly over time overall (Frintner et al., 2022). While 86 percent of pediatricians thought their work was personally rewarding, 37 percent were frustrated with their work situation. Over the study years, pediatricians with the strongest work satisfaction reported increased flexibility with work hours, support from colleagues, and time with patients while pediatricians who reported increased work hours and obstacles to balancing work and

---

[14] *Patient Protection and Affordable Care Act*, Section 5101.

personal responsibilities were more likely to report dissatisfaction (Frintner et al., 2022).

Clinician Burnout

The 2019 National Academies report *Taking Action Against Clinician Burnout* described burnout as "a syndrome characterized by high emotional exhaustion, high depersonalization (i.e., cynicism), and a low sense of personal accomplishments from work" (NASEM, 2019b, p. 1). Pediatric subspecialists may be at greater risk of burnout because of pressure to work longer hours (as a result of workforce shortages), and lower reimbursement compared with adult practice physicians (Kumar and Mezoff, 2020). As noted by Sallie Permar, Nancy C. Paduano Professor and chair of pediatrics at Weill Cornell Medicine, pediatrician-in-chief at New York Presbyterian/Weill Cornell Medical Center, and professor of immunology and microbial pathogenesis at Weill Cornell Graduate School of Medical Sciences, in one of the committee's public webinars:

> The low [compensation] tied to the low reimbursement rate really does hold us back in terms of not only being able to recruit pediatricians throughout the pipeline from before medical school, in medical school, but also what I've found to be a problem also in preventing burnout and retaining our faculty in those roles. And we know that the burnout issue does face women and minorities more intensely.[15]

Students, clinicians, and faculty from URiM backgrounds may experience burnout due to what has been described as the "minority tax"—that is, "extra responsibilities placed on minority faculty in the name of efforts to achieve diversity" such as through disproportionate involvement in community outreach efforts or diversity initiatives (Rodriguez et al., 2015). This burden is often compounded by a lack of value assigned to these activities by their employers (such as in comparison to pursuing research), feelings of exclusion or isolation within their institutions, and a lack of mentors (Rodriguez et al., 2015; Williamson et al., 2021).

Although there are few studies of burnout specific to pediatric subspecialists, burnout has been documented in pediatric emergency medicine physicians (Gorelick et al., 2016; Gribben et al., 2019), pediatric hematology/oncology fellows (Moerdler et al., 2020), and pediatric nephrology fellows and faculty (Halbach et al., 2022). Only 43 percent of early career pediatricians (including subspecialists) reported having an appropriate work–life

---

[15] The webinar recording can be accessed at https://www.nationalacademies.org/event/07-19-2022/the-pediatric-subspecialty-workforce-and-its-impact-on-child-health-and-well-being-webinar-1.

balance and 30 percent reported feeling burned out (Starmer et al., 2016). Burnout among pediatric subspecialists results in feeling less compassionate, a perception of higher stress and lower quality of life, and lower job satisfaction (Gorelick et al., 2016; Gribben et al., 2019; Halbach et al., 2022; Moerdler et al., 2020). During the early stages of the COVID-19 pandemic, several factors were significant predictors of increased burnout levels among pediatric subspecialists, including high levels of compassion fatigue, self-care not being a priority, and emotional depletion (Kase et al., 2022).

Administrative demands and electronic health record (EHR) documentation requirements have grown over time and can contribute to burnout in primary care (Frintner et al., 2021b; Gardner et al., 2019). Three-quarters of general pediatricians report EHR documentation as a major or moderate burden (Frintner et al., 2021b). Overhage and Johnson (2020) found that the mean total active time for EHR users per patient encounter across all pediatric subspecialties was 16 minutes, with 12 percent of this time after-hours, and ranged across subspecialties, from 14.5 minutes (generalists) to 30.8 minutes (rheumatologists). Using the assumption that an average pediatrician might care for 25 patients per day, Overhage and Johnson (2020) estimated that pediatricians spend 6 hours and 40 minutes using their EHR per day. This is slightly more than the average of 5.9 hours found for family medicine physicians' EHR use per day (Arndt et al., 2017). This time-consuming documentation may contribute to pediatricians having or at least perceiving they have less time to address the needs of their patients.

Special Considerations for URiM

Discrimination in the workplace from co-workers, patients, families, and visitors has been documented among residents, practicing physicians, and faculty from URiM backgrounds (de Bourmont et al., 2020; Dyrbye et al., 2022; Filut et al., 2020; Lu et al., 2020; Nunez-Smith et al., 2009; Osseo-Asare et al., 2018; Serafini et al., 2020). Examples of discrimination include refusal of care by patients, racial epithets, and structural biases preventing advancement. However, the role of the work environment itself has not been extensively studied, particularly on how it may affect career trajectories, including burnout and retention. As noted by the American Medical Association (2021):

> Concerted efforts toward increasing physician workforce diversity require an understanding of the workplace conditions that racially minoritized physicians face…[h]owever, little research exists documenting the experience of minoritized and marginalized physicians and how their experiences of racism may drive burnout, reduce well-being, and impact the practice of medicine.

Limited studies specific to pediatrics show similar concerns and the need to promote a more inclusive work environment (Kemper et al., 2020; March et al., 2018; Nfonoyim et al., 2020; Whitgob et al., 2016). Strategies to improve retention rates of URiM pediatricians will require a range of actions, but examining the culture of equity and inclusion in the workplace is a critical first step.

KEY FINDINGS AND CONCLUSIONS

Key Findings

Finding #5-1: Many factors can influence an individual's choice to pursue subspecialty training, including:
- Exposure to the complete array of board-certified pediatric subspecialties and subspecialists (e.g., before medical school, during medical school, during residency);
- The presence of role models from subspecialty fields, particularly for URiM trainees (which may be scarce due to the small numbers of subspecialists);
- The length of fellowship training;
- The requirement for scholarly activity during fellowship;
- The debt burden of education and training;
- Relatively lower salaries, particularly for some pediatric medical subspecialties compared with general pediatricians in outpatient practice and adult medical subspecialists; and
- Lifestyle factors (e.g., work–life balance, job satisfaction, burnout).

Finding #5-2: ABP/ACGME requires that all pediatric subspecialty fellows participate in scholarly activity (see also Chapter 4).

Finding #5-3: While ABP provides a limited number of alternate, streamlined pathways for fellowship training, these pathways are primarily for trainees who are committed to careers in research. Similar pathways do not exist for trainees who are committed to careers in clinical practice.

Finding #5-4: There is no consensus among fellows, fellowship directors, and practicing subspecialists as to the optimal length of clinical and scholarly training in pediatric fellowship programs. Furthermore, there is a lack of evidence on the optimal duration and model of subspecialty training to prepare the subspecialty workforce to deliver high-quality care and to develop the foundational scientific evidence for that care.

Finding #5-5: Funding for pediatric residency programs may be derived from different sources, including Medicare, Medicaid, the CHGME program, and the THCGME program. However, more than half of pediatric training positions rely on CHGME funding.

Finding #5-6: The CHGME program was established to provide GME payments to freestanding children's hospitals that only received minimal payments under the rules of Medicare GME. By contrast with Medicare GME, CHGME requires annual discretionary funding, and the payment levels are limited by the level of annual appropriations. On average, CHGME payments are less than half of the Medicare GME payment rate.

Finding #5-7: A 2014 IOM Committee concluded that the Medicare GME program is outdated and discourages training needed for modern health care, and recommended major reforms in the statutory payment formulas, accountability, and governance. These have not been implemented.

Finding #5-8: Female physicians tend to have lower starting salaries and earning potential than male physicians, which further exacerbates the financial disincentives in pursuing pediatric subspecialty careers because an increasingly larger portion of pediatricians are women.

Finding #5-9: Medical students from URiM backgrounds have higher levels of educational debt on average than other students.

Finding #5-10: Pediatricians are among the lowest paid specialists, even among primary care specialties.

Finding #5-11: While the Pediatric Specialty Loan Repayment Program was authorized at $30 million per year, it has not yet been fully funded at this level.

Finding #5-12: There are few examples of evidence-based models to inform the recruitment and retention needs of URiM physicians, specifically in pediatrics and subspecialties.

Finding #5-13: Efforts to date have not been effective in significantly increasing representation of URiM subspecialists.

Finding #5-14: There is minimal understanding of the impact of the work environment on URiM burnout and retention.

Conclusions

Conclusion #5-1: The current model of education and training for pediatric medical subspecialists focuses on the creation of subspecialists who demonstrate competency in all aspects of academic careers, including clinical care, research, and education (see also Chapter 4).

Conclusion #5-2: Flexibility in fellowship design and length could encourage more residents to pursue pediatric subspecialty training. This flexibility could encourage trainees to pursue different types of careers in accordance with their interests (e.g., clinical focus, research focus, education focus).

Conclusion #5-3: As a result of lower salaries for some subspecialties and longer training, pediatric subspecialists (particularly subspecialists from URiM, and economically disadvantaged backgrounds) may face a higher debt burden, which can discourage pediatricians from careers in lower paid subspecialties.

Conclusion #5-4: Loan repayment programs may help overcome some financial disincentives to pursuing a career in a pediatric subspecialty.

Conclusion #5-5: While pediatric subspecialty training is largely supported by the discretionary CHGME program, the lower level of funding places a disproportionate financial burden on freestanding children's hospitals compared with Medicare GME hospitals. This may limit the expansion and training of pediatric subspecialties.

Conclusion #5-6: Federal GME funding does not come with requirements or accountability related to physician workforce needs, such as specialty or geographic distribution. The current structures of Medicare GME and CHGME are barriers to producing a robust pediatric subspecialty workforce.

Conclusion #5-7: The workforce needs to evolve to meet the demands of the 21st century child population in the United States, including enhancing the number of URiM clinicians in the pediatric subspecialty workforce in order to mirror the diversity of the children and families it serves.

Conclusion #5-8: Strategies to improve recruitment and retention rates of URiM students, residents, fellows, and faculty will require a range of actions, but understanding the culture of equity and inclusion in the workplace is a critical first step.

Conclusion #5-9: *Recruitment efforts to increase representation will need to begin earlier in academic pathways to increase the numbers of trainees overall.*

RECOMMENDATIONS

Attracting sufficient numbers of physicians in many of the pediatric medical subspecialties has been problematic, and a variety of mechanisms will be necessary to generate and maintain a diverse array of subspecialists, particularly for high-priority subspecialties. As noted in Chapter 2, the preparation of the pediatric specialty workforce needs to evolve to meet the demands of the twenty-first century population of infants, children, and adolescents in the United States. This means, first, that the workforce must be diverse to mirror the demographic make-up of the children and families it serves, and that it will require special attention for the recruitment and retention of a diverse set of trainees. The workforce also needs to be diverse in the type of physicians being produced. Academic medical centers cannot fulfill their missions of clinical care, education, and research without a workforce that is differentiated in skills and efforts in each of these three mission areas. Residency and fellowship training needs to reflect this reality and abandon the inflexible approach of applying a single training model for the vast majority of graduates. Finally, as is discussed further in Chapter 5, the financial realities of educational debt coupled with the relatively low salaries for many specialists and the time demands for subspecialty training require consideration for ways to remove financial disincentives to entering pediatric subspecialty careers. Specifically, mechanisms such as loan repayment are needed to reduce financial burdens on trainees, and the funding of GME needs to be reexamined and the disparities between CHGME and Medicare-funded GME eliminated to encourage physicians to enter pediatrics.

Therefore, to achieve goals of **enhancing education, training, recruitment, and retention** and **reducing financial and payment disincentives**, the committee provides the following recommendations:

RECOMMENDATION 5-1 ABP, the American Osteopathic Board of Pediatrics, and ACGME should develop, implement, and evaluate distinct fellowship training pathways, including a 2-year option for those who aspire to a career with a primary focus on clinical care.

The committee emphasizes that multiple novel pathways should be considered, and that a pathway focused on clinical training, for example, does not mean that the trainees will receive no academic training or experience in research or research principles. Rather, distinct training pathways would allow for tailoring of training programs for specific career goals, as already exists for the alternative pathways for research.

RECOMMENDATION 5-2 Congress should reform GME and CHGME formulas and programs to ensure equitable and sufficient support for pediatric GME. Funding should be distributed to address priority pediatric workforce needs such as increased inclusion of URiM clinicians, high-priority subspecialty and geographic shortages, and enhanced training for new models of care.

RECOMMENDATION 5-3 Pediatric department chairs, medical school deans, and health systems should develop, implement, and publicly report on plans and outcomes to attract, support, and retain students, residents, fellows, and faculty from URiM backgrounds in pediatric subspecialties.
- These plans should include efforts to further the development and growth of recruitment programs for pre-college URiM students and initiatives to make learning and working environments more inclusive at all levels of the subspecialist career pathway.
- The responsible individuals and entities above should publicly report annual metrics on the demographics of their pediatric subspecialty workforce.

RECOMMENDATION 5-4 Congress should increase funding for the Pediatric Specialty Loan Repayment Program to $30 million as originally authorized. HRSA should focus on loan repayment for high-priority pediatric medical subspecialties as well as subspecialists from URiM and/or economically disadvantaged backgrounds.

REFERENCES

AAMC (Association of American Medical Colleges). 2022a. *Report on residents. Table A1. Continuity of specialty preference on the Matriculating Student Questionnaire and the 2021 Graduation Questionnaire.* https://www.aamc.org/data-reports/students-residents/data/report-residents/2022/table-a1-continuity-specialty-preference-matriculating-student-questionnaire (accessed May 4, 2023).

AAMC. 2022b. *Report on residents. Table C4. Physician retention in state of residency training, by last completed GME specialty.* https://www.aamc.org/data-reports/students-residents/data/report-residents/2022/table-c4-physician-retention-state-residency-training-last-completed-gme (accessed May 4, 2023).

AAMC. 2022c. *Report on residents. Table C5. Physician retention in state of residency training, by last completed GME specialty and gender.* https://www.aamc.org/data-reports/students-residents/data/report-residents/2022/table-c5-physician-retention-state-residency-training-last-completed-gme (accessed May 4, 2023).

AAMC. 2022d. *Report on residents. Table B3. Number of active residents, by type of medical school, GME specialty, and gender.* https://www.aamc.org/data-reports/students-residents/data/report-residents/2022/table-b3-number-active-residents-type-medical-school-gme-specialty-and-gender (accessed May 4, 2023).

AAMC. 2023. *Medicaid graduate medical education payments: Results from the 2022 50-state survey.* https://store.aamc.org/medicaid-graduate-medical-education-payments-results-from-the-2022-50-state-survey.html (accessed July 14, 2023).

AAMC and AAP (American Academy of Pediatrics). 2022. *Percentage of graduating pediatric residents who report they would choose a categorical pediatric residency again.* https://downloads.aap.org/AAP/Images/Slide%208.jpg?_ga=2.117569099.315331748.1672250570-2052152754.1670872831 (accessed December 28, 2022).

ABIM (American Board of Internal Medicine). 2023a. *Policies & procedures for certification.* https://www.abim.org/Media/splbmcpe/policies-and-procedures.pdf (accessed June 22, 2023).

ABIM. 2023b. *Research pathway policies and requirements.* https://www.abim.org/certification/policies/research-pathway (accessed May 4, 2023).

ABP (American Board of Pediatrics). 2004. *Training requirements for subspecialty certification.* https://www.abp.org/sites/abp/files/trainingrequirements.pdf (accessed November 28, 2022).

ABP. 2014. *Subspecialty survey results.* https://www.abp.org/content/subspecialty-survey-results (accessed December 18, 2022).

ABP. 2020. *Pediatric hospital medicine certification.* https://www.abp.org/content/pediatric-hospital-medicine-certification (accessed November 28, 2022).

ABP. 2022a. *General ABP FAQs.* https://www.abp.org/content/general-abp-faqs (accessed November 28, 2022).

ABP. 2022b. *Subspecialty certifications and admission requirements.* https://www.abp.org/content/subspecialty-certifications-and-admission-requirements (accessed November 21, 2022).

ABP. 2022c. *General criteria for subspecialty certification.* https://www.abp.org/content/general-criteria-subspecialty-certification (accessed November 18, 2022).

ABP. 2022d. *Non-standard pathways.* https://www.abp.org/content/non-standard-pathways (accessed November 28, 2022).

ABP. 2022e. *Accelerated research pathway (ARP) details.* https://www.abp.org/content/accelerated-research-pathway-arp-details (accessed November 28, 2022).

ABP. 2022f. *Integrated research pathway (IRP).* https://www.abp.org/become-certified/subspecialty-certification/non-standard-pathways/integrated-research-pathway-irp (accessed November 28, 2022).

ABP. 2022g. *Subspecialty fast-tracking.* https://www.abp.org/content/subspecialty-fast-tracking (accessed November 28, 2022).

ABP. 2022h. *Dual subspecialty certification policy for development of training proposals.* https://www.abp.org/content/dual-subspecialty-certification-policy-development-training-proposals (accessed November 28, 2022).

ABP. 2023a. *Comparison of ABP data to the NRMP match data.* https://www.abp.org/content/comparison-abp-data-nrmp-match-data (accessed July 18, 2023).

ABP. 2023b. *Yearly growth in general pediatrics residents by demographics and program characteristics: Residents by demographics.* https://www.abp.org/dashboards/yearly-growth-general-pediatrics-residents-demographics-and-program-characteristics (accessed April 23, 2023).

ABP. 2023c. *Yearly growth in pediatric fellows by demographics and program characteristics: Home, key findings, and summary of all fellows.* https://www.abp.org/dashboards/yearly-growth-pediatric-fellows-subspecialty-demographics-and-program-characteristics (accessed April 24, 2023).

Acevedo, N. 2023. *DeSantis' anti-DEI law is sparking 'confusion, anxiety and fear' among Florida faculty.* https://www.nbcnews.com/news/latino/desantis-anti-dei-education-law-chilling-effect-florida-rcna85646 (accessed July 18, 2023).

Alsan, M., O. Garrick, and G. Graziani. 2019. Does diversity matter for health? Experimental evidence from Oakland. *American Economic Review* 109(12):4071-4111.

AMA (American Medical Association). 2021. *Summary report: Experiences of racially and ethnically minoritized and marginalized physicians in the U.S. during the COVID-19 pandemic.* https://www.ama-assn.org/system/files/summary-report-covid-mmps-survey.pdf (accessed May 10, 2023).

Amoli, M. A., J. M. Flynn, E. W. Edmonds, M. P. Glotzbecker, D. M. Kelly, and J. R. Sawyer. 2016. Gender differences in pediatric orthopaedics: What are the implications for the future workforce? *Clinical Orthopaedics and Related Research* 474(9):1973-1978.

AMSPDC (Association of Medical School Pediatric Department Chairs). 2023. *Pediatrics 2025: AMSPDC Workforce Initiative.* https://amspdc.org/workforce (accessed May 5, 2023).

Arndt, B. G., J. W. Beasley, M. D. Watkinson, J. L. Temte, W. Tuan, C. A. Sinsky, and V. J. Gilchrist. 2017. Tethered to the EHR: Primary care physician workload assessment using EHR event log data and time-motion observations. *Annals of Family Medicine* 15(5):419-426.

CAMPP (Consortium of Accelerated Medical Pathway Programs). 2023. *Consortium of accelerated medical pathway programs: Making medical education more efficient and less expensive.* https://www.acceleratedmdpathways.org/ (accessed March 14, 2023).

Cangiarella, J. 2021. *Three-year medical school programs are growing. Here's why.* https://www.aamc.org/news-insights/three-year-medical-school-programs-are-growing-here-s-why (accessed March 14, 2023).

Cangiarella, J., K. Eliasz, A. Kalet, E. Cohen, S. Abramson, and C. Gillespie. 2022. A preliminary evaluation of students' learning and performance outcomes in an accelerated 3-year MD pathway program. *Journal of Graduate Medical Education* 14(1):99-107.

Catenaccio, E., J. M. Rochlin, and H. K. Simon. 2021a. Differences in lifetime earning potential between pediatric and adult physicians. *Pediatrics* 148(2).

Catenaccio, E., J. M. Rochlin, and H. K. Simon. 2021b. Differences in lifetime earning potential for pediatric subspecialists. *Pediatrics* 147(4).

Catenaccio, E., J. M. Rochlin, and H. K. Simon. 2022. Addressing gender-based disparities in earning potential in academic medicine. *JAMA Network Open* 5(2):e220067.

CRS (Congressional Research Service). 2021. *Children's hospitals graduate medical education (CHGME): R45067.* https://crsreports.congress.gov/product/pdf/R/R45067/9 (accessed April 26, 2023).

CRS. 2022. *Medicare graduate medical education payments: An overview.* https://crsreports.congress.gov/product/pdf/IF/IF10960 (accessed July 14, 2023).

CRS. 2023. *Children's hospitals graduate medical education (CHGME): R45067.* https://sgp.fas.org/crs/misc/R45067.pdf (accessed July 20, 2023).

Cull, W. L., S. K. Katakam, A. J. Starmer, E. A. Gottschlich, A. A. Miller, and M. P. Frintner. 2017. A study of pediatricians' debt repayment a decade after completing residency. *Academic Medicine* 92(11):1595-1600.

Curran, F. C. 2023. *Proposed legislation threatens viewpoint diversity in higher education.* https://www.brookings.edu/articles/proposed-legislation-threatens-viewpoint-diversity-in-higher-education (accessed July 18, 2023).

de Bourmont, S. S., A. Burra, S. S. Nouri, N. El-Farra, D. Mohottige, C. Sloan, S. Schaeffer, J. Friedman, and A. Fernandez. 2020. Resident physician experiences with and responses to biased patients. *JAMA Open Network* 3(11):e2021769.

Diekroger, E. A., C. Reyes, K. M. Myers, H. Li, S. K. Kralovic, and N. Roizen. 2017. Perceived mentoring practices in developmental-behavioral pediatrics fellowship programs. *Journal of Developmental & Behavioral Pediatrics* 38(4):269-275.

Dixon, G., T. Kind, J. Wright, N. Stewart, A. Sims, and A. Barber. 2021. Factors that influence underrepresented in medicine (UIM) medical students to pursue a career in academic pediatrics. *Journal of the National Medical Association* 113(1):95-101.

Donnelly, L. F., J. M. Racadio, and J. L. Strife. 2007. Exposure of first-year medical students to a pediatric radiology research program: Is there an influence on career choice? *Pediatric Radiology* 37:876-878.

Dorsey, E. R., D. Jarjoura, and G. W. Rutecki. 2003. Influence of controllable lifestyle on recent trends in specialty choice by US medical students. *JAMA* 290(9):1173-1178.

Doximity and Curative. 2023. *2023 physician compensation report.* https://press.doximity.com/reports/doximity-physician-compensation-report-2023.pdf (accessed May 5, 2023).

Drees, B. M., and K. Omurtag. 2012. Accelerated medical education: Past, present and future. *Missouri Medicine* 109(5):352.

Dugger, R. A., A. M. El-Sayed, A. Dogra, C. Messina, R. Bronson, and S. Galea. 2013. The color of debt: Racial disparities in anticipated medical student debt in the United States. *PloS One* 8(9):e74693.

Dyrbye, L. N., C. P. West, C. A. Sinsky, M. Trockel, M. Tutty, D. Satele, L. Carlasare, and T. Shanafelt. 2022. Discrimination by patients, families, and visitors and association with burnout. *JAMA Network Open* 5(5):e2213080.

Enoch, L., J. T. Chibnall, D. L. Schindler, and S. J. Slavin. 2013. Association of medical student burnout with residency specialty choice. *Medical Education* 47(2):173-181.

Fagan, E. B., C. Gibbons, S. C. Finnegan, S. Petterson, L. E. Peterson, R. L. Phillips, and A. W. Bazemore. 2015. Family medicine graduate proximity to their site of training: Policy options for improving the distribution of primary care access. *Family Medicine* 47(2):124-130.

Feldman, M. D., P. A. Arean, S. J. Marshall, M. Lovett, and P. O'Sullivan. 2010. Does mentoring matter: Results from a survey of faculty mentees at a large health sciences university. *Medical Education Online* 15.

Filut, A., M. Alvarez, and M. Carnes. 2020. Discrimination toward physicians of color: A systematic review. *Journal of the National Medical Association* 112(2):117-140.

Fraher, E. P., J. C. Spero, and T. Bacon. 2017. *State-based approaches to reforming Medicaid-funded graduate medical education.* https://www.shepscenter.unc.edu/wp-content/uploads/2017/01/ExecSumm_FraherGME_y3_final-1.pdf (accessed November 28, 2022).

Freed, G. L., K. M. Dunham, M. D. Jones, G. A. McGuinness, and L. Althouse. 2009. General pediatrics resident perspectives on training decisions and career choice. *Pediatrics* 123(Suppl 1):S26-S30.

Freed, G. L., K. M. Dunham, L. M. Moran, L. Spera, G. A. McGuinness, and D. K. Stevenson, on behalf of the Research Advisory Committee of the American Board on Pediatrics. 2014a. Pediatric subspecialty fellowship clinical training project: Current fellows. *Pediatrics* 133(Suppl 2):S58-S63.

Freed, G. L., K. M. Dunham, L. M. Moran, L. Spera, G. A. McGuinness, and D. K. Stevenson. 2014b. Fellowship program directors perspectives on fellowship training. *Pediatrics* 133(Suppl 2):S64-S69.

Freed, G. L., K. M. Dunham, L. M. Moran, L. Spera, G. A. McGuinness, and D. K. Stevenson, on behalf of the Research Advisory Committee of the American Board on Pediatrics. 2014c. Pediatric subspecialty fellowship clinical training project: Recent graduates and midcareer survey comparison. *Pediatrics* 133(Suppl 2):S70-S75.

Freed, G. L., K. M. Dunham, L. M. Moran, L. Spera, G. A. McGuinness, and D. K. Stevenson, on behalf of the Research Advisory Committee of the American Board on Pediatrics. 2014d. Specialty specific comparisons regarding perspectives on fellowship training. *Pediatrics* 133(Suppl 2):S76-S77.

Freed, G. L., L. M. Moran, L. A. Althouse, K. D. Van, L. K. Leslie, and Research Advisory Committee of American Board of Pediatrics. 2016. Jobs and career plans of new pediatric subspecialists. *Pediatrics* 137(3).

Freed, G. L., L. M. Moran, K. D. Van, and L. K. Leslie. 2017. Current workforce of pediatric subspecialists in the United States. *Pediatrics* 139(5).

Frintner, M. P., B. Sisk, B. J. Byrne, G. L. Freed, A. J. Starmer, and L. M. Olson. 2019. Gender differences in earnings of early- and midcareer pediatricians. *Pediatrics* 144(4).

Frintner, M. P., C. Somberg, and H. Haftel. 2021a. *Factors that are priorities in pediatric subspecialty choice.* https://www.aap.org/en/research/pas-abstracts/factors-that-are-priorities-in-pediatric-subspecialty-choice (accessed March 28, 2023).

Frintner, M. P., D. C. Kaelber, E. S. Kirkendall, E. M. Lourie, C. A. Somberg, and C. U. Lehmann. 2021b. The effect of electronic health record burden on pediatricians' work-life balance and career satisfaction. *Applied Clinical Informatics Journal* 12(3):697-707.

Frintner, M. P., L. K. Leslie, E. A. Gottschlich, A. J. Starmer, and W. L. Cull. 2022. Changes in work characteristics and pediatrician satisfaction: 2012–2020. *Pediatrics* 150(1).

Frugé, E., J. Margolin, T. Horton, L. Venkateswaran, D. Lee, D. L. Yee, and D. Mahoney. 2010. Defining and managing career challenges for mid-career and senior stage pediatric hematologist/oncologists. *Pediatric Blood & Cancer* 55(6):1180-1184.

FSMB (Federation of State Medical Boards). 2018. *State specific requirements for initial medical licensure.* https://www.fsmb.org/step-3/state-licensure (accessed November 28, 2022).

Fuentes-Afflick, E., S. A. Shipman, B. Dreyer, J. M. Perrin, and G. L. Freed. 2022. Engaging pediatricians to address workforce diversity. *Pediatric Research* https://doi.org/10.1038/s41390-022-02355-7. Epub ahead of print.

GAO (U.S. Government Accountability Office). 2018. *Physician workforce: HHS needs better information to comprehensively evaluate graduate medical education funding.* Washington, DC: U.S. Government Accountability Office.

GAO. 2021a. *Graduate medical education: Programs and residents increased during transition to single accreditor; distribution largely unchanged.* Washington, DC: U.S. Government Accountability Office.

GAO. 2021b. *Physician workforce: Caps on Medicare-funded graduate medical education at teaching hospitals.* Washington, DC: U.S. Government Accountability Office.

Gardner, R. L., E. Cooper, J. Haskell, D. A. Harris, S. Poplau, P. J. Kroth, and M. Linzer. 2019. Physician stress and burnout: The impact of health information technology. *Journal of the American Medical Informatics Association* 26(2):106-114.

Goodfellow, A., J. G. Ulloa, P. T. Dowling, E. Talamantes, S. Chheda, C. Bone, and G. Moreno. 2016. Predictors of primary care physician practice location in underserved urban or rural areas in the United States: A systematic literature review. *Academic Medicine* 91(9):1313-1321.

Gorelick, M. H., R. Schremmer, H. Ruch-Ross, C. Radabaugh, and S. Selbst. 2016. Current workforce characteristics and burnout in pediatric emergency medicine. *Academic Emergency Medicine* 23(1):48-54.

Gribben, J. L., S. A. MacLean, T. Pour, E. D. Waldman, and A. S. Weintraub. 2019. A cross-sectional analysis of compassion fatigue, burnout, and compassion satisfaction in pediatric emergency medicine physicians in the United States. *Academic Emergency Medicine* 26(7):732-743.

Guiot, A. B., R. C. Baker, and T. G. Dewitt. 2013. When and how pediatric history and physical diagnosis are taught in medical school: A survey of pediatric clerkship directors. *Hospital Pediatrics* 3(2):139-143.

Haftel, H. M., C. M. Somberg, and M. P. M. Frintner. 2020. 81. Factors that are priorities in pediatric subspecialty choice. *Academic Pediatrics* 20(7):e38-e39.

Halbach, S. M., K. Pillutla, P. Seo-Mayer, A. Schwartz, D. Weidemann, and J. D. Mahan. 2022. Burnout in pediatric nephrology fellows and faculty: Lessons from the sustainable pediatric nephrology workforce project (superpower). *Frontiers in Pediatrics* 10:488.

Harris, M. C., J. Marx, P. R. Gallagher, and S. Ludwig. 2005. General vs subspecialty pediatrics: Factors leading to residents' career decisions over a 12-year period. *Archives of Pediatrics and Adolescent Medicine* 159(3):212-216.

Hauer, K. E., S. J. Durning, W. N. Kernan, M. J. Fagan, M. Mintz, P. S. O'Sullivan, M. Battistone, T. DeFer, M. Elnicki, H. Harrell, S. Reddy, C. K. Boscardin, and M. D. Schwartz. 2008. Factors associated with medical students' career choices regarding internal medicine. *JAMA* 300(10):1154-1164.

HHS (U.S. Department of Health and Human Services). 2009. *Pipeline programs to improve racial and ethnic diversity in the health professions: An inventory of federal programs, assessment of evaluation approaches, and critical review of the research literature.* https://aapcho.org/wp/wp-content/uploads/2012/11/PipelineToImproveDiversityInHealthProfessions.pdf (accessed November 28, 2022).

Hoff, M. L., N. N. Liao, C. A. Mosquera, A. Saucedo, R. G. Wallihan, J. R. Walton, R. Scherzer, E. M. Bonachea, L. W. Wise, O. W. Thomas, J. D. Mahan, J. A. Barnard, and O. N. R. Bignall, II. 2021. An initiative to increase residency program diversity. *Pediatrics* 149(1).

HRSA (Health Resources and Services Administration). 2021. *NHSC loan repayment programs: One application, three programs.* https://nhsc.hrsa.gov/loan-repayment/nhsc-all-loan-repayment-programs-comparison (accessed March 15, 2023).

HRSA. 2022a. *Fiscal year 2023. Justification of estimates for appropriations committees.* https://www.hrsa.gov/sites/default/files/hrsa/about/budget/budget-justification-fy2023.pdf (accessed November 28, 2022).

HRSA. 2022b. *View grant opportunity: HRSA-23-012 Children's hospitals graduate medical education (CHGME) payment program: Related documents: Full announcement.* https://www.grants.gov/web/grants/view-opportunity.html?oppId=341227 (accessed July 13, 2023).

HRSA. 2022c. *Teaching health center graduate medical education (THCGME) academic year 2022–2023 awardees.* https://bhw.hrsa.gov/funding/apply-grant/teaching-health-center-graduate-medical-education/ay2022-2023-awardees (accessed July 14, 2023).

HRSA. 2023a. *Children's Hospital Graduate Medical Education Program.* https://bhw.hrsa.gov/sites/default/files/bureau-health-workforce/data-research/childrens-hospital-graduate-medical-education-annual-report-2021-2022.pdf (accessed May 4, 2023).

HRSA. 2023b. *Bureau of Health Workforce field strength and students and trainees dashboards.* https://data.hrsa.gov/topics/health-workforce/field-strength (accessed May 5, 2023).

HRSA. 2023c. *FY 2023 operating plan.* https://www.hrsa.gov/about/budget/operating-plan (accessed March 15, 2023).

HRSA. 2023d. *Pediatric specialty loan repayment program: Full-time service opportunities: Fiscal year 2023 application & program guidance. June 2023.* https://bhw.hrsa.gov/sites/default/files/bureau-health-workforce/funding/pediatric-specialty-lrp-application-guidance.pdf (accessed July 13, 2023).

HRSA. 2023e. *FY 2023 operating plan.* https://www.hrsa.gov/about/budget/operating-plan (accessed July 13, 2023).

IOM (Institute of Medicine). 2014. *Graduate medical education that meets the nation's health needs.* Washington, DC: The National Academies Press.

IWPR (Institute for Women's Policy Research). 2021. *The gender wage gap by occupation, race, and ethnicity, 2020.* https://iwpr.org/wp-content/uploads/2021/03/2021-Occupational-Wage-Gap-Brief-v2.pdf (accessed December 28, 2022).

Kane, L. 2022. *Medscape physician compensation report 2022: Income gain, pay gaps remain.* https://www.medscape.com/sites/public/physician-comp/2022 (accessed March 15, 2023).

Kase, S. M., J. L. Gribben, K. F. Guttmann, E. D. Waldman, and A. S. Weintraub. 2022. Compassion fatigue, burnout, and compassion satisfaction in pediatric subspecialists during the SARS-CoV-2 pandemic. *Pediatric Research* 91(1):143-148.

Keating, E. M., E. P. O'Donnell, and S. R. Starr. 2013. How we created a peer-designed specialty-specific selective for medical student career exploration. *Medical Teacher* 35(2):91-94.

Kemper, K. J., A. Schwartz, and the Pediatric Resident Burnout-Resilience Study Consortium. 2020. Bullying, discrimination, sexual harassment, and physical violence: Common and associated with burnout in pediatric residents. *Academic Pediatrics* 20(7):991-997.

Kistemaker, R., and K. Montez. 2022. Early specialization in medical education—a pathway to mitigate the growing physician deficit. *JAMA Pediatrics* 177(2):109-110.

Kumar, G., and A. Mezoff. 2020. Physician burnout at a children's hospital: Incidence, interventions, and impact. *Pediatric Quality and Safety* 5(5):e345.

Kumar, S., A. P. Ashraf, A. Lteif, J. Lynch, and T. Aye. 2021. Pediatric endocrinology: Perspectives of pediatric endocrinologists regarding career choice and recruitment of trainees. *Endocrine Practice* 27(7):743-748.

Laitman, B. M., A. Malbari, S. Friedman, S. Moerdler, S. Kase, and K. Gibbs. 2019. Preseason pediatrics: An interactive preclinical curriculum enhances knowledge and skills in medical students. *Medical Science Educator* 29(1):233-239.

Lauer, M. 2019. *Outcomes for NIH loan repayment program awardees: A preliminary look.* https://nexus.od.nih.gov/all/2019/05/21/outcomes-for-nih-loan-repayment-program-awardees-a-preliminary-look (accessed July 13, 2023).

LCME (Liaison Committee on Medical Education). 2023. *Functions and structure of a medical school: Standards for accreditation of medical education programs leading to the M.D. degree.* www.lcme.org/publications (accessed March 14, 2023).

Leong, S. L., C. Gillespie, B. Jones, T. Fancher, C. L. Coe, L. Dodson, M. Hunsaker, B. M. Thompson, A. Dempsey, R. Pallay, W. Crump, and J. Cangiarella. 2022. Accelerated 3-year MD pathway programs: Graduates' perspectives on education quality, the learning environment, residency readiness, debt, burnout, and career plans. *Academic Medicine* 97(2):254-261.

Levaillant, M., L. Levaillant, N. Lerolle, B. Vallet, and J.-F. Hamel-Broza. 2020. Factors influencing medical students' choice of specialization: A gender based systematic review. *eClinicalMedicine* 28:100589.

Levanon, A., P. England, and P. Allison. 2009. Occupational feminization and pay: Assessing causal dynamics using 1950–2000 U.S. Census data. *Social Forces* 88(2):865-891.

Lewin Group, Inc. 2016. *National Health Service Corps—an extended analysis.* https://aspe.hhs.gov/sites/default/files/private/pdf/255496/NHSCanalysis.pdf (accessed November 28, 2022).

Lindgren, A. M., and S. A. Shah. 2023. How to recruit and train diverse pediatric orthopaedic surgeons. *Journal of the Pediatric Orthopaedic Society of North America* 5(S1):Special Edition—February 15.

Lopez, K. N., and E. Fuentes-Afflick. 2022. Engaging pediatric subspecialists in pursuit of health equity—breaking out of the silo. *JAMA Pediatrics* 176(9):841-842.

Lopez, M. A., and J. L. Raphael. 2021. Increasing diversity in pediatric hospital medicine: An enduring priority for a young subspecialty. *Hospital Pediatrics* 11(8):e161-e163.

Lu, D. W., A. Pierce, J. Jauregui, S. Heron, M. D. Lall, J. Mitzman, D. M. McCarthy, N. D. Hartman, and T. D. Strout. 2020. Academic emergency medicine faculty experiences with racial and sexual orientation discrimination. *Western Journal of Emergency Medicine* 21(5):1160-1169.

Mabeza, R. M., B. Christophers, S. A. Ederaine, E. J. Glenn, Z. P. Benton-Slocum, and J. R. Marcelin. 2023. Interventions associated with racial and ethnic diversity in US graduate medical education. *JAMA Network Open* 6(1):e2249335.

Macy, M. L., L. K. Leslie, D. Boyer, K. D. Van, and G. L. Freed. 2018. Timing and stability of fellowship choices during pediatric residency: A longitudinal survey. *Journal of Pediatrics* 198:294-300.e291.

Macy, M. L., L. K. Leslie, A. Turner, and G. L. Freed. 2021. Growth and changes in the pediatric medical subspecialty workforce pipeline. *Pediatric Research* 89(5):1297-1303.

March, C., L. W. Walker, R. L. Toto, S. Choi, E. C. Reis, and S. Dewar. 2018. Experiential communications curriculum to improve resident preparedness when responding to discriminatory comments in the workplace. *Journal of Graduate Medical Education* 10(3):306-310.

Marrast, L. M., L. Zallman, S. Woolhandler, D. H. Bor, and D. McCormick. 2014. Minority physicians' role in the care of underserved patients: Diversifying the physician workforce may be key in addressing health disparities. *JAMA Internal Medicine* 174(2):289-291.

McDonough, J. E. 2021. *Old wine in a new bottle—time for a national health care workforce commission.* https://www.milbank.org/quarterly/opinions/old-wine-in-a-new-bottle-time-for-a-national-health-care-workforce-commission (accessed March 15, 2023).

MedPAC (Medicare Payment Advisory Committee). 2010. *June 2010 report to Congress: Aligning incentives in Medicare.* Washington, DC: Medicare Payment Advisory Commission.

Moerdler, S., Y. Li, S. Weng, and J. Kesselheim. 2020. Burnout in pediatric hematology oncology fellows: Results of a cross-sectional survey. *Pediatric Blood & Cancer* 67(11):e28274.

Morris, C. G., B. Johnson, S. Kim, and F. Chen. 2008. Training family physicians in community health centers: A health workforce solution. *Family Medicine* 40(4):271-276.

Mullan, F. 2005. The metrics of the physician brain drain. *New England Journal of Medicine* 353(17):1810-1818.

NASEM (National Academies of Sciences, Engineering, and Medicine). 2019a. *The science of effective mentorship in STEMM.* Washington, DC: The National Academies Press.

NASEM. 2019b. *Taking action against clinician burnout: A systems approach to professional well-being.* Washington, DC: The National Academies Press.

Nelson, B. A., J. A. Rama, P. Weiss, and L. J. Hinkle. 2020. How and why trainees choose a career in pediatric pulmonology. A qualitative study. *ATS Scholar* 1(4):372-383.

Newton, D. A., M. S. Grayson, and L. F. Thompson. 2005. The variable influence of lifestyle and income on medical students' career specialty choices: Data from two U.S. medical schools, 1998–2004. *Academic Medicine* 80(9):809-814.

Nfonoyim, B., A. Martin, A. Ellison, J. L. Wright, and T. J. Johnson. 2020. Experiences of underrepresented faculty in pediatric emergency medicine. *Academic Emergency Medicine* https://doi.org/10.1111/acem.14191.

NIH (National Institutes of Health). 2022a. *Extramural loan repayment program for pediatric research (LRP-PR).* https://grants.nih.gov/grants/guide/notice-files/NOT-OD-22-149.html (accessed May 7, 2023).

NIH. 2022b. *Summer internships in biomedical research for high school students.* https://www.training.nih.gov/programs/hs-sip (accessed November 28, 2022).

NIH. 2023. *LRP dashboard.* https://dashboard.lrp.nih.gov/app/#/ (accessed May 7, 2023).

NRMP (National Resident Matching Program). 2022. *Results and data: Specialties Matching Service: 2023 appointment year.* https://www.nrmp.org/wp-content/uploads/2022/03/2022-SMS-Results-Data-FINAL.pdf (accessed July 18, 2023).

Nunez-Smith, M., N. Pilgrim, M. Wynia, M. M. Desai, B. A. Jones, C. Bright, H. M. Krumholz, and E. H. Bradley. 2009. Race/ethnicity and workplace discrimination: Results of a national survey of physicians. *Journal of General Internal Medicine* 24:1198-1204.

Orr, C. J., A. L. Turner, V. S. Ritter, J. Gutierrez-Wu, and L. K. Leslie. 2023. Pursuing a career in pediatrics: Intersection of educational debt and race/ethnicity. *Journal of Pediatrics* 252:162-170.

Osseo-Asare, A. L. Balasuriya, S. J. Huot, D. Keene, D. Berg, M. Nunez-Smith, I. Genao, D. Latimore, and D. Boatright. 2018. Minority resident physicians' views on the role of race-ethnicity in their training experiences in the workplace. *JAMA Network Open* 1(5):e182723.

Overhage, J. M., and K. B. Johnson. 2020. Pediatrician electronic health record time use for outpatient encounters. *Pediatrics* 146(6).

Patel, S. J., J. Lynn, S. Varghese, R. D. Sanders, E. Zwemer, E. B. Seelbach, K. P. Patra, D. R. Mirchandani, E. Griego, and J. Beck. 2021. Preparing for a career in pediatric hospital medicine: A needs assessment and recommendations for individualized curricula. *Hospital Pediatrics* 12(1):e30-e37.

Pelley, E., 2020. When a specialty becomes "women's work": Trends in and implications of specialty gender segregation in medicine. *Academic Medicine* 95(10):1499-1506.

Petersen, T. L., J. C. King, J. J. Fussell, H. A. Gans, L. A. Waggoner-Fountain, D. Castro, M. L. Green, M. F. Hamilton, K. Marcdante, R. Mink, K. R. Nielsen, D. A. Turner, C. M. Watson, A. D. Zurca, and D. L. Boyer. 2022. Benefits and limitations of virtual recruitment: Perspectives from subspeciality directors. *Pediatrics* 150(4).

Pfarrwaller, E., J. Sommer, C. Chung, H. Maisonneuve, M. Nendaz, N. Junod Perron, and D. M. Haller. 2015. Impact of interventions to increase the proportion of medical students choosing a primary care career: A systematic review. *Journal of General Internal Medicine* 30(9):1349-1358.

Pfarrwaller, E., M.-C. Audétat, J. Sommer, H. Maisonneuve, T. Bischoff, M. Nendaz, A. Baroffio, N. Junod Perron, and D. M. Haller. 2017. An expanded conceptual framework of medical students' primary care career choice. *Academic Medicine* 92(11):1536-1542.

Phillips, J. P., S. M. Petterson, A. W. Bazemore, and R. L. Phillips. 2014. A retrospective analysis of the relationship between medical student debt and primary care practice in the United States. *Annals of Family Medicine* 12(6):542-549.

Phillips, R. L., S. Petterson, and A. Bazemore. 2013. Do residents who train in safety net settings return for practice? *Academic Medicine* 88(12):1934-1940.

Powell, W. T., K. M. W. Dundon, M. P. Frintner, K. Kornfeind, and H. M. Haftel. 2021. Parenthood, parental benefits, and career goals among pediatric residents: 2008 and 2019. *Pediatrics* 148(6).

Quigley, L. 2022. Whom do incentive program physicians serve? New measures for assessing program reach. *Journal of Ambulatory Care Management* 45(4):266-278.

Rao, R. D., O. N. Khatib, and A. Agarwal. 2017. Factors motivating medical students in selecting a career specialty: Relevance for a robust orthopaedic pipeline. *Journal of the American Academy of Orthopaedic Surgeons* 25(7):527-535.

Reddy, S., and V. Olivares. 2023. *Texas faculty, students worry about how dropping DEI policies will impact universities.* dallasnews.com/news/education/2023/03/23/texas-faculty-students-worry-about-how-dropping-dei-policies-will-impact-universities (accessed July 18, 2023).

Rochlin, J. M., and H. K. Simon. 2011. Does fellowship pay: What is the long-term financial impact of subspecialty training in pediatrics? *Pediatrics* 127(2):254-260.

Rodriguez, J. E., K. M. Campbell, and L. H. Pololi. 2015. Addressing disparities in academic medicine: What of the minority tax? *BMC Medical Education* 15(6). doi.org/10.1186/s12909-015-0290-9.

Rogo, T., S. Holland, M. Fassiotto, Y. Maldonado, T. Joseph, O. Ramilo, K. Byrd, and S. Delair. 2022. Strategies to increase workforce diversity in pediatric infectious diseases. *Journal of the Pediatric Infectious Diseases Society* 11(Suppl 4):S148-S154.

Russell, D. J., E. Wilkinson, S. Petterson, C. Chen, and A. Bazemore. 2022. Family medicine residencies: How rural training exposure in GME is associated with subsequent rural practice. *Journal of Graduate Medical Education* 14(4):441-450.

Saba, T. G., M. B. Hershenson, M. Arteta, I. A. Ramirez, P. B. Mullan, and S. T. Owens. 2015. Pre-clinical medical student experience in a pediatric pulmonary clinic. *Medical Education Online* 20:28654.

Saha, S., G. Guiton, P. F. Wimmers, and L. Wilkerson. 2008. Student body racial and ethnic composition and diversity-related outcomes in US medical schools. *JAMA* 300(10):1135-1145.

Salsberg, E., P. H. Rockey, K. L. Rivers, S. E. Brotherton, and G. R. Jackson. 2008. US residency training before and after the 1997 Balanced Budget Act. *JAMA* 300(10):1174-1180.

Scheurer, D., S. McKean, J. Miller, and T. Wetterneck. 2009. U.S. physician satisfaction: A systematic review. *Journal of Hospital Medicine* 4(9):560-568.

Seifer, S. D., K. Vranizan, and K. Grumbach. 1995. Graduate medical education and physician practice location: Implications for physician workforce policy. *JAMA* 274(9):685-691.

Serafini, K., C. Coyer, J. Brown Speights, D. Donova, J. Guh, J. Washington, and C. Ainsworth. 2020. Racism as experienced by physicians of color in the health care setting. *Family Medicine* 52(4):282-287.

Shen, M. J., E. B. Peterson, R. Costas-Muñiz, M. H. Hernandez, S. T. Jewell, K. Matsoukas, and C. L. Bylund. 2018. The effects of race and racial concordance on patient-physician communication: A systematic review of the literature. *Journal of Racial and Ethnic Health Disparities* 5(1):117-140.

Sozio, S. M., K. A. Pivert, H. H. Shah, H. A. Chakkera, A. R. Asmar, M. R. Varma, B. D. Morrow, A. B. Patel, K. Leight, and M. G. Parker. 2019. Increasing medical student interest in nephrology. *American Journal of Nephrology* 50(1):4-10.

Starmer, A. J., M. P. Frintner, and G. L. Freed. 2016. Work–life balance, burnout, and satisfaction of early career pediatricians. *Pediatrics* 137(4).

Starmer, A. J., M. P. Frintner, K. Matos, C. Somberg, G. Freed, and B. J. Byrne. 2019. Gender discrepancies related to pediatrician work-life balance and household responsibilities. *Pediatrics* 144(4).

Stevenson, D. K., G. A. McGuinness, J. D. Bancroft, D. M. Boyer, A. R. Cohen, J. T. Gilhooly, M. F. Hazinski, E. S. Holmboe, M. D. Jones, Jr, M. L. Land, Jr, S. S. Long, V. F. Norwood, D. J. Schumacher, T. C. Sectish, J. W. St Geme, III, and D. C. West. 2014. The initiative on subspecialty clinical training and certification (SCTC): Background and recommendations. *Pediatrics* 133(Suppl 2):S53-S57.

TAGGS (Tracking Accountability in Government Grants System). 2022. *Health professions recruitment program for Indians.* https://taggs.hhs.gov/Detail/CFDADetail?arg_CFDA_NUM=93970 (accessed November 28, 2022).

Tankwanchi, A. B. S., Ç. Özden, and S. H. Vermund. 2013. Physician emigration from sub-Saharan Africa to the United States: Analysis of the 2011 AMA physician masterfile. *PLoS Medicine* 10(9).

Toretsky, C., S. Mutha, and J. Coffman. 2018. *Breaking barriers for underrepresented minorities in the health professions.* University of California San Francisco: Healthforce Center.

Toretsky, C., S. Mutha, and J. Coffman. 2019. *Reducing educational debt among underrepresented physicians and dentists.* University of California San Francisco: Healthforce Center.

Tsai, K., C. Long, T. Z. Liang, J. Napolitano, R. Khawaja, and A. M. Leung. 2022. Driving factors to pursue endocrinology training fellowship: Empirical survey data and future strategies. *Journal of Clinical Endocrinology and Metabolism* 107(6):e2459-e2463.

Umoren, R. A., and M. P. Frintner. 2014. Do mentors matter in graduating pediatrics residents' career choices? *Academic Pediatrics* 14(4):348-352.

van Ryn, M., R. Hardeman, S. M. Phelan, D. J. Burgess, J. F. Dovidio, J. Herrin, S. E. Burke, D. B. Nelson, S. Perry, M. Yeazel, and J. M. Przedworski. 2015. Medical school experiences associated with change in implicit racial bias among 3547 students: A medical student changes study report. *Journal of General Internal Medicine* 30(12):1748-1756.

Vinci, R. J., L. Degnon, and S. U. Devaskar. 2021. Pediatrics 2025: The AMSPDC workforce initiative. *Journal of Pediatrics* 237:5-8.e1.

Weinstein, A. R., K. Reidy, V. F. Norwood, and J. D. Mahan. 2010. Factors influencing pediatric nephrology trainee entry into the workforce. *Clinical Journal of the American Society of Nephrology* 5(10):1770-1774.

Weyand, A. C., D. G. Nichols, and G. L. Freed. 2020. Current efforts in diversity for pediatric subspecialty fellows: Playing a zero-sum game. *Pediatrics* 146(5).

Whitgob, E. E., R. L. Blankenburg, and A. L. Bogetz. 2016. The discriminatory patient and family: Strategies to address discrimination towards trainees. *Academic Medicine* 91(11):S64-S69

Wiley, J. F., II, S. Fuchs, S. E. Brotherton, G. Burke, W. L. Cull, J. Friday, H. Simon, E. A. Jewett, and H. Mulvey. 2002. A comparison of pediatric emergency medicine and general emergency medicine physicians' practice patterns: Results from the Future of Pediatric Education II Survey of Sections project. *Pediatric Emergency Care* 18(3):153-158.

Williamson, T., C. R. Goodwin, and P. A. Ubel. 2021. Minority tax reform—Avoiding overtaxing minorities when we need them most. *New England Journal of Medicine* 384:1877-1879.

Women Chairs of the Association of Medical School Pediatric Department Chairs. 2007. Women in pediatrics: Recommendations for the future. *Pediatrics* 119(5):1000-1005.

Yang, Y., J. Li, X. Wu, J. Wang, W. Li, Y. Zhu, C. Chen, and H. Lin. 2019. Factors influencing subspecialty choice among medical students: A systematic review and meta-analysis. *BMJ Open* 9(3):e022097.

Youngclaus, J., and J. A. Fresne. 2020. *Physician education debt and the cost to attend medical school: 2020 update*. Washington, DC: Association of American Medical Colleges.

Zhao, C., P. Dowzicky, L. Colbert, S. Roberts, and R. R. Kelz. 2019. Race, gender, and language concordance in the care of surgical patients: A systematic review. *Surgery (United States)* 166(5):785-792.

6

Trends in the Pediatric Physician–Scientist Workforce

Pediatric subspecialty physicians play a critical role in pursuing the research that leads to advances in child health. The robustness and endurance of the pediatric physician–scientist workforce pathway can have long-lasting effects on child and adolescent health through research to prevent, diagnose, and treat diseases that occur specifically in children or begin in childhood and affect the life course. As a result, advances in pediatric research have improved the lives of both children and adults. This chapter summarizes the pediatric research landscape in general, including examples of previous successes and unique challenges inherent to pediatric research. The chapter then delves into factors and barriers that affect the pediatric physician–scientist pathway and impact the ability of the physician subspecialty workforce to pursue a robust research portfolio that advances the care of all children and youth. There is limited available information specific to pediatric subspecialists, so much of this chapter is on the overall pediatric research workforce while considering the implications for research by physician–scientists in the pediatric medical subspecialties specifically. The challenges faced by the pediatric physician–scientist workforce are further compounded given the smaller numbers of pediatric subspecialists. Additionally, while other clinician scientists[1] and non-clinician scientists (i.e., Ph.D. scientists who study pediatric subspecialty conditions and treatments) are discussed as relevant, the focus of this chapter is on the pediatric physician–scientist workforce.

---

[1] For more information on the National Pediatric Nurse Scientists Collaborative, see https://npnsc.org/ (accessed May 3, 2023).

THE IMPORTANCE OF PEDIATRIC RESEARCH

In 1979, James B. Wyngaarden described "The Clinical Investigator as an Endangered Species" in his presidential address to the Association of American Physicians (Wyngaarden, 1979). Since then, discussions have continued about the plight of the physician–scientist, including pediatric physician–scientists specifically (Alvira et al., 2018; Daye et al., 2015; Milewicz et al., 2015; Rubenstein and Kreindler, 2014; Salata et al., 2018; Schafer, 2010; Zemlo et al., 2000). The scope of the pediatric research enterprise is transdisciplinary and has broadened to include the full spectrum of basic science, translational, community-based, population health, health services, health equity, and child health policy research (AAMC, 2023a; COPR, 2014; Williams et al., 2022). Furthermore, the development, recruitment, and retention of pediatric physician–scientists is critical to accelerate advances in wide-ranging fields such as molecular biology, genetics, genomics, precision medicine, health care delivery, health services research, and injury prevention (Alvira et al., 2018).

Pediatric Research Successes

Improving children's health is essential to developing a productive and healthy population (NRC and IOM, 2004), and research is the foundation of evidence-based innovation in pediatric care. Recent developments in research and clinical care include the increasing application of genome sequencing to diagnosis, clinical monitoring, and treatment; progress in developing cell therapy for cancers that are resistant to treatment; advances in developing gene therapy for a growing number of single gene disorders; targeted research on surfactant therapies for pediatric and neonatal acute respiratory distress syndrome; immunotherapeutic modalities for the treatment of pediatric malignancies; and a clearer understanding of the relationship between the microbiome and specific diseases (Baruteau et al., 2017; Bick et al., 2019; De Luca et al., 2021; Gilbert et al., 2018; Holstein and Lunning, 2020; Hutzen et al., 2019; Janssens et al., 2018). Some examples of notable pediatric scientific achievements are listed in Box 6-1.

Success stories serve as testimony to the transformative impact of scientific discovery on clinical care, but such discoveries require ongoing efforts and partnerships among medical schools, hospitals, payers, advocates, clinicians, and researchers to address rising challenges and to optimize access of therapeutics to children as early as possible. Boxes 6-2 and 6-3 highlight two specific case studies of pediatric research success: spinal muscular atrophy (SMA) and the Children's Oncology Group (COG). Challenges and controversy have unfolded as health systems navigate this era of precision health in pediatric disease, including access, handling, and delivery of

> **BOX 6-1**
> **Selected Examples of Notable Pediatric Scientific Achievement**
>
> - Eradication of invasive Haemophilus influenzae type B (Hib) infection, once the leading cause of mortality and acquired intellectual disability, due to the development of the Hib vaccine (NICHD, 2017b);
> - Elimination of phenylketonuria, congenital hypothyroidism, and other disorders that once caused intellectual disabilities through the development and implementation of widespread newborn screening and therapies (NICHD, 2017a, 2017c);
> - Reduced risk of sudden infant death with the *Back to Sleep* and *Safe to Sleep* public education campaigns (NICHD, 2017d, 2022e; Trachtenberg et al., 2012);
> - Improved survival rates for childhood acute lymphoblastic leukemia to 90 percent through clinical trials for combination chemotherapies (Hunger et al., 2012);
> - Improved life expectancy and quality of life for children with cystic fibrosis and sickle cell disease due to screening panels, effective medications, preventative care, and standardized medical management (CFF, 2022; SCDAA, 2021); and
> - Decreased risk of transmission of HIV from mother to infant (to less than 1 percent) in the United States due to antiretroviral therapy, universal HIV testing for pregnant women, avoidance of breastfeeding, and scheduled cesarean delivery in mothers at high risk of HIV transmission (Branson et al., 2006; CDC, 2022; Cheng et al., 2016; Lampe et al., 2023).

these drugs, particularly in the context of their high cost (zolgensma, used to treat SMA, costs $2.1 million per dose). These precision health opportunities also have motivated expansion of the newborn screening program and development of scalable assays to accelerate timely diagnosis of these now-curable conditions.

There has also been advancement in research, evaluation, and measurement infrastructure for child health services research, such as the increased representation of children in the National Patient-Centered Clinical Research Network (PCORnet) (Forrest et al., 2021) and the establishment of the National Cancer Institute Childhood Cancer Data Initiative (NCI, 2023a). Other examples of success can be seen in the substantial advancements in the care of prematurely born infants. Use of intrapulmonary surfactant and improvements in ventilation strategies, external environment

BOX 6-2
Pediatric Research Success Case Study: SMA

Spinal muscular atrophy (SMA), a once-fatal pediatric condition, is a group of genetic conditions that cause motor neuron loss in the spinal cord and brainstem. Historically SMA was the leading genetic cause of infant death in the first few years of life because of weakness in respiratory muscles (Farrar and Kiernan, 2015; Tisdale and Pellizzoni, 2015). Extensive preclinical research with cellular and animal models focused on understanding and then modulating the survival motor neuron (SMN) gene mutation, which led to the development of an antisense oligonucleotide (ASO) that promotes increased production of SMN. The ASO trial showed that treated infants were reaching unprecedented motor milestones (Finkel et al., 2017), and through rapid U.S. Food and Drug Administration (FDA) designation, the drug nusinersin was approved in 2016. ASO treatment requires continued intrathecal injections, which are both invasive and labor intensive. Therefore, in parallel, a gene replacement therapy was developed and results from a phase 2 safety trial demonstrated both treatment safety and efficacy in improving motor function in infants with SMA (Mendell et al., 2017). In 2019, FDA approved the gene therapy zolgensma, which requires only a single administration (FDA, 2019a). SMA is now considered a chronic illness that requires specialty care and monitoring, but with close to normal quality of life for children and adults. More than 11,000 patients have been treated with nusinersin worldwide (Jedrzejowska, 2020). ASOs and gene therapies are being developed and tested in many other childhood neurological conditions.

BOX 6-3
Pediatric Research Success Case Study: COG

The Children's Oncology Group (COG) is a National Cancer Institute-supported clinical trials network that has created a robust research infrastructure to design, study, and rapidly implement proven therapies to improve children's survival and quality of life (COG, 2023). Ninety percent of the approximately 16,000 children diagnosed with cancer each year receive care at COG member hospitals and are enrolled in one of more than 100 active clinical trials. Childhood cancer has evolved from a nearly "incurable disease 50 years ago to one with a combined 5-year survival rate of 80 percent today" (COG, 2023; NCI, 2023b).

management, and neuromonitoring devices have improved viability (defined as the gestational age at which there is a 50 percent chance of survival with or without medical care) from 25 to 26 weeks' gestation in the mid-1990s to 23–24 weeks gestation by the mid-2000s (Glass et al., 2015). Innovative research also has been applied to directly improving patient outcomes through the development of pediatric learning health systems (Forrest et al., 2021; Varnell et al., 2023) and uncovered insights related to implicit bias and racism on child and adolescent health (Goyal et al., 2020, 2015; Johnson et al., 2017a; Priest et al., 2013; Puumala et al., 2016; Trent et al., 2019). In addition to improved pediatric patient outcomes, pediatric research has far-reaching impacts on both children and adults' life course health related to health equity, social and structural determinants of health, and other pressing issues that can improve health across the lifespan (Braveman et al., 2009; Cheng et al., 2022; Halfon et al., 2022; Woodward et al., 2022). (See Chapter 2 for more information on additional emerging health needs for pediatric patients that could be supported by pediatric research.)

UNIQUE CHALLENGES OF PEDIATRIC RESEARCH

Pediatric studies bring specific challenges, including ethical considerations, logistical and technical factors in administering interventions, smaller population size (especially for subspecialty care), developmental considerations in studying children across ages, reluctance to include pregnant women and their fetuses in clinical intervention research, and financial disincentives related to the limited commercial market potential for pediatric drugs compared with adult drugs (Blehar et al., 2013; Burckart, 2020; Caldwell et al., 2004; Kern, 2009; Rees et al., 2021; Shakhnovich et al., 2019; Steinbrook, 2002). As a result, despite the potential for lifelong benefit, fewer studies are conducted in children, even for diseases and conditions that are common in pediatrics, and children tend to be underrepresented in randomized clinical trials for diseases that affect both adults and children (Groff et al., 2020; Hwang et al., 2020; Thomson et al., 2010). Similarly, fewer clinical trials are performed in children compared with other patient populations (Bourgeois et al., 2014; Viergever and Rademaker, 2014), and "while as much as 65 percent of funding for studies in adult populations is provided by the pharmaceutical industry, nearly 60 percent of pediatric clinical trials are sponsored primarily by government and nonprofit organizations" (Rees et al., 2021, p.1237), showcasing the lack of financial incentives for robust industry participation in pediatric research.

Historical Limitations of Pediatric Research Compared with Adult Research

Historically there has been a mismatch between the number of pediatric randomized controlled trials (RCTs) and pediatric disease burden (Groff et al., 2020). Older studies have noted this paucity of pediatric RCTs in published literature (Cohen et al., 2007, 2010; Thomson et al., 2010). Bourgeois et al. (2012) reviewed the clinical trial landscape for conditions known to have pediatric involvement and found that nearly 60 percent of the disease burden was attributable to children, but only 12 percent of trials were pediatric. The authors concluded that the significant disparity between pediatric burden of disease and the level of clinical trial research devoted to pediatric populations may be due in part to having to rely on non-industry funding sources.

The evidence base for treatment and health research and development in children also lags behind that for adults (Viergever and Rademaker, 2014). A major contributor is the lack of pediatric natural history and clinical registry data due to the logistic, ethical, and legal challenges of performing clinical investigations in children (Brussee et al., 2016; Goulooze et al., 2020). Current data collection methods are based on experience with adult populations and do not sufficiently capture the effects of family, environment, and biological factors on children's health and development. Specific aspects of pediatric RCTs that can undermine recruitment, retention, and trial success include ethical considerations around parental consent and child assent, scientific challenges in the paucity of well-validated clinical endpoints or biomarkers in children, and logistical issues such as the time and financial resources needed for participation. Overall consent rates in pediatric RCTs have improved, but are still not optimal (Groff et al., 2020; Lonhart et al., 2020), especially among minoritized groups.

A review of pediatric studies in ClinicalTrials.gov[2] from 2008 to 2019 found a total of 36,136 clinical trials and 16,692 observational studies, with the number of pediatric clinical trials nearly doubling over this period (from 7,000 to almost 12,000), and with an overall decrease in drug trials, but an increase in behavioral trials (Zhong et al., 2021). Pediatric trials were mostly small scale, single site, and usually not funded by industry or the National Institutes of Health (NIH).

---

[2] ClinicalTrials.gov is a database of clinical studies around the world and is provided by the U.S. National Library of Medicine.

Regulatory Landscape and Historical Efforts to Improve Pediatric Drug Development

Largely due to the challenges in pediatric research described previously, far more drugs have been approved for clinical use in adults than for pediatric populations, which leads to a significant proportion of drugs in children being an "off label" use for various medical conditions (Sachs et al., 2012). As a result, most drugs used to treat children are used without an adequate understanding of appropriate pharmacokinetics, dose, safety, or efficacy (NICHD, 2022a). Among other legislative attempts, two laws have aimed to address the study of drugs in pediatric populations—the *Pediatric Research Equity Act* (PREA)[3] and the *Best Pharmaceuticals for Children Act* (BPCA), which provide requirements and incentives with the aim to expand the study of drugs in children (IOM, 2012).[4] Specifically, PREA authorized the Food and Drug Administration (FDA) "to require pediatric studies in certain drugs and biological products. Studies must use appropriate formulations for each age group. The goal of the studies is to obtain pediatric labeling for the product" (FDA, 2019b). BPCA's aim is to (1) "encourage the pharmaceutical industry to perform pediatric studies to improve labeling for patented drug products used in children by granting an additional 6 months of patent exclusivity," and (2) "authorize NIH…to prioritize needs in various therapeutic areas and sponsor clinical trials of off-patent drug products that need further study in children, as well as training and other research that addresses knowledge gaps in pediatric therapeutics" (NICHD, 2022c). The two acts together contributed to the safe and effective use of more than 400 drugs within the first 5 years of implementation (Burckart, 2020), and today there are more than 1,050 small-molecule and biologic products with pediatric labeling from the results of these acts.[5] However, Benning et al. (2021) found that pediatric label changes were not associated with subsequent changes in pediatric drug use, and although some drugs had increased pediatric use after gaining new pediatric indications, the pattern was not consistent.

Recent policy efforts to improve pediatric drug development also include the *Research to Accelerate Cures and Equity for Children (RACE) Act*, which requires evaluation of new drugs and biologics "substantially relevant to growth or progression" of pediatric cancer (Caruso, 2020), and the establishment of the Rare Pediatric Disease Priority Voucher Program,

---

[3] *Pediatric Research Equity Act of 2003*, Public Law 108-155, 108th Congress.

[4] *Best Pharmaceuticals for Children Act of 2002*, Public Law 107-109, 107th Congress.

[5] Current as of June 27, 2023. See https://www.fda.gov/science-research/pediatrics/pediatric-labeling-changes (accessed June 27, 2023) to see access the Pediatric Labeling Changes Spreadsheet.

which awards companies with priority review for drugs targeting a list of rare diseases (Coppes et al., 2022; Hwang et al., 2019).

Diversity and Inclusion in Pediatric Research Populations

Representative and inclusive clinical trials include people's heterogeneous lived experiences and living conditions, as well as demographic characteristics such as race and ethnicity, age, sex, and sexual orientation/gender identification (NIH, 2022a). The efficacy of treatments is best assessed when a diverse population is included in clinical trials (Masters et al., 2022). As with adult research, pediatric clinical trials have not always been appropriately inclusive of populations experiencing health disparities (Aristizabal et al., 2015; Faulk et al., 2020; Lund et al., 2009; Walsh and Ross, 2003; Winestone et al., 2019). Rees et al. (2022) found that most racial and ethnic groups were underrepresented in the trials conducted in the United States.

In recent years, the Eunice Kennedy Shriver National Institute of Child Health and Human Development (NICHD) and NIH have made explicit efforts to increase inclusion of pregnant and lactating people, children, and people with intellectual disabilities in their research (Spong and Bianchi, 2018); however, there is still work to be done. For example, Chen et al. (2022) found that non-English-speaking communities were underrepresented in pediatric health research from 2012 to 2021, and only one in 10 pediatric research studies included patients with limited English proficiency. In addition, Watson et al. (2022) found that children in rural settings are underrepresented in clinical trials, potentially contributing to rural health disparities. As the pediatric population of the United States continues to become more diverse, including diverse populations in pediatric clinical trials is critical. Furthermore, Popkin et al. (2022) emphasized that meaningful inclusion in clinical research begins with training diverse medical and scientific workforces and enhancing the diversity of research and clinical teams. See later section on increasing the diversity of pediatric researchers, Chapter 4 for the current demographics of pediatric subspecialists, and Chapter 5 for influences on career choice for individuals who are underrepresented in medicine.

THE PEDIATRIC PHYSICIAN–SCIENTIST WORKFORCE

No single term defines a pediatric researcher, as individuals with a variety of professional backgrounds can engage in investigational activities. Physician–scientists possess a unique combination of clinical and research expertise based on their education and training that enables them to identify knowledge gaps in clinical care and research questions, gain a comprehensive understanding of critical aspects of medical physiology through clinical epidemiology and disease-specific features, act as a bridge between basic science researchers and clinicians, and develop research strategies aimed at uncovering breakthroughs that can enhance clinical care (Singh et al., 2018; Williams et al., 2022; Yap, 2012). For the purposes of this report, the committee focused on the pediatric physician–scientists, namely those with M.D., D.O.,[6] M.D./Ph.D., or M.D./MPH degrees who perform biomedical, behavioral science, health services research, or public health research of any type as their primary professional activity. This definition includes physician–scientists who are conducting "basic research" (fundamental investigations not specific to disease or patient population), "disease-oriented research" (investigations into the causes or treatments of diseases, with no patient involvement), or "patient-oriented research" (clinically oriented studies with direct patient contact) (Zemlo et al., 2000).

The Physician–Scientist Pathway

The decision to pursue a career as a physician–scientist can be made at many points in an individual's training. The physician–scientist pathway has been described as "long and leaky" (Milewicz et al., 2015). Figure 6-1 highlights the physician–scientist workforce pathway and points of attrition, with best known estimates of losses, as well as the entry points for recruitment, though data are lacking across the continuum. There are various ways in which individuals may experience research career attrition, and each stage can have a cumulative effect. Researchers may choose not to return to research, pursue full-time clinical practice outside of academia, become assistant professors within academia but predominantly focus on patient care, obtain tenure but allocate little time to research, or substantially reduce the amount of research effort at varying points in their academic careers (Milewicz et al., 2015; NIH, 2014). Unfortunately, data on attrition rates specific to pediatric subspecialties are unknown. Across all disciplines, the numbers of physician–scientists have diminished, and the length of their productive scientific careers has decreased, with the average age of first independent funding at 46 years old (Daniels, 2015; Kerschner et al., 2018).

There are two major ways that pediatrician physician–scientists begin their career: directly following completion of an M.D. or D.O. program, and

---

[6] The research literature primarily focuses on those with M.D. or M.D./Ph.D. and less on physician–scientists with D.O. degrees. However, there are increasing numbers of D.O. degrees among physician-scientists.

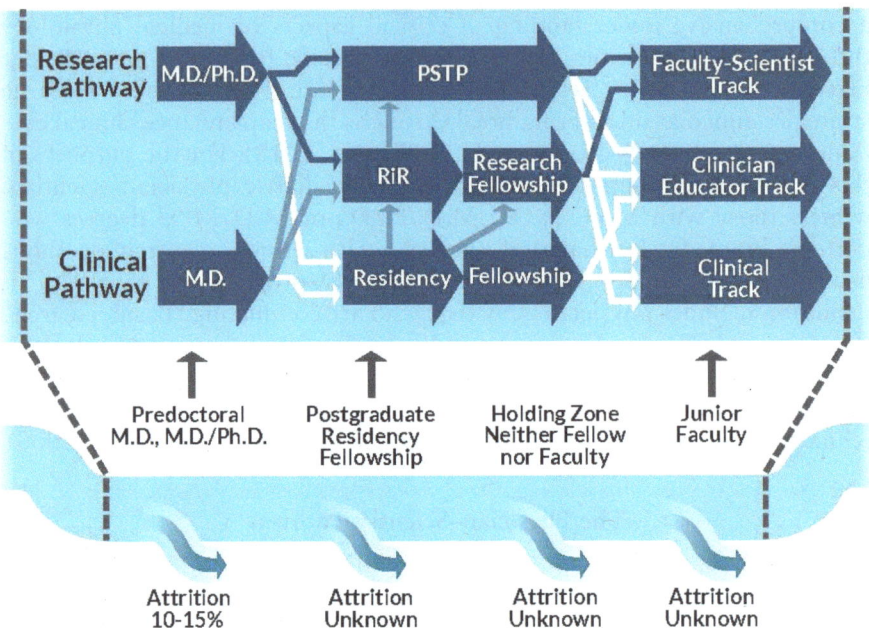

FIGURE 6-1 The physician–scientist career path.
NOTES: Labeled block arrows represent training opportunities. Arrows indicate options for transitions between training programs, with solid navy arrows denoting the standard research-based physician–scientist training pathway, solid blue arrows indicating on-ramps, and solid white arrows showing points of physician–scientist loss, where trainees opt not to pursue research-based careers. PSTP: physician–scientist training program; RiR: research in residency.
SOURCES: Adapted from Williams et al., 2018; Milewicz et al., 2015. Used with permission of JCI Insight, permission conveyed through Copyright Clearance Center, Inc.

through M.D.-Ph.D. programs. Additionally, international medical graduates may be a resource for increasing the number of physician–scientists.

Following M.D./D.O. Programs

As mentioned in Chapters 4 and 5, the conventional pathway for a pediatric subspecialist involves completing a pediatric residency and then pursuing a subspecialty fellowship. During this fellowship, the trainee selects an academic focus that will serve as the foundation of their career development. Scholarly activity is a required component of most residency training programs as well as pediatric fellowship programs. In most pediatric fellowship programs, the initial year of training is largely clinical; trainees rarely have an opportunity to experience a research setting until their second year of training. As a result, by the time they become fully integrated into a laboratory or clinical research program, establish a research focus, and begin to acquire the necessary tools to test hypotheses, they are often well into their second or third year of training. This can make it challenging to complete an independent research project—typically defined as a first author, peer-reviewed publication—by the end of a 3-year fellowship, let alone develop the skills and focus to be successful as a physician–scientist (Rubenstein and Kreindler, 2014).

Evidence shows that formal, structured research tracks have led to greater trainee research engagement (Ercan-Fang et al., 2017). As noted in Chapter 5, the American Board of Pediatrics (ABP) has developed several specialized physician–scientist training structures to speed up the time to become a pediatric physician–scientist, which reflect the frequent calls to reduce training time for physician–scientists (Blish, 2018; Milewicz et al., 2015). These integrated clinical and research pathways are also used by the American Board of Internal Medicine and the American Board of Family Medicine (Doubeni et al., 2017; Todd et al., 2013). There are also several institutional physician–scientist training initiatives (e.g., "umbrella" programs) that include seminars and research forums, along with providing research funding (Permar et al., 2020; Williams et al., 2022).

Following fellowship training, the most common pathway to an independent, academic career for pediatric subspecialty fellows is the transition from fellowship to junior faculty by way of a mentored physician–scientist award, usually in the NIH K series. The competition for these awards is high (see section on NIH funding later in this chapter), though the success rates between "M.D.-only" researchers and Ph.D.s or M.D.-Ph.D.s is comparable (Ley and Hamilton, 2008; NIH, 2014) (see section on M.D.-Ph.D.s).

International Medical Graduates

International medical graduates are individuals who received their primary medical degree from a medical school outside the United States and Canada. There have been proposals to better integrate international medical graduates into the research workforce to address the physician–scientist shortages (Muraro, 2002; Vidyasagar, 2007). However, while international medical graduates represent nearly one-fourth of the pediatric workforce, less than 1 percent designate research as their major professional activity (Duvivier et al., 2020).

M.D.-Ph.D. programs

M.D.-Ph.D. programs combine medical and graduate school within an integrated curriculum in order to train physicians for a career that combines clinical perspectives with research (Akabas et al., 2018). The number of students entering M.D.-Ph.D. programs has been slowly rising, and most graduates become academic physician–scientists (Garrison and Ley, 2022). A 2010 study by Brass and colleagues showed that attrition rates from M.D.-Ph.D. programs averaged 10 percent, and suggested the low rate might be because trainees typically receive tuition waivers for both medical school and graduate school plus a stipend. At that time, most of those who withdrew completed medical school or graduate school; approximately 80 percent of M.D.-Ph.D. program graduates worked in academia, industry, or research institutes (Brass et al., 2010). Over the past 50 years, the M.D.-Ph.D. training time in the United States has steadily increased, increasing from just over 6 years before 1975 to over 8 years in 2014, with no evidence that spending more time as an M.D.-Ph.D. student resulted in a greater research effort years later (Brass and Akabas, 2019).

M.D.-Ph.D. students represent approximately 3 percent of all medical students graduating each year (Akabas et al., 2018). In 2022, M.D.-Ph.D. programs matriculated 709 students and had an enrollment totaling 6,005 trainees in 155 medical schools across all disciplines (AAMC, 2022a). Roughly half of the programs are supported by NIH through a T32[7] mechanism from the National Institute of General Medical Sciences, which provides financial support and consistency in training activities (Williams et al., 2022). According to survey data from 2015, approximately 13 percent of M.D.-Ph.D. program graduates chose residency training in pediatrics (Akabas et al., 2018). Among those that chose to pursue a pediatrics residency, approximately 82 percent reported a subspecialty fellowship choice, with the largest percentages in hematology/oncology (21 percent), medical genetics (10 percent), endocrinology (7 percent), and infectious disease (7 percent) (Akabas et al., 2018). Table 6-1 includes the most recent data of M.D.-Ph.D. dual-degree program graduates from U.S. M.D.-granting medical schools in pediatric subspecialties.

Historically, M.D.-Ph.D. graduates have tended to cluster in certain fields, including pediatrics (Andriole et al., 2008; Paik et al., 2009). However, more recent data have indicated a trend away from the historical trends of internal medicine, pediatrics, neurology, and pathology (Akabas et al., 2018; Brass et al., 2010). This trend of decreasing M.D.-Ph.D. graduates in pediatrics may have implications for the overall pediatric research workforce.

---

[7] An NIH T32 award is an Institutional Training Grant that is made to institutions to support groups of pre- and/or postdoctoral fellows, including trainees in basic, clinical, and behavioral research. Purpose: Ensures that a diverse and highly trained workforce is available to assume leadership roles in biomedical, behavioral, and clinical research. Issued to eligible institutions to support research training for groups of pre- and/or postdoctoral fellows. The number of positions or "slots" varies with each award (NICHD, 2023a).

TABLE 6-1 M.D.-Ph.D. Residents by Subspecialty, 2019–2021

Subspecialty	2019	2020	2021
Adolescent Medicine	1	2	1
Child Abuse Pediatrics	1	1	0
Developmental-Behavioral Pediatrics	4	4	2
Neonatal-Perinatal Medicine	15	18	15
Pediatric Cardiology	15	12	7
Pediatric Critical Care Medicine	8	6	9
Pediatric Emergency Medicine	4	4	1
Pediatric Endocrinology	5	5	6
Pediatric Gastroenterology	5	5	8
Pediatric Hematology/Oncology	36	27	25
Pediatric Infectious Diseases	21	18	17
Pediatric Nephrology	5	5	6
Pediatric Pulmonology	2	1	0
Pediatric Rheumatology	10	10	9

NOTE: *Hospital medicine excluded as there were no M.D.-Ph.D. graduates as active residents from 2019 through 2021.
SOURCE: AAMC, 2022b.

Data Limitations and Effect on Pediatric Physician–Scientist Workforce Projections

It is difficult to characterize the pediatric physician–scientist workforce overall (including numbers) due to data limitations and little to no coordination between the funders and other parties involved in the pediatric research workforce. For example, data from NIH on the number of physicians supported on T32 institutional training grants, receiving K01 Mentored Research Career Development Awards,[8] and awarded R01[9]-Equivalent research grants are currently unavailable (Garrison and Ley,

---

[8] "K awards provide support for senior postdoctoral fellows or faculty-level candidates. The objective of these programs is to bring candidates to the point where they are able to conduct their research independently and are competitive for major grant support." A K01 award is the colloquial name for the Mentored Research Scientist Development Award, which "supports 3 to 5 years of mentored research training experience in the biomedical, behavioral, or clinical sciences. NICHD accepts K01 applications for only three research areas: Rehabilitation Research, Child Abuse and Neglect, and Population Research" (NICHD, 2023b).

[9] The R01 is historically the oldest and most common grant mechanism used by NIH; R01s are for "mature research projects that are hypothesis-driven with strong preliminary data" and provide up to 5 years of support (NIH, 2023a).

2022; see section on NIH funding). The NIH Physician–Scientist Working Group last met in 2013 and there has not been an updated report since then, let alone one specific to the pediatric physician–scientist workforce. There is also a stark lack of communication and collaboration among funding agencies and other participants in the research enterprise to target important areas of pediatric research.

More information on the composition of career development awards and tracking of research careers by demographic factors such as sex, race and ethnicity, disability status, geography, type of science across the continuum (e.g., basic, clinical, implementation), topic/subspecialty, and professional background of the principal investigator (PI) is needed to truly quantify the pediatric physician–scientist workforce and to understand trends. There is also little to no tracking of outcomes from pediatric physician–scientist career development pathway programs. In addition to these quantitative data, qualitative data (e.g., on successful researchers as well as those researchers who leave the research track, including quality of relationship with mentors, satisfaction with career progression, reasons for attrition or retention) will be critical for retention of successful pediatric physician–scientists. During one of the committee's public webinars, Ericka Boone, director for the Division of Biomedical Research Workforce, Office of Extramural Research, NIH, highlighted the need for data on the workforce and barriers to the pathway:

> The only way we can have a clear understanding of what these barriers are is if we ask the individuals that are engaging in these research careers, especially those individuals who have exited out of the research career. What were those things? What were those barriers that just said, I can't do this anymore?...Why are we losing postdocs? Why are we losing early career investigators? Why are they exiting out of these careers? And then doing something to keep them in.[10]

See Box 6-4 for clinician perspectives on the need for physician–scientists.

Trends in Research Work Profiles by Subspecialty

There are considerable disparities in the proportion of physicians who spend a significant amount of time in research activities across the pediatric subspecialties, and the data available are mostly self-reported (typically through ABP's maintenance of certification process). As noted in Chapter 4, data from 2018–2022 reveal that among the ABP-certified pediatric

---

[10] The webinar recording can be accessed at https://www.nationalacademies.org/event/11-02-2022/the-pediatric-subspecialty-workforce-and-its-impact-on-child-health-and-well-being-webinar-3.

> **BOX 6-4**
> **Clinician Perspectives—Need for**
> **Pediatric Physician–Scientists**
>
> "We need more clinician-scientists across the board, especially in critical care medicine. Our patients are becoming more complex, but our diagnostic tests are also becoming more sophisticated."
> **– Practicing Physician–Scientist for over 10 Years, Houston, TX**
>
> "There is a crisis with regard to the decreasing number of individuals who wish to pursue a career as a physician–scientist in a pediatric subspecialty. The duration of training to achieve this goal, coupled with the burden of debt from medical school, the work–life balance expectations of current trainees, the low funding rate for grant submissions, and annual income for the additional training years to pursue a career as a physician–scientist are all factors that have driven some of the best and the brightest to clinical practice or positions with industry."
> **– Faculty Member, Houston, TX**
>
> "Pediatric subspecialty training allows for the leaders in the specialty to drive the important knowledge that disseminates to the pediatric workforce. It is imperative for excellent quality care and separates the [United States] from other countries in their degree of research and knowledge about the specialty."
> **– Experienced Clinician from Hollywood, FL**
>
> *These quotes were collected from the committee's online call for trainee, clinician, patient, and family perspectives.*

subspecialists overall, less than 8 percent reported spending more than 50 percent of their time on research, and 48 percent reported not being involved in any research activities (ABP, 2023). Additionally, the amount of time dedicated to research varies across the subspecialties. ABP-certified subspecialties with the highest percentage of clinicians spending 50 percent or more of their time to research include hematology/oncology (21.6 percent), infectious disease (19.3 percent), rheumatology (14.2 percent), pulmonology (10.8 percent), and endocrinology (10.6 percent) (ABP, 2023). At the extremes, nearly 12 percent of hematology/oncology subspecialists spent 75 percent or more of their time on research while 69 percent of hospital medicine subspecialists reported spending no time on research. Macy et al. (2020) examined ABP's maintenance of certification data from 2009–2016 and found that the number and proportion of pediatric subspecialists engaged in research has not increased or decreased over the study time period, suggesting that previous efforts to bolster the pediatric physician–scientist workforce have not made a difference in increasing this segment of the workforce.

CHALLENGES TO THE PHYSICIAN–SCIENTIST WORKFORCE AND INTERVENTIONS TO SUPPORT PEDIATRIC RESEARCHERS

Pediatric physician–scientists continue to accelerate new basic science and medical insights, behavioral discoveries, and organizational effectiveness. However, the system for producing and nurturing physician–scientists has been inadequate, with limited funding, and heightened clinical and teaching demands (Salata et al., 2018; Williams et al., 2022). The shortage of resources available to support early career pediatric physician–scientists, combined with the multitude of influences on personal career decisions (see Chapter 5) and the demands of clinical practice, has resulted in a decreasing and aging workforce of pediatric researchers, with concerns for the viability of the workforce (Speer et al., 2023). Additionally, retention of physician–scientists in the mid-career space is also a major concern. While the committee has recommended increased flexibility in training curriculum including clinical-only tracks (see Chapter 5), it is critical to also continue to invest in pediatric researchers and to use strategies for improved recruitment and retention of pediatric physician–scientists. For example, flexible training curricula might allow for earlier exposure to research to help support the pediatric physician–scientist pathway.

Since 2017, *Pediatric Research* has published a series of commentaries that provide an opportunity for early career investigators to share experiences or inspirations that influenced their career path, thoughts on what contributed to their success or choices, and advice to others who are in early stages of their career (El-Khuffash, 2017; Guttmann, 2022; Harshman, 2021; Lovinsky-Desir, 2019; Menon, 2021; Salas, 2020; Sun, 2021). For many, early encounters with the medical or the health field, formative research experiences, patient encounters that informed research questions, and inspiring mentors helped fuel and define interest in medicine and/or research careers. Other key factors that influence early career physician–scientists include acquiring the needed academic and professional skills and training, resources, and protected time, and learning from failure (Christou et al., 2016; Flores et al., 2019; Ragsdale et al., 2014).

Threats to the sustainability and growth potential of the physician–scientist workforce and to pediatric research more broadly include: (1) lack of structured and sufficient mentorship and training, most significantly, but not exclusively, for fellows and early career investigators; (2) financial considerations (e.g., educational debt) that impact trainees' decision to pursue research; (3) protection of time for physician–scientists to engage in research; and (4) adequate funding (both extramural and institutional) for research (Alganabi and Pierro, 2021; Permar et al., 2020).

Specific efforts are needed to encourage and facilitate entry into research careers and foster the early phases of career development for pediatric physician–scientists. This is especially true for physician–scientists from populations underrepresented in the extramural scientific workforce (including the biomedical, clinical, behavioral, and social sciences workforces) (NIH, 2022b), which includes certain racial and ethnic groups, individuals with disabilities, individuals from economically disadvantaged backgrounds, and others (depending upon the discipline).

Academic physician–scientist retention is also distressingly low regardless of the mechanism of training (Williams et al., 2022), so efforts for retention of pediatric physician–scientists are also critical. The following sections provide an overview of several of the challenges faced by the pediatric research workforce, including mentorship financial considerations and protection of time, as well as interventions to increase representation in the research workforce. The adequacy and distribution of funding for research itself is discussed after this section.

Mentorship and Training

The importance of mentorship in career success and in advice to new researchers are highlighted in the *Pediatric Research* commentaries discussed above. The authors advise being intentional about seeking out skilled mentors to support the growth and development of the early career investigator, in addition to building a network of support that includes other investigators, peer mentors, and family and friends (El-Khuffash, 2017; Guttmann, 2022; Harshman, 2021; Lovinsky-Desir, 2019; Menon, 2021; Salas, 2020; Sun, 2021). Gaps in mentorship for physician–scientists exist across the entire professional timeline.

Medical School

In medical school, research often is introduced later in training, often too late for an individual to develop strong mentorship and pursue an area of scholarly interest in depth prior to the start of residency training. In 2020, medical school curriculum pathways from 145 schools were reviewed, and numerous examples of research opportunities for medical students were highlighted (McOwen et al., 2020). Some of the opportunities were explicitly research while others were a component of an optional or required scholarly concentration program rather than research in the traditional sense (McOwen et al., 2020; Thompson et al., 2020). Overall, there has been a decline in the aspirations of graduating medical students to pursue research, which may be a result of curricular reforms that place increased emphasis on clinical decision making, and a decreased emphasis on foundations in basic science (Buja, 2019; Garrison and Ley, 2022). However, medical schools have also developed initiatives to bolster the number of physician–scientists. More than 30 medical schools have Physician–Scientist Training Programs (PSTPs) that integrate residency, fellowship, and postdoctoral training for trainees that commit to a physician–scientist career path (Garrison and Ley, 2022; Muslin et al., 2009), though only a small proportion of medical school graduates enter PSTPs (NRMP, 2023).

Residency and Fellowship Training

Not all residency training programs or specialty fellowships provide focused mentorship opportunities for research, which can limit the exposure of trainees to adequate career mentors. "In certain large non-university medical centers with expansive clinical outlays—which focus predominantly on the clinical mission as a driver (and determinant) of research activities—it is relatively rare to have physician–scientists on faculty in clinical departments, further limiting the role models for this career" (Williams et al., 2022). Residents are immersed in intense clinical training with relatively little time for or training in research, with a curriculum that emphasizes information relevant to clinical care and is largely defined by national medical board standards. Many residency programs lack a dedicated research track for physician–scientists, and there are insufficient guidelines, or dissemination of best practices, from the pediatric research community on research training and mentorship. The PSTP programs provide research training opportunities for both M.D. and M.D.-Ph.D. trainees both during or after the completion of clinical training (Williams et al., 2022). Some fellowship programs provide more comprehensive research experiences. While clinical competency must be ensured, greater exposure to research at this stage increases the chance of developing into a successful physician–scientist (Rubenstein and Kreindler, 2014). One possible solution is to encourage trainees to participate in extra years of fellowship; however, there are significant financial disincentives to remaining in training (at fellowship income levels) by comparison to opportunities for faculty or clinical positions (Rubenstein and Kreindler, 2014).

In 2022, the National Pediatric Scientist Collaborative Workgroup, a collaborative of leaders in pediatric research and medical education, surveyed pediatric residency program directors about barriers to developing physician–scientists. Three priority areas were identified: (1) institutional infrastructure, human resources, and financial resources to develop physician–scientist training; (2) "dual professional identity formation" of the pediatric physician–scientist; and (3) input and pathway of candidates into this career path (Burns et al., 2022). This workgroup has begun to develop efforts to address these areas by creating guidelines for best practices in physician–scientist training. Other organizations, such as the Burroughs Wellcome Trust,[11] also have invested resources into bolstering the M.D.-only researcher pathway through early career awards and career development workshops. There are other programs as well, such as the consortium funded National Clinician Scholars Program,[12] which supports physicians and nurses through a two-year site-based research training fellowship (NCSP, 2023) and the Doris Duke Physician Scientists Fellowship program, which provides grants to physician–scientists at the subspecialty fellowship level who are seeking to conduct additional years of research beyond their subspecialty requirement (Doris Duke Foundation, 2023).

The relatively new NIH pilot program, "Stimulating Access to Research in Residency (StARR)" (R38) was initiated in 2017 to create new research opportunities for residents during their clinical training in efforts to recruit resident investigators and increase the body of clinician investigators. Hurst et al. (2019) describes a single institution's pediatric physician–scientist development program, supported in part by an NIH R38 StARR award, that affords research-integrated training across the spectrum of research, for trainees interested in academic general pediatrics or a pediatrics subspecialty and includes support regarding mentor and mentorship teams, scholarly oversight committees, research productivity, educational enrichment, and professional development. The National R38 Consortium consists of principal investigators (PIs) and multiple principal investigators from the first round of R38 awards that were granted in 2018. In a report of early outcomes, PIs endorsed institutional commitment of new resources to support the program and viewed the program positively regarding enhancing research opportunities and recruitment, although there is a need to increase the pool and appointees from populations underrepresented in the extramural scientific workforce (Price Rapoza et al., 2022). After R38 appointment, resident investigator respondents reported a number of positive outcomes, including likelihood of pursuing a physician–scientist career, clarity of research direction, and expanded mentorship.

---

[11] For more information about the Burroughs Wellcome Trust, see https://www.bwfund.org/ (accessed June 27, 2023).

[12] This consortium was grown out of the previous Robert Wood Johnson Foundation Clinical Scholars program.

Early Career

Mentored time immediately after completion of fellowship during the first years of faculty appointment is critical. Mentored research training programs with a focus on fellows and/or early career faculty are offered in multiple settings, including individual institutions, national NIH or foundational programming, and pediatric specialty or subspecialty societies (Badawy et al., 2017; Chen et al., 2016; Cranmer et al., 2018; Kashiwagi et al., 2013; Vasylyeva et al., 2019). Of note, NIH has an embedded component of mentorship through the K-series awards with a requirement that applicants designate mentors and specify a formal mentoring plan (DeCastro et al., 2013; NIAID, 2021). Chen et al. (2016) described the multifaceted "Pediatric Mentoring Program" implemented for instructors and assistant professors in an academic pediatrics department with the goal of promoting retention and job satisfaction. The program consisted of mandatory annual/biannual mentor meetings as well as grant review assistance and peer-group mentoring and annual evaluations. The majority of participants described benefits related to understanding of criteria for advancement or progress toward career goals, but only a minority reported developing collaborations with peers or improved work–life balance. King et al. (2021) described self-reported benefits of participation in a one-year mentored clinical research training program for hematology/oncology fellows and early career faculty (pediatric and adult). Most participants endorsed the program as instrumental to retention in hematological research and facilitation of career development in research; those who endorsed a positive program impact performed better on conventional research metrics such as first author publications and percentage of effort in research when compared with the minority of participants who did not endorse positive program impact.

Mid-Career

While most formal mentoring programs are targeted towards early-career researchers and junior faculty, mentorship is also important in the mid-career space, particularly for female researchers and other populations underrepresented in the extramural scientific workforce (Bora, 2023; Lewiss et al., 2020; Sotirin and Goltz, 2023; Teshima et al., 2019). In academic medicine overall, high-quality mentorship is essential to faculty productivity, job satisfaction, and retention, as well as academic advancement (AAMC, 2023b; Bland et al., 2010; Mylona et al., 2016; Walensky et al., 2018). However, few universities have instituted formal mid-career mentoring programs, let alone mid-career programs specific to the pediatric scientific workforce, and mid-career physician–scientists have reported a lack of high-quality mentoring (Bora, 2023; Pololi et al., 2023). Specific to pediatrics, a discussion-based workshop at the American Society of Pediatric Hematology/Oncology annual meeting found that mid-career participants frequently lacked mentors and thought that "mentors did not appreciate the complexity of the mid-career role" (Frugé et al., 2010).

Financial Considerations

Choosing a career as a physician–scientist is likely influenced by the loss of opportunities for higher salaries both because of extended periods of training (leading to deferred entry into faculty positions) and comparatively higher salaries for private practice (Donath et al., 2009; Pickering et al., 2014; Rosenberg, 1999; Somekh et al., 2019). For example, Zemlo et al. (2000) found that a rising level of student debt in the 1990s was correlated with a declining proportion of physicians choosing research careers. Physician–scientists can incur major debts because of the extra training time needed to gain expertise for both research and clinical care. As mentioned earlier, M.D.-Ph.D. programs may be more attractive for trainees due to the free tuition and avoidance of medical school debt. This incentive is not typically given for M.D.-only investigators, though several medical schools have begun to cover some or all of the cost of tuition through dedicated endowments. Additionally, salaries for pediatric physician–scientists can also be negatively affected by less clinical incentive income and low pay lines in awards. For example, career development awards (e.g., K-series awards) cover some salary support, but this often needs to be supplemented with cost sharing by the physician–scientists' institutions (Daniels, 2015; Garrison and Deschamps, 2014; NIH, 2017a). Given the relatively lower clinical margin in pediatric departments, this issue may be particularly difficult for pediatric physician–scientists. (See Chapter 8 for more information.) During one of the committee's public webinars, Mary Leonard, Arline and Pete Harman Professor and Chair of the Department of Pediatrics at Stanford University, director of the Stanford Maternal and Child Health Research Institute, and physician-in-chief of Lucile Packard Children's Hospital, highlighted how financial considerations play a role in pursuing a pediatric research career: "Going the physician–scientist route defers compensation even further. You have longer trained intervals. In some places, you have lower salaries."[13] See Box 6-5 for clinician perspectives on the financial challenges for pediatric physician–scientists.

---

[13] The webinar recording can be accessed at https://www.nationalacademies.org/event/07-19-2022/the-pediatric-subspecialty-workforce-and-its-impact-on-child-health-and-well-being-webinar-1.

> **BOX 6-5**
> **Clinician Perspectives—Financial Challenges**
> **for Pediatric Physician–Scientists**
>
> "As a physician–scientist, I have always been interested in viruses and trying to understand how they cause disease. However, the fact that we earn less money than nearly or all other pediatric subspecialties, and certainly less than generalists, has made maintaining the culture of a rigorous and exciting academic environment challenging."
> – **Pediatric Infectious Disease Attending from Chapel Hill, NC**
>
> "[I] chose subspecialty because I was really fascinated by the pathophysiology and because I primarily wanted to do research. I do not necessarily regret the decision, but the opportunity cost has been MASSIVE in terms of lost salary...the salary is so much poorer than being a general pediatrician, and I do not see how or why anyone who has medical school or college loans would choose to do this."
> – **Physician-Investigator from Boston, MA**
>
> *These quotes were collected from the committee's online call for trainee, clinician, patient, and family perspectives.*

NIH Loan Repayment Programs (LRPs) and Impact on Research Careers

Loan repayment for pediatric researchers is one approach to overcome financial barriers to entering or remaining in pediatric subspecialty research careers. During the committee's public webinars, Stephanie Lovinsky-Desir, assistant professor and chief of the Pediatric Pulmonary Division at Columbia University Irving Medical Center, Morgan Stanley Children's Hospital of New York Presbyterian discussed the role of loan repayment to help alleviate financial disincentives to pursuing a pediatric research career:

> I applied for the NIH loan repayment program...it was really instrumental toward me staying in a field of pediatric research...a loan repayment that could help offset some of the burden that I have actually was helpful in making the decision to be able to remain in academia and remain in a research-intensive tract...loan repayment is super important for someone like me who didn't benefit from generational wealth, and I have a ton of

debt, and so I'm not quite finished, I'm 10 years out of fellowship training, paying down all of those loans, even with the loan repayment.[14]

Since 1988, the NIH LRPs have supported early-stage investigator awardees in their pursuit of biomedical and behavioral research, including repaying up to $50,000 in educational loans per year in exchange for a commitment to research for at least 20 hours per week for at least 2 years (with possibility for renewal) (Lauer, 2019; NIH, 2022c). From FY2013 to FY2022, there were 3,105 LRP awards in pediatric research, with a 52 percent success rate overall (40 percent for new awards and 71 percent for renewal awards) and total funding of $177,264,184 (with over $105 million of that going to new awards) (NIH, 2023d). In FY2022, the mean award for new pediatrics applications was $88,669 while the mean for renewals was $47,720; the mean age of new awardees was 36 years (NIH, 2023d).

Lauer (2019) compared research-related outcomes between applicants who received and did not receive an LRP award (during fiscal years 2003–2009) with follow-up of research productivity through 2017 (see Figure 6-2). The author reported that receipt of an LRP award was associated with higher levels of "persistence in research" (composite measure including

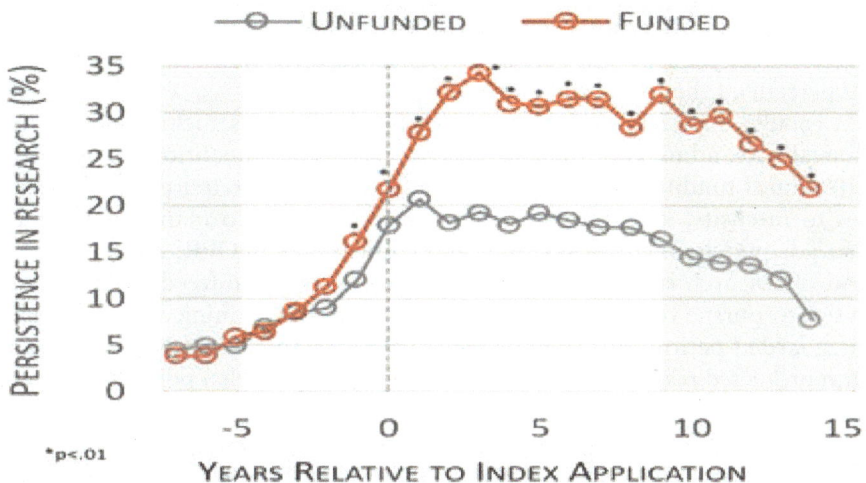

FIGURE 6-2 Annual persistence in research for funded and unfunded applicants.
SOURCE: Adapted from Lauer, M. 2019. Reproduced with permission from the NIH Open Mike Blog.

---

[14] The webinar recording can be accessed at https://www.nationalacademies.org/event/07-19-2022/the-pediatric-subspecialty-workforce-and-its-impact-on-child-health-and-well-being-webinar-1.

submission or receipt of grant or fellowship awards and publications) over a decade after initial application. Although confounding factors may contribute to findings, Lauer noted the NIH LRP Program is an important potential strategy for retention of early career investigators in the research workforce.

Across all NIH LRPs (including non-pediatric awards) in 2022, more than half of awardees had a total education-related debt of over $200,000 (NIH, 2023d). The NIH LRP is an attractive option to encourage the pursuit of a research career.

Protection of Research Time

The time required for pediatric subspecialists to be successful as physician–scientists can be substantial. Historically, a physician–scientist profile has required that 50 percent of one's professional time be focused on research, but with increasing clinical demands and the need to fund this protected research time, a growing number of physicians are conducting research with less time allocated to the effort. NIH requires K-awardees to devote at least 75 percent FTE to research. However, only 3.4 percent of subspecialists report spending at least 75 percent of their time in research (ABP, 2023). Most individuals with R-level grants are devoting at least 50 percent of their time and often much more to research in order to be successful and competitive, yet only 7.6 percent of subspecialists report working at least 50 percent of their time on research (ABP, 2023).

Faculty physician–scientists balance many priorities, including teaching, clinical care, administration, and research. As the competition for securing extramural funding and meeting clinical productivity requirements continues to intensify, it has become increasingly difficult to maintain a career that adequately balances research and clinical care (COPR, 2014). Protection of research time allows physician–scientists to be freed from clinical duties to pursue research. Career development and training awards offer a safeguarded period for emerging scientists to establish a research program with protected research time in order to ultimately reach a point where they can independently conduct research with their own funding support (Garrison and Ley, 2022). Training awards, either institutional (e.g., T32/K12 grants) or individual (e.g., K series grants), require protection of at least 75 percent of their time.

T32 institutional training program grants are made to institutions to support groups of pre- and/or postdoctoral fellows and K12 institutional career development institutional grants (e.g., for PDSPs) aim to prepare newly trained physicians who have made a commitment to independent research careers by providing support to institutions that mentor clinical fellows and scientists (Garrison and Levy, 2022; NICHD, 2023a). Success of a T32 program can be difficult to measure. A NICHD task force that conducted an in-depth review of its extramural training programs and mechanisms found that individuals supported by T32 programs had less-favorable outcomes when compared with individuals supported at the career level (either through individual K or institutional K12 grants) (NICHD, 2015; Steinbach et al., 2018). On the other hand, Abramson et al. (2021) found that having a T32 training grant doubled the probability that pediatric subspecialty fellows published during their fellowship. Historically, NICHD has "emphasized the institutional training and career development awards to a greater degree than many other NIH institutes and centers" and strongly invested in K12 development programs (Twombly et al., 2018).

However, the NICHD task force that reviewed its extramural training programs recommended placing more emphasis on individual awards compared with institutional training awards (NICHD, 2015; Steinbach et al., 2018), and NICHD announced their intention to allocate a greater proportion of its career development fund allocation to individual awards (Twombly et al., 2018). There are a variety of individual K programs targeting specific career stages and research areas. The largest programs are:

- K01 Mentored Research Scientist Career Development Award,
- K08 Mentored Clinical Scientist Research Career Development Award,
- K23 Mentored Patient-Oriented Research Career Development Award, and
- K99 Pathway to Independence Award.

While M.D.s can apply for any of these awards, they are most often supported by the K08 and K23 mechanisms, which comprise approximately half of all K awards (Garrison and Ley, 2022). Estimates suggest that at least 3,000 physicians were supported on career development awards each year from 2011 through 2020, though there has not been an increase in career development awards targeted to physicians (Garrison and Ley, 2022). The number of pediatricians, let alone pediatric subspecialists, is unknown. (See the section on NIH in the funding section in this chapter for more information.)

Previous reports that have looked at bolstering the physician–scientist workforce have proposed increases in the number of career development awards so that early career physician–scientists have the necessary supports to initiate successful research programs (Jain et al., 2019; NIH, 2014; Salata et al., 2018). Multiple studies across different specialties have shown that NIH K awardee are more likely to receive subsequent, independent NIH awards than medical school graduates without them (Jeffe et al., 2018; King et al., 2013; Nikaj and Lund, 2019; Okeigwe et al., 2017). Funding rates for K-series awards vary widely by NIH institute and federal agencies (e.g., the Agency for Healthcare Research and Quality [AHRQ]) and by year, with success rates typically ranging from 20 to 40 percent in a given cycle and many investigators requiring multiple submissions before receiving funding (AHRQ, 2016; Conte and Omary, 2018; NIH, 2023c). Those engaged in research without such funding sources may struggle to allocate sufficient time for investigation, leading to increased burden of professional responsibilities and risk for burnout. Most pediatric departments do not have the resources to support a sizeable amount of research time for more than a limited number of years. As careers progress, the cost of providing the "over the NIH cap" component of the salary can lead to increased pressure to perform clinical work instead of research, unless discretionary funds such as endowed professorships are provided to cover these costs, but these clinical requirements erode protected time.

Increasing the Diversity of Pediatric Researchers

As discussed in Chapter 5, to mirror the demographic make-up of the children and families it serves, the pediatric workforce will require special attention for the recruitment and retention of a diverse set of trainees; this is especially true for the pediatric research workforce. There is evidence that "scientific teams that are composed of diverse individuals with diverse perspectives, backgrounds, and mental models are better positioned to solve complex problems among children and their families" (Guevara et al., 2023), and are more likely to engage in research with diverse groups and communities and generate higher quality research (Ayedun et al., 2023; Campbell et al., 2013; Page, 2007). However, the number of pediatric physician–scientists from populations underrepresented in the extramural scientific workforce is small and growing at a slow rate (AAMC, 2019; Guevara et al., 2023; Lett et al., 2018), though exact statistics are not available. A principal recommendation of the NIH Physician–Scientist Workforce Working Group Report was to improve diversity among all researchers (NIH, 2014). However, structural, systemic, and cultural barriers exist for trainees and faculties from populations underrepresented in the extramural scientific workforce that limit entry or reduce retention in this career path (Behera et al., 2019), including limited opportunities for mentorship and mentorship training, bias and discrimination, and systemic factors at the institutional level (Kalet et al., 2022; Siebert et al., 2020). Minority academic pediatricians have identified a range of obstacles that impede the successful recruitment and retention of minority physicians, including insufficient financial resources, ineffective recruitment strategies, limited opportunities for career advancement, fewer research resources, and inadequate research support (Johnson et al., 2017b; Saboor et al., 2022). Other key issues that threaten the retention of physician–scientists from populations underrepresented in the extramural scientific workforce include disparities in personal wealth, excessive service demands to provide diverse perspectives in committees and conferences, feelings of isolation arising from intersectionality, and apprehensions regarding reinforcing stereotypes (Kalet et al., 2022).

Strategies that have been suggested to promote representation in the research workforce include institutional antiracism policies; support for trainees and faculty from populations underrepresented in the extramural scientific workforce; encouraging diversity in public engagements and institutional leadership; providing child/elder care subsidies; tracking diversity outcome measures; and developing "diversity aware" training curricula (Williams et al., 2022). Interventions include faculty development programs like the Research in Pediatrics Initiative on Diversity, which is a national program of the Academic Pediatrics Association that provides mentoring, research training, and career development for URiM junior pediatrics faculty, and has resulted in increased grant productivity and promotion of participants (Flores et al., 2021). Pediatric departments and children's hospitals, especially with national discussions of racism in society and medicine after the May 2020 murder of George Floyd, have recognized the need to address equity, diversity, and inclusion in all their activities, including the composition of faculty investigators (Pursley et al., 2020; Walker-Harding et al., 2020; Wright et al., 2020). Institutions are addressing diversity in a number of ways, all of which have the potential to be accelerated:

- Recruiting a much more diverse residents' workforce, realizing that their own residency program is an important source of potential fellows.
- Recruiting more diverse fellows, recognizing that graduating fellows are an important source of future faculty.
- Creating fellowship opportunities specifically for populations underrepresented in the extramural scientific workforce.
- Creating internal K-12–like individual career development programs specifically for populations underrepresented in the extramural scientific workforce.
- Providing start-up packages for faculty that increase the chance of success in their research.
- Ensuring that appropriate and intensive mentoring is available for populations underrepresented in the extramural scientific workforce at each stage in their careers.

Given the importance of mentoring in the professional growth, development, and success of trainees and early career investigators—and the potential impact on racial disparities in R01 success (Ginther et al., 2011)—it is important to support mentors in their efforts to gain the knowledge and skills needed to be effective mentors for trainees from diverse backgrounds, particularly for trainees from backgrounds underrepresented in the biomedical research workforce, as well as recognizing mentoring efforts and excellence (NASEM, 2019). Efforts such as the National Research Mentoring Network created/fostered opportunities for mentors and mentees to improve relationships through competency-based trainings offered in multiple types of settings and platforms, including Culturally Aware Mentoring (Byars-Winston et al., 2018; Sorkness et al., 2017).

Across all disciplines, there has been evidence that Black scientists are less likely to receive NIH funding when compared with White scientists (Ginther at al., 2011; Ginther, 2022). As discussed previously, career development awards are an important lever to support early career researchers. An analysis of the race-ethnicity of NIH K awardees from 2010 to 2022 found that while the numbers of Black and Hispanic applicants and awardees have steadily increased over time, the total number of Black and Hispanic applicants remains "quite low" (Lauer and Bernard, 2023). Notably, K award funding rates for Black applicants have increased over the past 3 years. NIH has taken steps to address racism in the scientific workforce and improve diversity, equity, and inclusion efforts (NIH, 2021). For example, the NIH UNITE Initiative was established to address structural racism and establish equity within the biomedical research enterprise (NIH, 2022d). The Extramural Research Ecosystem: Changing Policy, Culture and Structure to Promote Workforce Diversity Committee is charged with performing systematic reviews of NIH extramural policies and processes to identify areas for policy change to address the lack of diversity and inclusivity within the extramural research ecosystem. Priorities include supporting career pathways, research resources, and capacity at minority-serving institutions,[15] promoting equity at extramural institutions in regard to environment and culture, and encouraging equity in policies and procedures at NIH.

Mid-Career Concerns and Retention

This chapter largely focuses on the early phases of the pediatric physician–scientist pathway, emphasizing that early career mentorship, protected research time, and funding are critical supports for entry into a research career, and these can lay a foundation to promote longevity over time. However, mid-career retention of physician–scientists and difficulties during the transition from career development (K series) awards to

---

[15] MSIs are institutions of higher education that serve minority populations. See https://www.doi.gov/pmb/eeo/doi-minority-serving-institutions-program (accessed July 18, 2023).

independent research grants (R series) (the 'K to R transition') remain a major area of challenge (Daye et al., 2015; Good et al., 2018a; Yin et al., 2015), although exact data on attrition rates by pediatric subspecialists during this transition are lacking. Retention of pediatric physician–scientists is threatened by burnout, inadequate mentoring, an increasingly competitive funding environment, financial pressures related to loan repayment and salary, inadequate institutional support and protected time for scholarship, and difficulties balancing clinical and research demands, among other factors (Alvira et al., 2018; Bauserman et al., 2022; Christou et al., 2016; Rosenthal et al., 2020; Salata et al., 2018; Shafer, 2010). (See Chapter 5 for more information on clinician burnout.)

The K to R transition has been described as "tortuous and prolonged," due to low success rates for R series awards and funding gaps (Yin et al., 2015). Women tend to be disproportionately affected at this transition point (Jagsi et al., 2009, 2011; Ghosh-Choudhary et al., 2022; NIH, 2014). Nguyen et al. (2023) found that women received 43 percent of all K awards from 1997–2011 and 34 percent of awards from 2012–2021. Funding rates were lower than faculty representation rates in 5 of the 13 departments assessed, including pediatrics. Regarding K to R transition, 37.7 percent of women who received mentored K awards between 1997 and 2011 successfully applied for R01-equivalent grants within 10 years, compared to 41.5 percent of men (Nguyen et al., 2023).

NIH has created a K99/R00 funding mechanism that incorporates the transition into the funding period (NCI, 2023c), but much of the burden of supporting this transition period falls on institutions, as the investigators require protection of time and financial resources to maintain a research team and program. Many institutions hold K to R transition workshops with programs such as mock grant review/study sections, structured mentoring for grant and manuscript preparation, and information about securing ancillary funding[16] (Jones et al., 2011; Yin et al., 2015). While such guidance is helpful, physician–scientists often require protection of time from clinical activities and bridge funding to ensure that their research can continue if there is a lapse in funding. This is a substantial financial investment to which pediatric departments often cannot commit due to financial pressures, so pediatric physician–scientists may be particularly vulnerable during the K to R transition period. Given the current data limitations, it is important to collect more data on the rates of attrition across the pediatric

---

[16] For examples, see https://ictr.johnshopkins.edu/education-training/seminars-courses/k-to-r/ (accessed July 18, 2023), https://learn.partners.org/courseversion/922/ (accessed July 18, 2023), https://catalyst.harvard.edu/courses/grasp (accessed July 18, 2023), and https://tracs.unc.edu/index.php/services/education/r-writing-group (accessed July 18, 2023).

subspecialties, as well as evidence-based interventions for a successful K to R transition, in order to develop data-driven policies to address these issues.

THE PEDIATRIC RESEARCH FUNDING LANDSCAPE: ADEQUACY AND DISTRIBUTION

Funding is the greatest challenge to the physician–scientist workforce. The federal government—particularly NIH—is a significant funder of child health research in the United States. Other major sources of funding for pediatric research include other federal agencies, private foundations, state and local governments, pharmaceutical companies, device manufacturers, and biotechnology firms. Academic medical centers also bear many of the costs of training physician–scientists and supporting their research efforts. There is an increasing move to align efforts across various funding organizations to maximize resources and avoid redundancy, although currently there is little coordination or collaboration among funders. Additionally, as discussed in more detail below, physician–scientists rely on institutional support to build and maintain the basic infrastructure (e.g., personnel, space, equipment, and salary) for a sustainable research program.

NIH

NIH remains the largest government funding source for global biomedical research (Rees et al., 2021). Historically, pediatric research funding has been low compared with funding for adult diseases, though it has been increasing along with the requirements for NIH to report pediatric research spending annually (Gitterman et al., 2004, 2018a, 2023; Speer et al., 2023). Nearly all of NIH's 27 institutes and centers fund child health research, with NICHD supporting the largest proportion of the pediatric portfolio (approximately 18 percent in 2021–2022[17]) (Gitterman et al., 2018b; NICHD, 2022d; NIH, 2017b). Since 2013, annual NIH support for pediatric research has increased, with $5.7 billion allocated in 2022 (see Figure 6-3). NIH funding for child health has generally kept pace with overall NIH funding increases in absolute dollar amounts[18] (Boat and Whitsett, 2021). While the total dollars spent on pediatric research has increased, the percentage of total NIH funding specific to pediatric research has remained steady at approximately 11 to 12 percent of the total NIH

---

[17] Estimate provided to the committee by Rohan Hazra, NICHD, on May 11, 2023.

[18] The overall NIH budget increased from $29 billion for FY2013 to $49 billion for FY2023. NIH funding adjusted for inflation (in projected constant FY2022 dollars) using the Biomedical Research and Development Price Index showed a smaller overall increase, from $36 billion in FY2015 to $47 billion in FY2023 (Sekar, 2023).

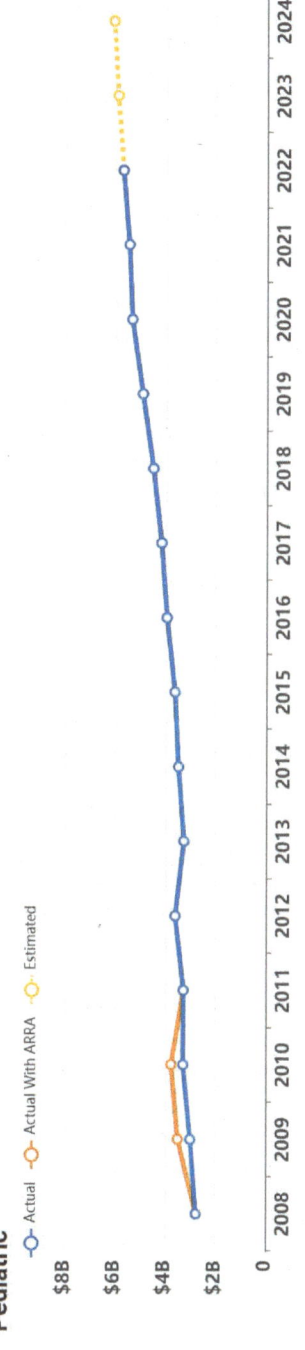

FIGURE 6-3 NIH pediatric research funding, 2008–2024.
NOTES: 2023–2024 are estimates. ARRA = *American Recovery and Reinvestment Act* (American Recovery and Reinvestment Act of 2009, Public Law No. 111-5, 111th Congr., H.R. 1 (February 17, 2009)).
SOURCE: NIH, 2023b.

budget for the past decade (not adjusted for inflation).[19] The number of applications for NIH awards by medical school pediatric departments has been steady from 2012 to 2019 (approximately 1,400 per year, with 16 to 21 percent of applications funded) (NIH, 2023c). There was a drop in applications in 2020 and 2021, with a rebound in the number of applications in 2022 to approximately 1,300 applications and a 20 percent success rate (NIH, 2023c).

NIH Research Funding by Subspecialty

NICHD funding for principal investigators with pediatric subspecialty fellowship training has risen steadily over time, with the largest increases coming in the past 4 years (see Figure 6-4).

Objective data on funding by pediatric subspecialty are not readily available, but self-reported survey data suggest that NIH research funding is not equally distributed across the different subspecialties in terms of total funding, proportion of R01-equivalent investigators, and other indicators (Good et al., 2018b). Good et al. (2018b) found that among the 907 R01-Equivalent Pediatric Physician–Scientist Awardees from 2012 to 2017, the highest percentages were in hematology/oncology, academic general pediatrics, and infectious disease (see Table 6-2). These differences across subspecialties warrant further exploration as they likely reflect a variety of factors, including the foundational tradition that these subspecialties have of doing research, uneven funding allocations for research in certain subspecialties, and the weakened research workforce pathway in certain subspecialties.

The critical role of the home institution in supporting research limits the scope of research activities in smaller, less academic institutions. Eligibility for some NIH awards requires institutions of higher education, often compelling freestanding children's hospitals to apply through other institutions which, in turn, creates more administrative inefficiencies, costs, and hurdles. Furthermore, the lower reimbursement rates for pediatric clinical care (see Chapter 8) leaves limited resources for institutions to support research. These funding challenges have resulted in major disparities in the distribution of research activities across institutions, with the largest children's hospitals with the strongest institutional infrastructure for research accounting for the majority of NIH-funded activities (see Table 6-3) (Good et al., 2018b). This disparity undermines the physician–scientist pathway in smaller institutions, especially those not associated with large academic centers, even though children in these locales would benefit equally (and

---

[19] Estimate calculated using pediatric funding data from NIH (2023b) and overall NIH budget data from Sekar (2023); estimates not adjusted for inflation.

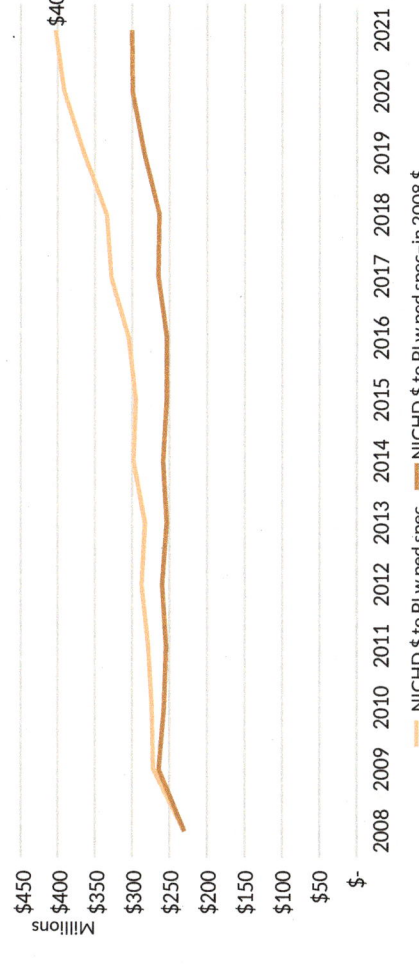

FIGURE 6-4 NICHD funding directly to PIs with pediatric medical subspecialty training; 2008–2021.
NOTES: Figure includes dollars from the *American Recovery and Reinvestment Act*. (American Recovery and Reinvestment Act of 2009, Public Law No. 111-5, 111th Congr., H.R. 1 (February 17, 2009)). Funding levels were adjusted for inflation in research costs using the Biomedical Research and Development Price Index (BRDPI). For more information on BRDPI, see https://officeofbudget.od.nih.gov/gbiPriceIndexes.html.
SOURCE: Provided to the committee by Rohan Hazra, NICHD, on September 9, 2022. NICHD's Child Health Information Retrieval Program (CHIRP): These are not official NIH-wide data.

TABLE 6-2 Pediatric Division Representation Among the 907 R01-Equivalent Physician–Scientist Awardees, 2012–2017

Pediatric Subspecialty	R01-Equivalent Awardees, No. (%)
Hematology/oncology	146 (16.1)
Academic general	109 (12.02)
Infectious disease	93 (10.25)
Neonatology	82 (9.04)
Endocrinology	49 (5.4)
Neurology	46 (5.07)
Pulmonology	45 (4.85)
Gastroenterology	44 (4.85)
Genetics	39 (4.3)
Cardiology	36 (3.97)
Nephrology	32 (3.53)
Critical care	31 (3.42)
Allergy and immunology	31 (3.42)
Rheumatology	15 (1.65)
Adolescent	14 (1.54)
Behavioral and development	10 (1.1)
Emergency medicine	10 (1.1)
Non-pediatric primary training	75 (8.27)

NOTE: Physician–scientists who had not completed a residency in pediatrics were considered "non-pediatric primary training."
SOURCE: Good et al., 2018b. Reproduced with permission from *JAMA Pediatrics*. Copyright ©2018 American Medical Association. All rights reserved.

perhaps more) from enrollment in investigational efforts, such as natural history studies, interventions, and clinical trials.

NIH funding to pediatric institutions and programs continues to be increasingly concentrated in a few sites. Boat and Whitsett (2021) analyzed the 2020 NIH Reporter data and found that 30 percent of NIH's $1.96 billion funding to pediatric institutions and programs went to 3 children's hospitals and 57 percent to the top 10 NIH grant recipients. Between 2013 and 2020, NIH funding of research to the top 10 grant recipients increased 93 percent while funding to those in the third and fourth deciles increased by about 10 percent (Boat and Whitsett, 2021). About one-third of pediatric departments have no NIH funding and more than half (57 percent) have five or fewer NIH grants. Factors differentiating the more and less well-funded programs include local institutional investments in research training, research leadership, and research faculty (Boat and Whitsett, 2021).

TABLE 6-3 Institutional Distribution of Pediatric R01-Equivalent Awards, 2012–2017

Institutions with R0-1 Equivalent Awards	Number of Awards
Boston Children's Hospital	326
Cincinnati Children's Hospital	289
Children's Hospital of Philadelphia	184
Seattle Children's Hospital	103
Baylor College of Medicine	78
Nationwide Children's Hospital	73
Emory University	68
Indiana University-Purdue University at Indianapolis	65
University of California, San Diego	64
University of Colorado, Denver	61
Stanford University	58
University of Pittsburgh	57
Vanderbilt University	46
University of Minnesota	45
Johns Hopkins University	44

NOTE: The top 15 institutions that accounted for 1,561 (63 percent) of the 2,471 individual Pediatric R01 awards from January 2012 to May 17, 2017.
SOURCE: Good et al., 2018b. Reproduced with permission from *JAMA Pediatrics*. Copyright ©2018 American Medical Association. All rights reserved.

Trans-NIH Pediatric Research Consortium

In recognition of the need for a collaborative effort in cataloging and then supporting pediatric research across NIH, in 2018 the NIH Pediatric Research Consortium (N-PeRC) was developed. This trans-NIH initiative, led by NICHD, includes a representative from each of NIH's 27 institutes and centers (NICHD, 2022d). The goal of N-PeRC is to "harmonize [pediatric research] activities across institutes, explore gaps in the overall pediatric research portfolio, and share best practices to advance science. The consortium meets several times a year to discuss scientific opportunities and potential new areas of collaboration, including efforts to enhance research training for the next generation of pediatricians [and pediatric surgeons]" (NICHD, 2022d). Other current priorities of the group include the COVID-19 pandemic and its impact on children and youth, pediatric medical devices, and aligning pediatric clinical trial and other research networks. As of the writing of this report, N-PeRC is still in the early stages of development and has not released any publicly available reports or quantified the total amount of trans-NIH pediatric funding.

Other Federal Funders

Although NIH is the largest federal funder of child research, other federal funders also fund pediatric research, though the breadth and exact numbers are difficult to determine. For example, since 2015, AHRQ has given out $817 million in grants, with approximately $82.8 million to projects that include pediatrics[20] (AHRQ, 2020). AHRQ has funded several projects related to pediatric telehealth implementation.[21] The Centers for Disease Control and Prevention (CDC) funds various grants and cooperatives related to pediatrics through its various offices, though it is difficult to quantify exactly how much of the total CDC funding is for pediatric research. Programs of the Maternal and Child Health Bureau within the Health Resources and Services Administration improve the health and well-being of America's mothers, children, and families (HRSA, 2023). These other federal funders are critical for pediatric research, but it is difficult to quantify the amounts specific to pediatric subspecialty research. There is also little coordination, transparency, or standardized metrics among federal pediatric research funders to prioritize specific areas for federal pediatric research support.

The Patient Centered Outcomes Research Institute

The Patient Centered Outcomes Research Institute (PCORI) is an independent nonprofit organization that funds comparative clinical effectiveness

---

[20] The amount of pediatric funding was calculated by searching "pediatrics" in the AHRQ grants by state.

[21] These include: Improving Recognition and Management of Hypertension in Youth: Comparing Approaches for Extending Effective [Clinical Decision Support] for use in a Large Rural Health System: This project is focused on using clinical decision support within the electronic health record to identify elevated blood pressure and hypertension in children and adolescents in primary care and subspecialty clinics at a large health system. Specifically, the grant notes that research on these tools is "crucial in rural areas where adolescent obesity is high and access to pediatric subspecialists is low" (AHRQ, 2023b); Feasibility Study of a Mobile Digital Personal Health Record for Family-Centered Care Coordination for Children and Youth with Special Healthcare Needs: This project aims to evaluate the feasibility of a digital personal health record mobile application to help coordinate care for children and youth with special health care needs (AHRQ, 2023a); and Telehealth Education for Asthma Connecting Hospital and Home (TEACHH): This project aims to determine the feasibility and acceptability, as well as impact on patient-reported outcomes, of implementing TEACHH for children with asthma throughout the hospital-to-home transition. If successful, the researchers hypothesize that TEACHH could also be used for other chronic childhood diseases, such as diabetes and sickle cell anemia.

research, meaning research in which two or more treatments or health practices are compared to help guide patient decision making. PCORI has funded more than 100 studies and projects focused on pediatric health (as of February 2022), with initiatives such as delivery of mental health services to children in underserved areas, evaluation of treatments for infantile spasms, improving access to hearing care for children in rural areas through telehealth visits, and psychotropic medication use in foster youth (PCORI, 2023).

Industry

In 2020, industry accounted for nearly two thirds of U.S. medical and health investment in research and development (Research America, 2022). However, as discussed previously, progress in pediatric pharmaceutical research has historically lagged that in adults due to the scarcity of available pediatric populations, physiologic differences between children and adults, ethical concerns about research involving children, highly competitive therapeutic domains, and lack of financial incentives with minimal financial returns on investment (given the lower market appeal for drugs for relatively rare pediatric conditions) (Benning et al., 2021; Bucci-Rechtweg, 2017; Cheng et al., 2022; Milne and Davis, 2014). Industry-sponsored trials involving children remain limited due to expected lower profitability (Speer et al., 2023). However, biopharmaceutical research companies are evaluating existing medicines that have already received approval for use in adults with the aim of ascertaining safe and effective dosages and methods of administration for children (PhRMA, 2020). In 2020, there were more than 2,100 industry-sponsored pediatric clinical trials underway,[22] testing 580 investigational medicines[23] in infants, children, and adolescents (PhRMA, 2020).

Foundations

Several foundations support pediatric research. For example, the Burroughs Wellcome Fund provides competitive peer-reviewed awards to both institutions and researchers, with an increasing focus on early career physician–scientists, physician-only scientists, and pediatric research. It has invested $250 million into support of physician–scientists

---

[22] Clinicaltrials.gov with search terms Recruiting, Not Yet Recruiting, Active, Not Recruiting, Interventional Studies, Child and Industry (accessed June 7, 2019).

[23] Number of medicines obtained through government and industry sources, and the Springer "AdisInsight" database. Current as of January 10, 2020.

since its inception in 1955.[24] In collaboration with the Coalition for Medical Research, the Burroughs Wellcome Fund held a summit in 2022 and produced a policy brief on *Developing the Next Generation of Diverse Pediatric Researchers* (BWF, 2022). Some key themes that were discussed in the summit and policy brief include articulation of barriers to pediatric research, summary of legislative priority areas of focus for pediatric research, including the *Pediatricians Accelerate Childhood Therapies (PACT) Act of 2021*,[25] and the Pediatric Subspecialty Loan Repayment Program. Other large foundations that support pediatric research include the Annie E. Casey Foundation, the Bill and Melinda Gates Foundation, the Cystic Fibrosis Foundation, the David & Lucile Packard Foundation, the Doris Duke Charitable Foundation,[26] the Juvenile Diabetes Research Foundation, the Pritzker Traubert Foundation, the Robert Wood Johnson Foundation, and the Thrasher Fund, among others. The Damon Runyon Cancer Research Foundation also funds the Damon Runyon Clinical Investigator Award, which is a program that is exclusive to M.D.-only would-be physician–scientists.

The Role of Academic Medical Centers in Cultivating Physician–Scientists

While NIH and private foundations persist in investing in the development of the physician–scientist workforce, academic medical centers bear a significant responsibility for cultivating and recruiting the next generation of physician–scientists (Brown, 2018). Academic medical centers (AMCs) have historically emphasized the education of physicians, relying on the hospital's inpatient and outpatient settings as primary training sites, and have made significant contributions to pediatric research (IOM, 2004; see Chapter 4 for more information on education and training). While research in AMCs brings in grant dollars, even with indirect cost funds, grants do not fully support the research conducted. Research funding has often relied

---

[24] Data provide during a presentation at an information gathering session by Louis J. Muglia, President and CEO of the Burroughs Wellcome Fund. The webinar recording can be accessed at https://www.nationalacademies.org/event/11-02-2022/the-pediatric-subspecialty-workforce-and-its-impact-on-child-health-and-well-being-webinar-3.

[25] *PACT Act of 2021*, S 1357, 117th Cong. (2021–2022).

[26] Related to retention and prevention attrition, the Doris Duke Fund to Retain Clinical Scientists awards 5-year grants of $540,000 each to medical schools and affiliated hospitals to retain early-career physician–scientists who are facing extraprofessional demands of caregiving such as childcare and eldercare. Building on this program, the Doris Duke Foundation, the American Heart Association, the Burroughs Wellcome Fund, Rita Allen Foundation, and Walder Foundation collaborated in 2021 to offer a one-time COVID-19 Fund to Retain Clinical Scientists funding opportunity. See https://www.dorisduke.org/funding-areas/medical-research/fund-to-retain-clinical-scientists (accessed July 21, 2023).

on the cross-subsidization of clinical revenue, as well as philanthropic funding (Kerschner et al., 2018). However, with increasing costs of providing clinical care, along with the increasing proportion of patients insured by Medicaid (see Chapter 8), the ability for this cross-subsidization is decreasing (Lakshminrusimha et al., 2022). In smaller academic medical centers, it is likely impossible, resulting in even less ability to support early career researchers and compelling faculty to focus on generating more clinical revenue (Garrison and Ley, 2022). Children's hospitals often prioritize clinical programs, with less investment in research, and training programs in freestanding children's hospitals often have less opportunity for interaction with a broader array of both clinicians and researchers (as compared with programs in university settings) (Boat and Whitsett, 2021). During one of the committee's public webinars, Sallie Permar (Nancy C. Paduano Professor and Chair of Pediatrics at Weill Cornell Medicine and pediatrician-in-chief at New York-Presbyterian/Weill Cornell Medical Center) highlighted the difficulties that AMCs and pediatric departments face in developing pediatric physician–scientists:

> Our departments [have] a challenge in covering junior faculty years that are needed for that ongoing research training before a physician–scientist can become independently funded. There is not as much margin as adult departments and surgical departments to continue allowing for research, training, and development of that independence. What this leaves us with is a therapeutic pipeline for children that's really threatened by not having enough bright new minds going into the field and really leaves out children when it comes to early adoption of novel therapies…we're really limiting the therapeutic opportunities that we bring to children by not attracting more and speaking to not only the enthusiasm of these pediatric subspecialists, but their earning potential for the long term.[27]

KEY FINDINGS AND CONCLUSIONS

Key Findings

<u>Finding #6-1</u>: Unique aspects of pediatric clinical trials can affect recruitment, retention, and trial success, including ethical considerations, logistical and technical factors in administering interventions, smaller population size (especially for subspecialty care), and financial disincentives related to the limited commercial market potential for pediatric drugs compared with adult drugs. These challenges in the

---

[27] The webinar recording can be accessed at https://www.nationalacademies.org/event/07-19-2022/the-pediatric-subspecialty-workforce-and-its-impact-on-child-health-and-well-being-webinar-1.

pediatric clinical trial enterprise present disadvantages to pursuing careers in pediatric research compared to adult research.

Finding #6-2: There is a limited number of pediatric researchers, with a variable and leaky pathway by subspecialty. The number and proportion of pediatric subspecialists engaged in research has remained steady over the past decade.

Finding #6-3: The paucity of objective data—including the exact number of researchers by subspecialty, percentage of time spent on research, and attrition across the research pathway (e.g., K to R transition)—makes it difficult to characterize the pediatric physician–scientist workforce.

Finding #6-4: The unequal distribution of funding across institutions—with funding for basic and clinical research concentrated in a small number of large U.S. pediatric medical centers and unequally distributed across the country—means that many institutions do not have the financial resources to provide adequate support to pediatric physician–scientists, particularly during the early phase of career development.

Finding #6-5: There is little coordination among pediatric research funders.

Finding #6-6: NIH funding for early career awards does not provide adequate support for investigator salary, mentorship nor research project expenses, thereby creating financial stress for institutions and departments, which are expected to cover the financial gaps.

Finding #6-7: Challenges to the growth of the pediatric physician–scientist workforce include the lack of a robust mentorship environment at different levels, particularly for fellows and early career investigators; financial considerations that impact trainees' decisions to pursue research; protection of time for physician–scientists to engage in research; and adequate extramural and intramural funding for research.

Finding #6-8: Receipt of an NIH Loan Repayment Program award is associated with higher levels of persistence in research over a decade after initial application.

Conclusions

<u>Conclusion #6-1</u>: To improve the quantity and quality of pediatric health research, a robust pediatric physician–scientist pathway and workforce are critical.

<u>Conclusion #6-2</u>: More evidence is needed on funding trends, unmet needs, quality of research mentorship, and outcomes from pediatric physician–scientist career development pathway programs.

<u>Conclusion #6-3</u>: There is a need for improved communication and collaboration among funding agencies and other participants in the research enterprise to target important areas of research need and the development of metrics to quantify the impact of pediatric research, including long-term health outcomes.

<u>Conclusion #6-4</u>: Specific and intentional efforts are needed to encourage and facilitate entry into research careers and foster the early phases of career development for pediatric physician–scientists. This is especially true for physician–scientists from populations underrepresented in the extramural scientific workforce.

<u>Conclusion #6-5</u>: Partnerships between government, public, and industry organizations can play a key role in building career pathways for pediatric researchers to help push the frontiers in clinical trials, drug discovery, and health services research.

<u>Conclusion #6-6</u>: Mentorship is key for pediatric research career advancement. It is critical for pediatric departments to recognize, reward, and incentivize exceptional research mentorship at the individual level.

<u>Conclusion #6-7</u>: Salaries for pediatric physician–scientists are negatively affected by less clinical incentive income, in addition to already the low salaries of many of the pediatric subspecialties. The NIH LRP Program is an important policy lever for retention of early career investigators in the research workforce and may be especially important for pediatric subspecialist physician–scientists.

RECOMMENDATIONS

The continued advances in child health require continued scientific discovery from T0 to T4.[28] This requires a highly skilled workforce in which the pediatric physician–scientist plays a crucial role. For the purposes of this report, the committee focused on the role of the pediatric subspecialty physician–scientists who are crucial in research to improve subspecialty care and related health and organizational outcomes. Training this workforce cannot be fully accomplished during the 12 months of scholarly activity required within a 3-year overall fellowship. Rather, physician–scientists need extended training accompanied by adequate research support at the beginning of their careers. Intentional efforts are needed to encourage and facilitate entry into research careers and foster the early phases of career development for pediatric physician–scientists, especially those from populations underrepresented in the extramural scientific workforce. The current system for producing and nurturing pediatric physician–scientists has been inadequate and needs to be improved. However, more evidence is needed on funding trends, unmet needs, quality of research mentorship, and outcomes from pediatric physician–scientist career development pathway programs to inform future efforts to support careers in research. Therefore, to achieve a goal of **supporting the pediatric physician–scientist pathway,** the committee makes the following recommendations.

RECOMMENDATION 6-1 The National Institutes of Health (NIH) Pediatric Research Consortium, with leadership from the National Institute of Child Health and Human Development and input from the NIH's Scientific Workforce Diversity Office, and with appropriate additional funding, should engage with other government and nongovernment pediatric research funders to create and maintain a publicly

---

[28] "The T0 pillar anchors basic science bench research, whereas T1 work extends basic science discovery to the first in human trials looking for safety and efficacy endpoints, proof-of-concept, and phase 1 clinic trials. T2 science includes the phase 2 and 3 clinical trials of diagnostics, therapeutics, devices, and other interventions for human health. The physician–scientist [needs] a different educational focus for this pillar than the T0/T1 physician–scientist. Education [needs to] cover clinical trials science, observational studies, meaningful endpoint detection, statistical methods focused on human populations, and human behavior. T3 science extends to phase 4 clinical trials and other observational studies such as health services and clinical outcomes research. Physician–scientists in this arena need education in community-based participatory research and cost-effectiveness and comparative effectiveness research methods. T4 science looks at population-level outcomes and how social determinants of health significantly influence health. Physician–scientists [need to] gain specialization in public policy and health disparities research to include population health guideline development and rigorous meta-analytic strategies" (Williams et al., 2022).

available central repository for qualitative and quantitative data on pediatric physician–scientists' funding and success throughout their careers (e.g., tracking funding rates and attrition by pediatric subspecialty), including the development of new measures as needed to understand the initial success and retention of pediatric physician–scientists. The Association of Medical School Pediatric Department Chairs should provide supplemental data as needed.

Examples of data needed include the following:

- Quantitative data on the funding rates of career development and subsequent awards and the tracking of research careers by demographic factors such as sex/gender, race and ethnicity, disability status, geography, type of science across the continuum (e.g., basic, clinical, translational, implementation, health services research), topic/subspecialty, and professional background of the PI; and
- Qualitative data on successful researchers and those who leave the research track, including the quality of relationship with mentors; types of support received from their institutions; availability of statistical, epidemiologic, academic and grant writing training and support; availability of funding to present and publish research; satisfaction with career progression; and reasons for attrition or retention.

RECOMMENDATION 6-2 The National Institutes of Health and the Agency for Healthcare Research and Quality should increase the number of career development grants in pediatrics, particularly institutional training awards (e.g., the Pediatric Scientist Development Program), the Pediatric Loan Repayment Program, and K awards, with attention to providing such grants to physician–scientists from backgrounds that are underrepresented in the scientific workforce[29] and for high-priority subspecialties in pediatric research. Funding for individual K awards should be increased to reflect current salaries and research project expenses and should include additional explicit funding for mentorship.

---

[29] See Chapter 1 of this report for a discussion of underrepresentation in the scientific workforce.

REFERENCES

AAMC (Association of American Medical Colleges). 2019. *Diversity in medicine: Facts and figures 2019*. https://www.aamc.org/data-reports/workforce/report/diversity-medicine-facts-and-figures-2019 (accessed May 3, 2023).

AAMC. 2022a. 2022 FACTS: Enrollment, Graduates, and MD-PhD Data. Table B-11.2. https://www.aamc.org/data-reports/students-residents/data/2022-facts-enrollment-graduates-and-md-phd-data (accessed June 27, 2023).

AAMC. 2022b. *Report on residents. Table B4. MD-PhD residents, by GME specialty. 2019–21 active residents*. https://www.aamc.org/data-reports/students-residents/data/report-residents/2022/table-b4-md-phd-residents-gme-specialty (accessed June 27, 2023).

AAMC. 2023a. *Physician-scientists*. https://www.aamc.org/what-we-do/mission-areas/medical-research/physician-scientist (accessed March 8, 2023).

AAMC. 2023b. *Mentoring*. https://www.aamc.org/professional-development/affinity-groups/gfa/mentoring (accessed July 17, 2023).

ABP (American Board of Pediatrics). 2023. *Survey results: 2018–2022 maintenance of certification enrollment surveys: Hours worked and work profiles*. https://www.abp.org/dashboards/results-continuing-certification-moc-enrollment-surveys-2018-2022 (accessed April 27, 2023).

Abramson, E. L., P. Weiss, M. Naifeh, M. D. Stevenson, J. G. Duncan, J. A. Rama, E. Mauer, L. M. Gerber, and S.-T. T. Li. 2021. Scholarly activity during pediatric fellowship. *Pediatrics* 147(1).

AHRQ (Agency for Healthcare Research and Quality). 2016. *Meeting minutes, November 2016*. https://www.ahrq.gov/news/events/nac/2016-11-nac/nacmtg1116-minutes.html (accessed May 1, 2023).

AHRQ. 2020. *AHRQ grants by state*. https://www.ahrq.gov/funding/grant-mgmt/grants-by-state.html (accessed February 7, 2023).

AHRQ. 2023a. *Feasibility study of a mobile digital personal health record for family-centered care coordination for children and youth with special healthcare needs*. https://digital.ahrq.gov/ahrq-funded-projects/feasibility-study-mobile-digital-personal-health-record-family-centered-care-coordination-children (accessed April 3, 2023).

AHRQ. 2023b. *Improving recognition and management of hypertension in youth: Comparing approaches for extending effective CDs for use in a large rural health system*. https://digital.ahrq.gov/ahrq-funded-projects/improving-recognition-and-management-hypertension-youth-comparing-approaches (accessed April 3, 2023).

Akabas, M., I. Tartakovsky, and L. Brass. 2018. *The national MD-PhD program outcomes study*. American Association of Medical Colleges Reports. https://store.aamc.org/national-M.D.-Ph.D.-program-outcomes-study.html (acessed May 2, 2023).

Alganabi, M., and A. Pierro. 2021. Becoming an academic pediatric surgeon scientist in Canada. *Seminars in Pediatric Surgery* 30(1):151015.

Alvira, C. M., R. H. Steinhorn, W. F. Balistreri, J. R. Fineman, P. E. Oishi, J. F. Padbury, J. P. Kinsella, and S. H. Abman. 2018. Enhancing the development and retention of physician-scientists in academic pediatrics: Strategies for success. *Journal of Pediatrics* 200:277-284.

Andriole, D. A., A. J. Whelan, and D. B. Jeffe. 2008. Characteristics and career intentions of the emerging M.D./Ph.D. workforce. *JAMA* 300(10):1165-1173.

Aristizabal, P., J. Singer, R. Cooper, K. J. Wells, J. Nodora, M. Milburn, S. Gahagan, D. E. Schiff, and M. E. Martinez. 2015. Participation in pediatric oncology research protocols: Racial/ethnic, language and age-based disparities. *Pediatric Blood & Cancer* 62(8):1337-1344.

Ayedun, A., V. Agbelese, L. Curry, R. Gotian, L. Castillo-Page, M. White, A. D. Antwi, M. Buchanan, M. Girma, D. Kline, C. Okeke, A. Raghu, H. Saleh, A. Schwartz, and D. Boatright. 2023. Perspectives on National Institutes of Health funding requirements for racial and ethnic diversity among medical scientist training program leadership. *JAMA Network Open* 6(5):e2310795-e2310795.

Badawy, S. M., V. Black, E. R. Meier, K. C. Myers, K. Pinkney, C. Hastings, J. M. Hilden, P. Zweidler-McKay, L. C. Stork, and T. S. Johnson. 2017. Early career mentoring through the American Society of Pediatric Hematology/Oncology: Lessons learned from a pilot program. *Pediatric Blood & Cancer* 64(3):e26252.

Baruteau, J., S. N. Waddington, I. E. Alexander, and P. Gissen. 2017. Gene therapy for monogenic liver diseases: Clinical successes, current challenges and future prospects. *Journal of Inherited Metabolic Disease* 40(4):497-517.

Bauserman, M., M. Vasquez, P. R. Chess, M. Carbajal, H. French, K. Reber, E. Cicalese, K. Lawrence, B. Schwarz, A. Payne, R. Angert, M. Gillam-Krakauer, J. Sharma, E. Bonachea, J. Trzaski, L. Johnston, R. Dadiz, J. Enciso, A. Falck, M. Frost, M. Gray, S. Izatt, S. Kane, A. Kiefer, K. Leeman, S. Malik, P. Myers, J. Nair, D. O'Reilly, T. Sawyer, M. C. Smith, K. Stanley, J. Wambach, C. L. Wraight, M. Good, and O. F. D. W. Group. 2022. Essentials of neonatal-perinatal medicine fellowship: Scholarship perspective. *Journal of Perinatology* 42(4):528-533.

Behera, A., J. Tan, and H. Erickson. 2019. Diversity and the next-generation physician-scientist. *Journal of Clinical and Translational Science* 3(2-3):47-49.

Benning, T. J., N. D. Shah, J. W. Inselman, H. K. Van Houten, J. S. Ross, and K. D. Wyatt. 2021. Drug labeling changes and pediatric hematology/oncology prescribing: Measuring the impact of U.S. legislation. *Clinical Trials* 18(6):732-740.

Bick, D., M. Jones, S. L. Taylor, R. J. Taft, and J. Belmont. 2019. Case for genome sequencing in infants and children with rare, undiagnosed or genetic diseases. *Journal of Medical Genetics* 56(12):783-791.

Bland, C., Taylor, A., and S. Shollenberger. 2010. *Mentoring systems: Benefits and challenges of diverse mentoring partnerships.* https://www.aamc.org/professional-development/affinity-groups/gfa/faculty-vitae/mentoring-systems-benefits-challenges (accessed July 17, 2023).

Blehar, M. C., C. Spong, C. Grady, S. F. Goldkind, L. Sahin, and J. A. Clayton. 2013. Enrolling pregnant women: Issues in clinical research. *Womens Health Issues* 23(1):e39-e45.

Blish, C. A. 2018. Maintaining a robust pipeline of future physician-scientists. *Journal of Infectious Diseases* 218(Suppl 1):S40-S43.

Boat, T. F., and J. A. Whitsett. 2021. How can the pediatric community enhance funding for child health research? *JAMA Pediatrics* 175(12):1212-1214.

Bora, S. 2023. *Strategic recommendations to promote justice, equity, diversity, and inclusion principles in the pediatric scientific workforce.* https://www.societyforpediatricresearch.org/jedi-toolbox-faculty-mentoring/ (accessed July 17, 2023).

Bourgeois, F. T., S. Murthy, C. Pinto, K. L. Olson, J. P. Ioannidis, and K. D. Mandl. 2012. Pediatric versus adult drug trials for conditions with high pediatric disease burden. *Pediatrics* 130(2):285-292.

Bourgeois, F. T., K. L. Olson, J. P. Ioannidis, and K. D. Mandl. 2014. Association between pediatric clinical trials and global burden of disease. *Pediatrics* 133(1):78-87.

Branson, B. M., H. H. Handsfield, M. A. Lampe, R. S. Janssen, A. W. Taylor, S. B. Lyss, and J. E. Clark. 2006. Revised recommendations for HIV testing of adults, adolescents, and pregnant women in health-care settings. *Morbidity and Mortality Weekly Report: Recommendations and Reports* 55(14):1-CE-4.

Brass, L. F., and M. H. Akabas. 2019. The national MD-PhD program outcomes study: Relationships between medical specialty, training duration, research effort, and career paths. *JCI Insight* 4(19).

Brass, L. F., M. H. Akabas, L. D. Burnley, D. M. Engman, C. A. Wiley, and O. S. Andersen. 2010. Are MD-PhD programs meeting their goals? An analysis of career choices made by graduates of 24 MD-PhD programs. *Academic Medicine* 85(4):692-701.

Braveman, P., and C. Barclay. 2009. Health disparities beginning in childhood: A life-course perspective. *Pediatrics* 124(Supplement_3):S163-S175.

Brown, N. J. 2018. Developing physician-scientists. *Circulation Research* 123(6):645-647.
Brussee, J. M., E. A. Calvier, E. H. Krekels, P. A. Välitalo, D. Tibboel, K. Allegaert, and C. A. Knibbe. 2016. Children in clinical trials: Towards evidence-based pediatric pharmacotherapy using pharmacokinetic-pharmacodynamic modeling. *Expert Review of Clinical Pharmacology* 9(9):1235-1244.
Bucci-Rechtweg, C. 2017. Enhancing the pediatric drug development framework to deliver better pediatric therapies tomorrow. *Clinical Therapeutics* 39(10):1920-1932.
Buja, L. M. 2019. Medical education today: All that glitters is not gold. *BMC Medical Education* 19(1):1-11.
Burckart, G. J. 2020. The revolution in pediatric drug development and drug use: Therapeutic orphans no more. *Journal of Pediatric Pharmacology and Therapeutics* 25(7):565.
Burns, A. M., D. J. Moore, C. S. Forster, W. Powell, S. Thammasitboon, M. K. Hostetter, P. Weiss, D. Boyer, M. A. Ward, and R. Blankenburg. 2022. Physician-scientist training and programming in pediatric residency programs: A national survey. *Journal of Pediatrics* 241:5-9. e3.
Burroughs Wellcome Fund (BWF). 2022. *Developing the next generation of diverse pediatric researchers*. https://www.dropbox.com/s/n07jtt0x0kcnq8k/May-5th-Convening-Program-FINAL.pdf?dl=0 (accessed 2023, April 28).
Byars-Winston, A., V. Y. Womack, A. R. Butz, R. McGee, S. C. Quinn, E. Utzerath, C. L. Saetermoe, and S. Thomas. 2018. Pilot study of an intervention to increase cultural awareness in research mentoring: Implications for diversifying the scientific workforce. *Journal of Clinical and Translational Science* 2(2):86-94.
Caldwell, P. H. Y., S. B. Murphy, P. N. Butow, and J. C. Craig. 2004. Clinical trials in children. *Lancet* 364(9436):803-811.
Campbell, L. G., S. Mehtani, M. E. Dozier, and J. Rinehart. 2013. Gender-heterogeneous working groups produce higher quality science. *PLoS ONE* 8(10):e79147.
Caruso, C.. 2020. RACE Act poised to advance pediatric cancer research. *Cancer Discovery* 10(10):1434.
CDC (Centers for Disease Control and Prevention). 2022. *HIV and perinatal transmission*. https://www.cdc.gov/hiv/group/pregnant-people/index.html (accessed December 19, 2022).
CFF (Cystic Fibrosis Foundation). 2022. *Intro to CF*. https://www.cff.org/intro-cf (accessed December 19, 2022).
Chen, A., S. Demaestri, K. Schweiberger, J. Sidani, R. Wolynn, D. Chaves-Gnecco, R. Hernandez, S. Rothenberger, E. Mickievicz, J. D. Cowden, and M. I. Ragavan. 2022. Inclusion of non–English-speaking participants in pediatric health research: A review. *JAMA Pediatrics* 177(1):81-88.
Chen, M. M., C. I. Sandborg, L. Hudgins, R. Sanford, and L. K. Bachrach. 2016. A multifaceted mentoring program for junior faculty in academic pediatrics. *Teaching and Learning in Medicine* 28(3):320-328.
Cheng, T. L., N. Monteiro, L. A. DiMeglio, A. T. Chien, E. S. Peeples, E. Raetz, B. Scheindlin, and S. C. Denne. 2016. Seven great achievements in pediatric research in the past 40 y. *Pediatric Research* 80(3):330-337.
Cheng, T. L., C. Russo, C. Cole, D. A. Williams, S. Shah, M. Patel, J. Raphael, J. Davis, D. Pursley, T. Cheng, S. U. Devaskar, J. Javier, L. Lee, and Council on Behalf of the Pediatric Policy. 2022. Advocacy for research starting early in the life course. *Pediatric Research* 91(6):1312-1314.
Christou, H., M. L. V. Dizon, K. N. Farrow, S. R. Jadcherla, K. T. Leeman, A. Maheshwari, L. P. Rubin, B. K. Stansfield, and D. H. Rowitch. 2016. Sustaining careers of physician-scientists in neonatology and pediatric critical care medicine: Formulating supportive departmental policies. *Pediatric Research* 80(5):635-640.

COG (Children's Oncology Group). 2023. *Children's oncology group (COG): Who we are.* https://childrensoncologygroup.org/childrens-oncology-group (accessed April 3, 2023).
Cohen, E., E. Uleryk, M. Jasuja, and P. C. Parkin. 2007. An absence of pediatric randomized controlled trials in general medical journals, 1985–2004. *Journal of Clinical Epidemiology* 60(2):118-123.
Cohen, E., R. D. Goldman, A. Ragone, E. Uleryk, E. G. Atenafu, U. Siddiqui, N. Mahmoud, and P. C. Parkin. 2010. Child vs adult randomized controlled trials in specialist journals: A citation analysis of trends, 1985–2005. *Archives of Pediatric & Adolescent Medicine* 164(3):283-288.
Conte, M. L., and M. B. Omary. 2018. NIH career development awards: Conversion to research grants and regional distribution. *Journal of Clinical Investigation* 128(12):5187-5190.
Coppes, M. J., C. Jackson, and E. M. Connor. 2022. I-act for children: Helping close the gap in drug approval for adults and children. *Pediatric Research*. https://doi.org/10.1038/s41390-022-02349-5.
COPR (Committee on Pediatric Research), M. D. Cabana, T. L. Cheng, A. J. Bauer, C. W. Bogue, A. T. Chien, J. M. Dean, B. Scheindlin, and A. Kelle. 2014. Promoting education, mentorship, and support for pediatric research. *Pediatrics* 133(5):943-949.
Cranmer, J. M., A. M. Scurlock, R. B. Hale, W. L. Ward, P. Prodhan, J. L. Weber, P. H. Casey, and R. F. Jacobs. 2018. An adaptable pediatrics faculty mentoring model. *Pediatrics* 141(5).
Daniels, R. J. 2015. A generation at risk: Young investigators and the future of the biomedical workforce. *Proceedings of the National Academy of Sciences* 112(2):313-318.
Daye, D., C. B. Patel, J. Ahn, and F. T. Nguyen. 2015. Challenges and opportunities for reinvigorating the physician-scientist pipeline. *Journal of Clinical Investigation* 125(3):883-887.
DeCastro, R., D. Sambuco, P. A. Ubel, A. Stewart, and R. Jagsi. 2013. Mentor networks in academic medicine: Moving beyond a dyadic conception of mentoring for junior faculty researchers. *Academic Medicine* 88(4):488-496.
De Luca, D., P. Cogo, M. C. Kneyber, P. Biban, M. G. Semple, J. Perez-Gil, G. Conti, P. Tissieres, and P. C. Rimensberger. 2021. Surfactant therapies for pediatric and neonatal ARDs: Espnic expert consensus opinion for future research steps. *Critical Care* 25(1):75.
Dermody, T. S., R. Hirsch, M. K. Hostetter, J. S. Orange, and J. W. St. Geme, III. 2019. Expanding the pipeline for pediatric physician-scientists. *Journal of Pediatrics* 207:3-7.e1.
Donath, E., K. B. Filion, and M. J. Eisenberg. 2009. Improving the clinician-scientist pathway: A survey of clinician-scientists. *Archives of Internal Medicine* 169(13):1241-1247.
Doris Duke Foundation. 2023. *Physician Scientist Fellowship.* https://www.dorisduke.org/funding-areas/medical-research/physician-scientist-fellowship/ (accessed June 27, 2023).
Doubeni, C. A., A. Davis, J. L. Benson, and B. Ewigman. 2017. From the Association of Departments of Family Medicine: A physician scientist pathway in family medicine residency training programs. *Annals of Family Medicine* 15(6):589.
Duvivier, R. J., M. E. Gusic, and J. R. Boulet. 2020. International medical graduates in the pediatric workforce in the United States. *Pediatrics* 146(6).
El-Khuffash, A. F. 2017. Early career investigator highlight–November. *Pediatric Research* 82(5):722.
Ercan-Fang, N. G., D. C. Rockey, C. J. Dine, S. Chaudhry, and T. Arayssi. 2017. Resident research experiences in internal medicine residency programs—a nationwide survey. *American Journal of Medicine* 130(12):1470-1476. e1473.
Farrar, M. A., and M. C. Kiernan. 2015. The genetics of spinal muscular atrophy: Progress and challenges. *Neurotherapeutics* 12(2):290-302.
Faulk, K. E., A. Anderson-Mellies, M. Cockburn, and A. L. Green. 2020. Assessment of enrollment characteristics for Children's Oncology Group (COG) upfront therapeutic clinical trials 2004–2015. *PLoS ONE* 15(4):e0230824.

FDA. (U.S. Food and Drug Administration). 2019a. *FDA approves innovative gene therapy to treat pediatric patients with spinal muscular atrophy, a rare disease and leading genetic cause of infant mortality.* https://www.fda.gov/news-events/press-announcements/fda-approves-innovative-gene-therapy-treat-pediatric-patients-spinal-muscular-atrophy-rare-disease (accessed June 27, 2023).

FDA. 2019b. *Pediatric research equity act: PREA.* https://www.fda.gov/drugs/development-resources/pediatric-research-equity-act-prea (accessed May 8, 2023).

Finkel, R. S., E. Mercuri, B. T. Darras, A. M. Connolly, N. L. Kuntz, J. Kirschner, C. A. Chiriboga, K. Saito, L. Servais, E. Tizzano, H. Topaloglu, M. Tulinius, J. Montes, A. M. Glanzman, K. Bishop, Z. J. Zhong, S. Gheuens, C. F. Bennett, E. Schneider, W. Farwell, and D. C. De Vivo. 2017. Nusinersen versus sham control in infantile-onset spinal muscular atrophy. *New England Journal of Medicine* 377(18):1723-1732.

Flores, G., F. S. Mendoza, M. R. DeBaun, E. Fuentes-Afflick, V. F. Jones, J. A. Mendoza, J. L. Raphael, and C. J. Wang. 2019. Keys to academic success for under-represented minority young investigators: Recommendations from the research in academic pediatrics initiative on diversity (RAPID) national advisory committee. *International Journal for Equity in Health* 18(1):93.

Flores, G., F. Mendoza, M. B. Brimacombe, and W. Frazier III. 2021. Program evaluation of the Research in Academic Pediatrics Initiative on Diversity (RAPID): Impact on career development and professional society diversity. *Academic Medicine* 96(4):549-556.

Forrest, C. B., K. M. McTigue, A. F. Hernandez, L. W. Cohen, H. Cruz, K. Haynes, R. Kaushal, A. N. Kho, K. A. Marsolo, V. P. Nair, R. Platt, J. E. Puro, R. L. Rothman, E. A. Shenkman, L. R. Waitman, N. A. Williams, and T. W. Carton. 2021. PCORnet 2020: Current state, accomplishments, and future directions. *Journal of Clinical Epidemiology* 129:60-67.

Frugé, E., J. Margolin, T. Horton, L. Venkateswaran, D. Lee, D. L. Yee, and D. Mahoney. 2010. Defining and managing career challenges for mid-career and senior stage pediatric hematologist/oncologists. *Pediatric Blood & Cancer* 55(6):1180-1184.

Garrison, H. H., and A. M. Deschamps. 2014. NIH research funding and early career physician scientists: Continuing challenges in the 21st century. *Federation of American Societies for Experimental Biology Journal* 28(3):1049-1058.

Garrison, H. H., and T. J. Ley. 2022. Physician-scientists in the United States at 2020: Trends and concerns. *FASEB Journal* 36(5):e22253.

Ghosh-Choudhary, S., N. Carleton, S. M. Nouraie, C. R. Kliment, and R. A. Steinman. 2022. Predoctoral MD-PhD grants as indicators of future NIH funding success. *JCI Insight* 7(6).

Gilbert, J. A., M. J. Blaser, J. G. Caporaso, J. K. Jansson, S. V. Lynch, and R. Knight. 2018. Current understanding of the human microbiome. *Nature Medicine* 24(4):392-400.

Ginther, D. K. 2022. Reflections on race, ethnicity, and NIH research awards. *Molecular Biology of the Cell* 33(1):ae1.

Ginther, D. K., W. T. Schaffer, J. Schnell, B. Masimore, F. Liu, L. L. Haak, and R. Kington. 2011. Race, ethnicity, and NIH research awards. *Science* 333(6045):1015-1019.

Gitterman, D. P., R. S. Greenwood, K. C. Kocis, B. R. Mayes, and A. N. McKethan. 2004. Did a rising tide lift all boats? The NIH budget and pediatric research portfolio. *Health Affairs* 23(5):113-124.

Gitterman, D. P., W. S. Langford, and W. W. Hay, Jr. 2018a. The uncertain fate of the National Institutes of Health (NIH) pediatric research portfolio. *Pediatric Research* 84(3):328-332.

Gitterman, D. P., W. S. Langford, and W. W. Hay, Jr. 2018b. The fragile state of the National Institutes of Health pediatric research portfolio, 1992-2015: Doing more with less? *JAMA Pediatrics* 172(3):287-293.

Gitterman, D. P., W. W. Hay, and W. S. Langford. 2023. Making the case for pediatric research: A life-cycle approach and the return on investment. *Pediatric Research* 93(4):797-800.

Glass, H. C., A. T. Costarino, S. A. Stayer, C. M. Brett, F. Cladis, and P. J. Davis. 2015. Outcomes for extremely premature infants. *Anesthesia and Analgesia* 120(6):1337-1351.

Good, M., S. J. McElroy, J. N. Berger, D. J. Moore, and J. L. Wynn. 2018a. Limited achievement of NIH research independence by pediatric K award recipients. *Pediatric Research* 84(4):479-480.

Good, M., S. J. McElroy, J. N. Berger, and J. L. Wynn. 2018b. Name and characteristics of National Institutes of Health R01-funded pediatric physician–scientists: Hope and challenges for the vanishing pediatric physician–scientists. *JAMA Pediatrics* 172(3):297-299.

Goulooze, S. C., L. B. Zwep, J. E. Vogt, E. H. Krekels, T. Hankemeier, J. N. van den Anker, and C. A. Knibbe. 2020. Beyond the randomized clinical trial: Innovative data science to close the pediatric evidence gap. *Clinical Pharmacology & Therapeutics* 107(4):786-795.

Goyal, M. K., T. J. Johnson, J. M. Chamberlain, L. Cook, M. Webb, A. L. Drendel, E. Alessandrini, L. Bajaj, S. Lorch, and R. W. Grundmeier. 2020. Racial and ethnic differences in emergency department pain management of children with fractures. *Pediatrics* 145(5).

Goyal, M. K., N. Kuppermann, S. D. Cleary, S. J. Teach, and J. M. Chamberlain. 2015. Racial disparities in pain management of children with appendicitis in emergency departments. *JAMA Pediatrics* 169(11):996-1002.

Groff, M. L., M. Offringa, A. Ein, Q. Mahood, P. C. Parkin, and E. Cohen. 2020. Publication trends of pediatric and adult randomized controlled trials in general medical journals, 2005-2018: A citation analysis. *Children (Basel)* 7(12).

Guevara, J. P., J. Aysola, R. Wade, B. Nfonoyim, M. Qiu, M. Reece, and K. N. Carroll. 2023. Diversity in the pediatric research workforce: A scoping review of the literature. *Pediatric Research* 94(3):904–914. https://doi.org/10.1038/s41390-023-02603-4.

Guttmann, K. F. 2022. Early career investigator biocommentary: Katherine Guttmann. *Pediatric Research* 92(4):916.

Halfon, N., S. A. Russ, and E. L. Schor. 2022. The emergence of life course intervention research: Optimizing health development and child well-being. *Pediatrics* 149(Supplement 5).

Harshman, L. A. 2021. Early career investigator highlight: Lyndsay A. Harshman. *Pediatric Research* 89(3):402.

Holstein, S. A., and M. A. Lunning. 2020. CAR T-cell therapy in hematologic malignancies: A voyage in progress. *Clinical Pharmacology & Therapeutics* 107(1):112-122.

HRSA (Health Resources and Services Administration). 2023. *Maternal and Child Health Bureau (MCHB) awarded grants*. https://data.hrsa.gov/topics/mchb/mchb-grants (accessed April 3, 2023).

Hunger, S. P., X. Lu, M. Devidas, B. M. Camitta, P. S. Gaynon, N. J. Winick, G. H. Reaman, and W. L. Carroll. 2012. Improved survival for children and adolescents with acute lymphoblastic leukemia between 1990 and 2005: A report from the Children's Oncology Group. *Journal of Clinical Oncology* 30(14):1663-1669.

Hurst, J. H., K. J. Barrett, M. S. Kelly, B. B. Staples, K. A. McGann, C. K. Cunningham, A. M. Reed, R. A. Gbadegesin, and S. R. Permar. 2019. Cultivating research skills during clinical training to promote pediatric-scientist development. *Pediatrics* 144(2).

Hutzen, B., S. N. Paudel, M. Naeimi Kararoudi, K. A. Cassady, D. A. Lee, and T. P. Cripe. 2019. Immunotherapies for pediatric cancer: Current landscape and future perspectives. *Cancer and Metastasis Reviews* 38(4):573-594.

Hwang, T. J., F. T. Bourgeois, J. M. Franklin, and A. S. Kesselheim. 2019. Impact of the priority review voucher program on drug development for rare pediatric diseases. *Health Affairs* 38(2):313-319.

Hwang, T. J., A. G. Randolph, and F. T. Bourgeois. 2020. Inclusion of children in clinical trials of treatments for coronavirus disease 2019 (COVID-19). *JAMA Pediatrics* 174(9):825-826.

IOM (Institute of Medicine). 2004. *Academic health centers: Leading change in the 21st century.* Washington, DC: The National Academies Press. https://doi.org/10.17226/10734.
IOM. 2012. *Safe and effective medicines for children: Pediatric studies conducted under the Best Pharmaceuticals for Children Act and the Pediatric Research Equity Act.* Washington, DC: The National Academies Press. https://doi.org/10.17226/13311.
Jagsi, R., A. R. Motomura, K. A. Griffith, S. Rangarajan, and P. A. Ubel. 2009. Sex differences in attainment of independent funding by career development awardees. *Annals of Internal Medicine* 151(11):804-811.
Jagsi, R., R. DeCastro, K. A. Griffith, S. Rangarajan, C. Churchill, A. Stewart, and P. A. Ubel. 2011. Similarities and differences in the career trajectories of male and female career development award recipients. *Academic Medicine* 86(11):1415-1421.
Jain, M. K., V. G. Cheung, P. J. Utz, B. K. Kobilka, T. Yamada, and R. Lefkowitz. 2019. Saving the endangered physician-scientist—a plan for accelerating medical breakthroughs. *New England Journal of Medicine* 381(5):399-402.
Janssens, Y., J. Nielandt, A. Bronselaer, N. Debunne, F. Verbeke, E. Wynendaele, F. Van Immerseel, Y. P. Vandewynckel, G. De Tré, and B. De Spiegeleer. 2018. Disbiome database: Linking the microbiome to disease. *BMC Microbiology* 18(1):50.
Jędrzejowska, M. 2020. Advances in newborn screening and presymptomatic diagnosis of spinal muscular atrophy. *Degenerative Neurological and Neuromuscular Disease* 10:39-47.
Jeffe, D. B., and D. A. Andriole. 2018. Prevalence and predictors of US medical graduates' federal F32, mentored-K, and R01 awards: A national cohort study. *Journal of Investigative Medicine* 66(2):340-350.
Johnson, T. J., A. M. Ellison, G. Dalembert, J. Fowler, M. Dhingra, K. Shaw, and S. Ibrahim. 2017a. Implicit bias in pediatric academic medicine. *Journal of the National Medical Association* 109(3):156-163.
Johnson, T. J., D. G. Winger, R. W. Hickey, G. E. Switzer, E. Miller, M. B. Nguyen, R. A. Saladino, and L. R. Hausmann. 2017b. Comparison of physician implicit racial bias toward adults versus children. *Academic Pediatrics* 17(2):120-126.
Jones, D. R., M. J. Mack, G. A. Patterson, and L. H. Cohn. 2011. A positive return on investment: Research funding by the thoracic surgery foundation for research and education (TSFRE). *The Journal of Thoracic and Cardiovascular Surgery* 141(5):1103-1106.
Kalet, A., A. M. Libby, R. Jagsi, K. Brady, D. Chavis-Keeling, M. H. Pillinger, G. L. Daumit, A. F. Drake, W. P. Drake, V. Fraser, D. Ford, J. S. Hochman, R. D. Jones, C. Mangurian, E. A. Meagher, G. McGuinness, J. G. Regensteiner, D. C. Rubin, K. Yaffe, and J. E. Ravenell. 2022. Mentoring underrepresented minority physician-scientists to success. *Academic Medicine* 97(4):497-502.
Kashiwagi, D. T., P. Varkey, and D. A. Cook. 2013. Mentoring programs for physicians in academic medicine: A systematic review. *Academic Medicine* 88(7):1029-1037.
Kern, S. E. 2009. Challenges in conducting clinical trials in children: Approaches for improving performance. *Expert Review of Clinical Pharmacology* 2(6):609-617.
Kerschner, J. E., J. R. Hedges, K. Antman, E. Abraham, E. Colón Negrón, and J. L. Jameson. 2018. Recommendations to sustain the academic mission ecosystem at U.S. medical schools. *Academic Medicine* 93(7):985-989.
King, A., I. Sharma-Crawford, A. F. Shaaban, T. H. Inge, T. M. Crombleholme, B. W. Warner, H. N. Lovvorn III, and S. G. Keswani. 2013. The pediatric surgeon's road to research independence: Utility of mentor-based National Institutes of Health grants. *Journal of Surgical Research* 184(1):66-70.
King, A. A., S. K. Vesely, G. Dadzie, C. Calhoun, A. Cuker, W. Stock, A. Walker, J. Fritz, and L. Sung. 2021. Self-reported positive impact of mentored clinical research training is associated with academic success in hematology. *Blood Advances* 5(14):2919-2924.

Kliment, C. R., I. J. Barbash, J. S. Brenner, D. Chandra, K. Courtright, M. C. Gauthier, K. M. Robinson, L. P. Scheunemann, F. A. Shah, and J. D. Christie. 2021. COVID-19 and the early-career physician-scientist. Fostering resilience beyond the pandemic. *ATS Scholar* 2(1):19-28.

Lakshminrusimha, S., S. Murin, J. D. Kirk, Z. Mustafa, T. R. Maurice, N. Sousa, J. Lee, and D. A. Lubarsky. 2022. "Funds flow": implementation at academic health centers: Unique challenges to pediatric departments. *Journal of Pediatrics* 249:6-10.e14.

Lampe, M. A., S. R. Nesheim, K. L. Oladapo, A. C. Ewing, J. Wiener, and A. P. Kourtis. 2023. Achieving elimination of perinatal HIV in the United States. *Pediatrics* 151(5):e2022059604.

Lauer, M. 2019. *Outcomes for NIH loan repayment program awardees: A preliminary look.* https://nexus.od.nih.gov/all/2019/05/21/outcomes-for-nih-loan-repayment-program-awardees-a-preliminary-look (accessed December 5, 2022).

Lauer, M., and M. A. Bernard. 2023. *Mentored career development application (K) funding rates by race-ethnicity FY 2010-FY 2022.* https://nexus.od.nih.gov/all/2023/03/16/mentored-career-development-application-k-funding-rates-by-race-ethnicity-fy-2010-fy-2022/ (accessed May 2, 2023).

Lett, E., W. U. Orji, and R. Sebro. 2018. Declining racial and ethnic representation in clinical academic medicine: A longitudinal study of 16 US medical specialties. *PLoS ONE* 13(11):e0207274.

Lewiss, R. E., J. K. Silver, A. A. Bernstein, A. M. Mills, B. Overholser, and N. D. Spector. 2020. Is academic medicine making mid-career women physicians invisible? *Journal of Women's Health* 29(2):187-192.

Ley, T. J., and B. H. Hamilton. 2008. The gender gap in NIH grant applications. *Science* 322(5907):1472-1474.

Lonhart, J. A., A. R. Edwards, S. Agarwal, B. P. Lucas, and A. R. Schroeder. 2020. Consent rates reported in published pediatric randomized controlled trials. *Journal of Pediatrics* 227:281-287.

Lovinsky-Desir, S. 2019. Early career investigator biocommentary-pediatric research. *Pediatric Research* 85(1):6.

Lund, M. J., M. T. Eliason, A. E. Haight, K. C. Ward, J. L. Young, and R. D. Pentz. 2009. Racial/ethnic diversity in children's oncology clinical trials: Ten years later. *Cancer* 115(16):3808-3816.

Macy, M. L., K. D. Van, L. K. Leslie, and G. L. Freed. 2020. Engagement in research among pediatric subspecialists at the time of enrollment in maintenance of certification, 2009-2016. *Pediatric Research* 87(6):1128-1134.

Masters, J. C., J. A. Cook, G. Anderson, G. Nucci, A. Colzi, M.-P. Hellio, and B. Corrigan. 2022. Ensuring diversity in clinical trials: The role of clinical pharmacology. *Contemporary Clinical Trials* 118:106807.

McOwen, K. S., A. J. Whelan, and A. L. Farmakidis. 2020. Medical education in the United States and Canada, 2020. *Academic Medicine* 95(9S):S2-S4.

Mendell, J. R., S. Al-Zaidy, R. Shell, W. D. Arnold, L. R. Rodino-Klapac, T. W. Prior, L. Lowes, L. Alfano, K. Berry, K. Church, J. T. Kissel, S. Nagendran, J. L'Italien, D. M. Sproule, C. Wells, J. A. Cardenas, M. D. Heitzer, A. Kaspar, S. Corcoran, L. Braun, S. Likhite, C. Miranda, K. Meyer, K. D. Foust, A. H. M. Burghes, and B. K. Kaspar. 2017. Single-dose gene-replacement therapy for spinal muscular atrophy. *New England Journal of Medicine* 377(18):1713-1722.

Menon, S. 2021. Early career investigator: Biocommentary. *Pediatric Research* 89(5):1051.

Milewicz, D. M., R. G. Lorenz, T. S. Dermody, and L. F. Brass. 2015. Rescuing the physician-scientist workforce: The time for action is now. *Journal of Clinical Investigation* 125(10):3742-3747.

Milne, C.-P., and J. Davis. 2014. The pediatric studies initiative: After 15 years have we reached the limits of the law? *Clinical Therapeutics* 36(2):156-162.

Muraro, P. A. 2002. An international solution to recruiting physician-scientists? *Nature Medicine* 8(9):902-903.

Muslin, A. J., S. Kornfeld, and K. S. Polonsky. 2009. The physician scientist training program in internal medicine at Washington University School of Medicine. *Academic Medicine* 84(4):468-471.

Mylona, E., L. Brubaker, V. N. Williams, K. D. Novielli, J. M. Lyness, S. M. Pollart, V. Dandar, and S. A. Bunton. 2016. Does formal mentoring for faculty members matter? A survey of clinical faculty members. *Medical Education* 50(6):670-681.

NASEM (National Academies of Sciences, Engineering, and Medicine). 2019. *The science of effective mentorship in STEMM*, edited by M. L. Dahlberg and A. Byars-Winston. Washington, DC: The National Academies Press.

NCI (National Cancer Institute). 2023a. *Childhood Cancer Data Initiative (CCDI).* https://www.cancer.gov/research/areas/childhood/childhood-cancer-data-initiative (accessed March 8, 2023).

NCI. 2023b. *Children's Oncology Group.* https://datacatalog.ccdi.cancer.gov/resource/COG (accessed April 3, 2023).

NCI. 2023c. *K99/R00—The pathway to independence award.* https://www.cancer.gov/grants-training/training/funding/k99 (accessed July 18, 2023).

NCSP (National Clinician Scolars Program). *About Us.* https://nationalcsp.org/about-us (accessed June 27, 2023).

Nguyen, M., A. Panyadahundi, C. Olagun-Samuel, S. I. Chaudhry, M. M. Desai, A. Dardik, and D. Boatright. 2023. Transition from mentored to independent NIH funding by gender and department. *JAMA* 329(24):2189-2190.

NIAID (National Institute of Allergy and Infectious Diseases). 2021. *How to find the right mentor for early-career awards.* https://www.niaid.nih.gov/grants-contracts/find-early-career-awards-mentor (accessed July 17, 2023).

NICHD (National Institute of Child Health and Human Development). 2015. *Review of NICHD training and career development programs.* https://www.nichd.nih.gov/sites/default/files/2017-09/NICHD_training_review_091615_508.pdf (accessed July 18, 2023).

NICHD. 2017a. *Congenital hypothyroidism (CH).* https://www.nichd.nih.gov/about/accomplishments/contributions/hypothyroidism#:~:text=Building%20on%20the%20discoveries%20that%20allowed%20mass%20screening,that%20results%20from%20problems%20with%20the%20thyroid%20gland (accessed November 29, 2022).

NICHD. 2017b. *Hemophilus influenza type b (Hib) vaccine.* https://www.nichd.nih.gov/about/accomplishments/contributions/hib-vaccine# (accessed November 29, 2022).

NICHD. 2017c. *Phenylketonuria (PKU) and newborn screening.* https://www.nichd.nih.gov/about/accomplishments/contributions/pku (accessed November 29, 2022).

NICHD. 2017d. *Sudden infant death syndrome (SIDS).* https://www.nichd.nih.gov/health/topics/sids (accessed December 19, 2022).

NICHD. 2022a. *About BPCA.* https://www.nichd.nih.gov/research/supported/bpca/about (accessed December 1, 2022).

NICHD. 2022b. *Best Pharmaceuticals for Children Act (BPCA).* https://www.nichd.nih.gov/research/supported/bpca (accessed December 1, 2022).

NICHD. 2022c. *NIH Pediatric Research Consortium (N-PERC).* https://www.nichd.nih.gov/research/supported/nperc (accessed December 2, 2022).

NICHD. 2022d. *Safe to sleep.* https://safetosleep.nichd.nih.gov/ (accessed December 19, 2022).

NICHD. 2023a. *Institutional training grants (T32/K12).* https://www.nichd.nih.gov/grants-contracts/training-careers/extramural/institutional (accessed April 28, 2023).

NICHD. 2023b. *Career development (K) awards.* https://www.nichd.nih.gov/grants-contracts/training-careers/extramural/career (accessed April 28, 2023).
NIH (National Institutes of Health). 2014. *Physician-scientist workforce working group report.* https://acd.od.nih.gov/documents/reports/PSW_Report_ACD_06042014.pdf (accessed April 27, 2023).
NIH. 2017a. *Clarifying percent effort and support for career development (K) awardees.* https://nexus.od.nih.gov/all/2017/10/11/clarifying-percent-effort-and-support-for-career-development-k-awardees/ (accessed July 21, 2023).
NIH. 2017b. *Reporter.* https://projectreporter.nih.gov/reporter.cfm (accessed December 13, 2022).
NIH. 2021. *The Advisory Committee to the Director Working Group on Diversity Racism in Science Report.* https://www.acd.od.nih.gov/documents/presentations/02262021Diversity Report.pdf (accessed May 8, 2023).
NIH. 2022a. *Diversity and inclusion in clinical trials.* https://www.nimhd.nih.gov/resources/understanding-health-disparities/diversity-and-inclusion-in-clinical-trials.html (accessed December 21, 2022).
NIH. 2022b. *Populations underrepresented in the extramural scientific workforce.* https://diversity.nih.gov/about-us/population-underrepresented (accessed July 10, 2023).
NIH. 2022c. *Extramural loan repayment program for pediatric research (LRP-PR).* https://grants.nih.gov/grants/guide/notice-files/NOT-OD-22-149.html (accessed May 8, 2023).
NIH. 2022d. *UNITE.* https://www.nih.gov/ending-structural-racism/unite (accessed December 5, 2022).
NIH. 2023a. *Comparing popular research project grants—R01, R03, and R21.* https://www.niaid.nih.gov/grants-contracts/research-project-grants (accessed February 7, 2023).
NIH. 2023b. *Estimates of funding for various research, condition, and disease categories (RCDC).* https://report.nih.gov/funding/categorical-spending#/ (accessed April 3, 2023).
NIH. 2023c. *Success rates.* https://report.nih.gov/funding/nih-budget-and-spending-data-past-fiscal-years/success-rates (accessed April 4, 2023).
NIH. 2023d. *NIH LRP dashboard.* https://dashboard.lrp.nih.gov/app/#/ (accessed April 25, 2023).
Nikaj, S., and P. K. Lund. 2019. The impact of individual mentored career development (K) awards on the research trajectories of early-career scientists. *Academic Medicine* 94(5):708-714.
NRC (National Research Council) and IOM. 2004. *Children's health, the nation's wealth: Assessing and improving child health.* Washington, DC: The National Academies Press.
NRMP (National Resident Matching Program). 2023. *Results and data: 2023 main residency match.* https://www.nrmp.org/wp-content/uploads/2023/05/2023-Main-Match-Results-and-Data-Book-FINAL.pdf (accessed July 18, 2023).
Okeigwe, I., C. Wang, J. A. Politch, L. J. Heffner, and W. Kuohung. 2017. Physician-scientists in obstetrics and gynecology: Predictors of success in obtaining independent research funding. *American Journal of Obstetrics and Gynecology* 217(1):84. e81-84, e88.
Page, S. 2007. *The difference: How the power of diversity creates better groups, firms, schools, and societies.* Princeton, NJ: Princeton University Press.
Paik, J. C., G. Howard, and R. G. Lorenz. 2009. Postgraduate choices of graduates from medical scientist training programs, 2004–2008. *JAMA* 302(12):1271-1273.
Patient Centered Outcomes Research Institute (PCORI). 2023. *Children's health.* https://www.pcori.org/topics/childrens-health (accessed May 3, 2023).
Permar, S. R., R. A. Ward, K. J. Barrett, S. A. Freel, R. A. Gbadegesin, C. D. Kontos, P. J. Hu, K. E. Hartmann, C. S. Williams, and J. M. Vyas. 2020. Addressing the physician-scientist pipeline: Strategies to integrate research into clinical training programs. *Journal of Clinical Investigation* 130(3):1058-1061.

PhRMA (Pharmaceutical Research and Manufacturers of America). 2020. *Medicines in development | 2020 report*. https://phrma.org/-/media/Project/PhRMA/PhRMA-Org/PhRMA-Org/PDF/MID-Reports/MID-2020-Children_8_FINAL.pdf (accessed April 27, 2023).

Pickering, C. R., R. C. Bast, Jr., and K. Keyomarsi. 2015. How will we recruit, train, and retain physicians and scientists to conduct translational cancer research? *Cancer* 121(6): 806-816.

Pololi, L. H., A. T. Evans, J. T. Civian, L. A. Cooper, B. K. Gibbs, K. Ninteau, R. K. Dagher, K. Bloom-Feshbach, and R. T. Brennan. 2023. Are researchers in academic medicine flourishing? A survey of midcareer Ph.D. and physician investigators. *Journal of Clinical and Translational Science* 7(1):e105.

Popkin, R., P. Taylor-Zapata, and D. W. Bianchi. 2022. Physician bias and clinical trial participation in underrepresented populations. *Pediatrics* 149(2).

Price Rapoza, M., A. McElvaine, M. B. Conroy, K. Okuyemi, N. Rouphael, S. J. Teach, M. Widlansky, C. Williams, and S. R. Permar. 2022. Early outcomes of a new NIH program to support research in residency. *Academic Medicine* 97(9):1305-1310.

Priest, N., Y. Paradies, B. Trenerry, M. Truong, S. Karlsen, and Y. Kelly. 2013. A systematic review of studies examining the relationship between reported racism and health and wellbeing for children and young people. *Social Science & Medicine* 95:115-127.

Pursley, D. M., T. D. Coyne-Beasley, G. L. Freed, L. R. Walker-Harding, and J. L. Wright. 2020. "Organizational solutions: Calling the question" APS racism series: At the intersection of equity, science, and social justice. *Pediatric Research* 88(5):702-703.

Puumala, S. E., K. M. Burgess, A. B. Kharbanda, H. G. Zook, D. M. Castille, W. J. Pickner, and N. R. Payne. 2016. The role of bias by emergency department providers in care for American Indian children. *Medical Care* 54(6):562.

Ragsdale, J. R., L. M. Vaughn, and M. Klein. 2014. Characterizing the adequacy, effectiveness, and barriers related to research mentorship among junior pediatric hospitalists and general pediatricians at a large academic institution. *Hospital Pediatrics* 4(2):93-98.

Rees, C. A., M. C. Monuteaux, V. Herdell, E. W. Fleegler, and F. T. Bourgeois. 2021. Correlation between National Institutes of Health funding for pediatric research and pediatric disease burden in the US. *JAMA Pediatrics* 175(12):1236-1243.

Rees, C. A., A. Stewart, S. D. Mehta, E. Avakame, J. Jackson, J. McKay, E. N. Portillo, K. Michelson, C. P. Duggan, and E. W. Fleegler. 2022. Race and ethnicity in published pediatric clinical trial enrollment in the United States, 2011–2020. *Pediatrics* 149(1 Meeting Abstracts February 2022):629-629.

Research America. 2022. *U.S. investments in medical and health research and development: 2016-2020*. https://www.researchamerica.org/wp-content/uploads/2022/09/ResearchAmerica-Investment-Report.Final_.January-2022-1.pdf (accessed July 18, 2023).

Rosenberg, L. E. 1999. The physician-scientist: An essential—and fragile—link in the medical research chain. *Journal of Clinical Investigation* 103(12):1621-1626.

Rosenthal, S. L. 2020. Preventing burnout among academic medicine leaders: Experiencing leadership flow. *JAMA Pediatrics* 174(7):636-638.

Rubenstein, R., and J. Kreindler. 2014. On preventing the extinction of the physician-scientist in pediatric pulmonology. *Frontiers in Pediatrics* 2.

Saboor, S., S. Naveed, A. M. Chaudhary, M. Jamali, M. Hussain, J. Siddiqi, and F. Khosa. 2022. Gender and racial profile of the academic pediatric faculty workforce in the United States. *Cureus* 14(2):e22518.

Sachs, A. N., D. Avant, C. S. Lee, W. Rodriguez, and M. D. Murphy. 2012. Pediatric information in drug product labeling. *JAMA* 307(18):1914-1915.

Salas, A. A. 2020. Early career investigator highlight biocommentary. *Pediatric Research* 88(5):688.

Salata, R. A., M. W. Geraci, D. C. Rockey, M. Blanchard, N. J. Brown, L. J. Cardinal, M. Garcia, M. P. Madaio, J. D. Marsh, and R. F. Todd, III. 2018. US physician-scientist workforce in the 21st century: Recommendations to attract and sustain the pipeline. *Academic Medicine* 93(4):565.

SCDAA (Sickle Cell Disease Association of America). 2021. *FAQs: Sickle cell disease.* https://www.sicklecelldisease.org/sickle-cell-health-and-disease/faqs/ (accessed December 19, 2022).

Schafer, A. I. 2010. The vanishing physician-scientist? *Translational Research* 155(1):1-2.

Sekar, K. 2023. *National Institutes of Health (NIH) funding: FY1996-FY2023.* https://sgp.fas.org/crs/misc/R43341.pdf (accessed May 3, 2023).

Shakhnovich, V., C. P. Hornik, G. L. Kearns, J. Weigel, and S. M. Abdel-Rahman. 2019. How to conduct clinical trials in children: A tutorial. *Clinical and Translational Science* 12(3):218-230.

Siebert, A. L., S. Chou, O. Toubat, A. J. Adami, H. Kim, D. Daye, and J. M. Kwan. 2020. Factors associated with underrepresented minority physician scientist trainee career choices. *BMC Medical Education* 20(1):422.

Singh, U., J. Levy, W. Armstrong, R. Bedimo, C. B. Creech, E. Lautenbach, K. J. Popovich, J. Snowden, J. M. Vyas, H. M. A. Infectious Diseases Society of America, and P. I. D. Society. 2018. Policy recommendations for optimizing the infectious diseases physician-scientist workforce. *The Journal of Infectious Diseases* 218(suppl_1):S49-S54.

Somekh, I., E. Somekh, M. Pettoello-Mantovani, and R. Somech. 2019. The clinician scientist, a distinct and disappearing entity. *Journal of Pediatrics* 212:252-253.e252.

Sorkness, C. A., C. Pfund, E. O. Ofili, K. S. Okuyemi, J. K. Vishwanatha, and on behalf of the NRMN team. 2017. A new approach to mentoring for research careers: The national research mentoring network. *BMC Proceedings* 11(Suppl 12):22.

Sotirin, P., and S. M. Goltz. 2023. Mid-career faculty peer mentoring: Rationale and program design. *New Directions for Higher Education* 2023(201-202):5-19.

Speer, E. M., L. K. Lee, F. T. Bourgeois, D. Gitterman, W. W. Hay, Jr., J. M. Davis, and J. R. Javier. 2023. The state and future of pediatric research-an introductory overview: The state and future of pediatric research series. *Pediatric Research*:1-5.

Spong, C. Y., and D. W. Bianchi. 2018. Improving public health requires inclusion of underrepresented populations in research. *JAMA* 319(4):337-338.

Steinbach, W. J., D. K. Benjamin, Jr., and J. W. Sleasman. 2018. Funding pediatric subspecialty training: Are T32 grants the future? *The Journal of Pediatrics* 202:4-7.e1.

Steinbrook, R. 2002. Testing medications in children. *New England Journal of Medicine* 347(18):1462-1470.

Sun, L. R. 2021. Early career investigator highlight biocommentary. *Pediatric Research* 89(4):718.

Tejeda, H. A., S. B. Green, E. L. Trimble, L. Ford, J. L. High, R. S. Ungerleider, M. A. Friedman, and O. W. Brawley. 1996. Representation of African-Americans, Hispanics, and Whites in National Cancer Institute cancer treatment trials. *Journal of the National Cancer Institute* 88(12):812-816.

Teshima, J., A. J. S. McKean, M. T. Myint, S. Aminololama-Shakeri, S. V. Joshi, A. L. Seritan, and D. M. Hilty. 2019. Developmental approaches to faculty development. *Psychiatric Clinics of North America* 42(3):375-387.

Thompson, B. M., E. M. Moser, J. D. Gonzalo, D. R. Wolpaw, T. D. Dreibelbis, and T. M. Wolpaw. 2020. Penn State College of Medicine. *Academic Medicine* 95(9S):S434-S438.

Thomson, D., L. Hartling, E. Cohen, B. Vandermeer, L. Tjosvold, and T. P. Klassen. 2010. Controlled trials in children: Quantity, methodological quality and descriptive characteristics of pediatric controlled trials published 1948–2006. *PLoS One* 5(9).

Tisdale, S., and L. Pellizzoni. 2015. Disease mechanisms and therapeutic approaches in spinal muscular atrophy. *Journal of Neuroscience* 35(23):8691-8700.

Todd III, R. F., R. A. Salata, M. E. Klotman, M. L. Weisfeldt, J. T. Katz, S. X. Xian, D. P. Hearn, and R. S. Lipner. 2013. Career outcomes of the graduates of the American Board of Internal Medicine research pathway, 1995–2007. *Academic Medicine* 88(11):1747-1753.

Trachtenberg, F. L., E. A. Haas, H. C. Kinney, C. Stanley, and H. F. Krous. 2012. Risk factor changes for sudden infant death syndrome after initiation of Back-to-Sleep campaign. *Pediatrics* 129(4):630-638.

Trent, M., D. G. Dooley, J. Dougé, R. M. Cavanaugh, A. E. Lacroix, J. Fanburg, M. H. Rahmandar, L. L. Hornberger, M. B. Schneider, and S. Yen. 2019. The impact of racism on child and adolescent health. *Pediatrics* 144(2).

Twombly, D. A., S. L. Glavin, J. Guimond, S. Taymans, C. Y. Spong, and D. W. Bianchi. 2018. Association of National Institute of Child Health and Human Development career development awards with subsequent research project grant funding. *JAMA Pediatrics* 172(3):226-231.

Varnell, C. D., Jr., P. Margolis, J. Goebel, and D. K. Hooper. 2023. The learning health system for pediatric nephrology: Building better systems to improve health. *Pediatric Nephrology* 38(1):35-46.

Vasylyeva, T. L., M. E. Díaz-González de Ferris, D. S. Hains, J. Ho, L. A. Harshman, K. J. Reidy, T. M. Brady, D. M. Okamura, D. V. Samsonov, and S. E. Wenderfer. 2019. Developing a research mentorship program: The American Society of Pediatric Nephrology's experience. *Frontiers in Pediatrics* 7:155.

Vidyasagar, D. 2007. Integrating international medical graduates into the physician-scientist pool: Solution to the problem of decreasing physician-scientists in the United States. *Journal of Investigative Medicine* 55(8):406-409.

Viergever, R. F., and C. M. Rademaker. 2014. Finding better ways to fill gaps in pediatric health research. *Pediatrics* 133(4):e824-e826.

Wade, C. 2021. Physician–scientists in the era of COVID-19: Gone but not forgotten. *Academic Medicine* 96(1):e5-e6.

Walensky, R. P., Y. Kim, Y. Chang, B. C. Porneala, M. N. Bristol, K. Armstrong, and E. G. Campbell. 2018. The impact of active mentorship: Results from a survey of faculty in the department of medicine at massachusetts general hospital. *BMC Medical Education* 18(1):108.

Walker-Harding, L. R., C. W. Bogue, K. D. Hendricks-Munoz, J. L. Raphael, and J. L. Wright. 2020. "Challenges and opportunities in academic medicine" APS racism series: At the intersection of equity, science, and social justice. *Pediatric Research* 88(5):699-701.

Walsh, C., and L. F. Ross. 2003. Are minority children under-or overrepresented in pediatric research? *Pediatrics* 112(4):890-895.

Watson, S. E., P. Smith, J. Snowden, V. Vaughn, L. Cottrell, C. A. Madden, A. S. Kong, R. McCulloh, C. Stack Lim, M. Bledsoe, K. Kowal, M. McNally, L. Knight, K. Cowan, and E. Yakes Jimenez. 2022. Facilitators and barriers to pediatric clinical trial recruitment and retention in rural and community settings: A scoping review of the literature. *Clinical and Translational Science* 15(4):838-853.

Williams, C. S., A. N. Iness, R. M. Baron, O. A. Ajijola, P. J. Hu, J. M. Vyas, R. Baiocchi, A. J. Adami, J. M. Lever, P. S. Klein, L. Demer, M. Madaio, M. Geraci, L. F. Brass, M. Blanchard, R. Salata, and M. Zaidi. 2018. Training the physician-scientist: Views from program directors and aspiring young investigators. *JCI Insight* 3(23).

Williams, C. S., W. K. Rathmell, J. M. Carethers, D. M. Harper, Y. M. D. Lo, P. J. Ratcliffe, and M. Zaidi. 2022. A global view of the aspiring physician-scientist. *eLife* 11:e79738.

Winestone, L. E., K. D. Getz, P. Rao, Y. Li, M. Hall, Y.-S. V. Huang, A. E. Seif, B. T. Fisher, and R. Aplenc. 2019. Disparities in pediatric acute myeloid leukemia (AML) clinical trial enrollment. *Leukemia & Lymphoma* 60(9):2190-2198.

Woodward, L. J., L. J. Horwood, B. A. Darlow, and S. Bora. 2022. Visuospatial working memory of children and adults born very preterm and/or very low birth weight. *Pediatric Research* 91(6):1436-1444.

Wright, J. L., J. N. Jarvis, L. M. Pachter, and L. R. Walker-Harding. 2020. "Racism as a public health issue" APS racism series: At the intersection of equity, science, and social justice. *Pediatric Research* 88(5):696-698.

Wyngaarden, J. B. 1979. The clinical investigator as an endangered species. *New England Journal of Medicine* 301(23):1254-1259.

Yap, K. K. 2012. The clinician-scientist: Uniquely poised to integrate science and medicine. *Australian Medical Studies J* 3:10-11.

Yin, H. L., J. Gabrilove, R. Jackson, C. Sweeney, A. M. Fair, and R. Toto. 2015. Sustaining the clinical and translational research workforce: Training and empowering the next generation of investigators. *Academic Medicine* 90(7):861-865.

Zemlo, T. R., H. H. Garrison, N. C. Partridge, and T. J. Ley. 2000. The physician-scientist: Career issues and challenges at the year 2000. *FASEB Journal* 14(2):221-230.

Zhong, Y., X. Zhang, L. Zhou, L. Li, and T. Zhang. 2021. Updated analysis of pediatric clinical studies registered in clinicaltrials.gov, 2008–2019. *BMC Pediatrics* 21(1):1-14.

7

Innovations at the Pediatric Primary–Specialty Care Interface

The nation's primary care workforce for children comprises many clinicians, including general primary care pediatricians, family medicine physicians, general internists (particularly in rural areas and for adolescents and young adults), and advanced practice providers (e.g., nurse practitioners [NPs], and physician assistants). There is also an extended team of health care professionals that work with primary care clinicians. Depending on needs, these professionals can include professionals such as behavioral health specialists, social workers, community health workers, and care coordinators (NASEM, 2021b). (See Chapter 4 for a discussion of the overall pediatric workforce.) The *pediatric medical home* includes pediatric clinicians (known to the child and family) who deliver or direct primary medical care that is "accessible, continuous, comprehensive, patient- and family-centered, coordinated, compassionate, and culturally effective" while a *pediatric medical neighborhood* includes "pediatric medical subspecialists, surgical specialists, mental and behavioral health specialists, and other [community partners] who work collaboratively with the pediatric medical home" (Price et al., 2020 pg. 2).

Ideally, general primary care clinicians and pediatric subspecialty physicians work collaboratively at the interface of primary and specialty care to provide the full spectrum of care for children with more complicated and unusual acute and chronic disorders. Most health issues for children are initially addressed in pediatric primary care, which acts as the site of first contact for the full range of a child's new health needs and the site of comprehensive care for routine care, preventive services, and most disorders. Primary care clinicians coordinate referrals to specialists or subspecialists within a patient's medical neighborhood (Kirschner and Greenlee, 2010; Medical Home Initiatives for Children with Special Needs Project Advisory Committee, 2002; NASEM, 2021b; Starfield, 1998). This chapter examines the interaction of primary care and pediatric subspecialty care with a focus on the efficient use of both primary care and subspecialty care clinicians and innovative models at the interface of primary and specialty care so as to ensure the delivery of high-quality subspecialty care.

COLLABORATION AND COORDINATION BETWEEN PEDIATRIC PRIMARY AND SPECIALTY CARE

General primary care and subspecialty pediatric clinicians often work closely together to deliver comprehensive care for children with and without complex medical needs, along with other health care providers and community partners. Collaboration and coordination among all members of the health care team is a component of high-quality care (Eichner et al., 2012; Huang and Rosenthal, 2014; Lax et al., 2021). The 2001 Institute of Medicine report *Crossing the Quality Chasm: A New Health System for the 21st Century* emphasized the importance of an interprofessional team to meet the needs of patients with increasingly complex health care needs (IOM, 2001). Team-based care has been defined as:

> the provision of health services to individuals, families, and/or their communities by at least two health providers who work collaboratively with patients and their caregivers—to the extent preferred by each patient—to accomplish shared goals within and across settings to achieve coordinated, high-quality care. (Mitchell et al., 2012)

Team-based care has been associated with higher quality of care, higher patient satisfaction, lower use, and reduced clinician burnout (Meyers et al., 2019; NASEM, 2021b; Pany et al., 2021; Reiss-Brennan et al., 2016; Will et al., 2019; Willard-Grace et al., 2014). In children specifically, research reveals the impact of team-based care on health maintenance, prevention of disease, acute illness management, and chronic disease management (Burkhart et al., 2020; Katkin et al., 2017; McLeigh et al., 2022; Reiss-Brennan et al., 2016). Team-based care was included among recommendations in the 2021 report from the National Academies of Sciences, Engineering, and Medicine (National Academies) on high-quality primary care (NASEM, 2021b). For example, one study showed that among chronically ill children, team-based care resulted in fewer hospitalizations, emergency department visits, and urgent care visits (Meyers et al., 2019). A few studies of children and adolescents have evaluated co-management of conditions between primary and subspecialty care with generally positive results (Richardson et al., 2009; Van Cleave et al., 2018). A meta-analysis of integrated primary care–behavioral health models for children and adolescents demonstrated superior outcomes for the integrated care model when compared with conventional care, and collaborative care models with a team-based approach that included primary care clinicians, care managers, and mental health specialists showed the strongest effects (Asarnow et al., 2015; NASEM, 2021b). See Box 7-1 for clinician perspectives on team-based care among pediatric primary and specialty care clinicians.

However, current payment models for care generally do not reward aspects of primary care–subspecialty collaboration, creating a disincentive for further evaluation and implementation of collaborative models (Kuo et al., 2022; Landon, 2014; Price et al., 2020). In August 2022, the Centers for Medicare & Medicaid Services (CMS) released guidance on a new option for states to cover an optional health home plan benefit in their Medicaid programs for children with medically complex conditions (CMS, 2022c). This new option enables states to design coordinated care systems for Medicaid-eligible children with chronic or rare conditions and allows flexibility with respect to certain Medicaid provisions such as statewideness[1]

BOX 7-1
Clinician Perspectives—Team-Based Care

"Team care has expanded substantially in health care in the past several years, both in primary care and in subspecialty pediatric practice. Team care has many advantages over previous approaches, bringing attention to important aspects of care, including coordination across services, reengagement with community services, home nursing, greater attention to co-existing mental/behavioral health concerns, family impact and well-being, etc."
– Professor of Pediatrics, Boston, MA

"Pediatric critical care in particular is very much a "team sport" that requires exceptional coordination between trained physicians and well-trained, experienced nurses, therapists, and other ancillary providers."
– Attending Pediatric Intensivist, Houston, TX

These quotes were collected from the committee's online call for trainee, clinician, and family perspectives.

---

[1] Statewideness refers to a requirement that the managed care program must be operational statewide.

and, notably, payment methodology. For example, states can reimburse designated providers (including providing higher payment to compensate for coordination time) or can reimburse teams. The federal government provides enhanced matching funds for the first 2 years of such programs to support their implementation.

Care Plans

Evidence from behavioral health integration shows that shared plans of care can significantly enhance the quality of care, prevent duplication of services, and reduce risk of adverse events (Collins et al., 2010). However, fewer than half of pediatric primary care clinicians in one study reported that patient care plans were integrated with pediatric medical subspecialists (Stille et al., 2006). Furthermore, pediatric primary care clinicians and subspecialists who did not consistently receive communications were significantly more likely to report that their ability to provide high-quality care was compromised (Stille et al., 2006). This speaks to a need for better coordination to facilitate subspecialty care for the elements of care that only a subspecialist can perform while delegating some aspects of care for a condition to a primary care clinician. For example, pediatric subspecialty care has become more sophisticated in the use of therapeutics for chronic conditions that require expertise and facilities not typically available to primary care clinicians. The use of biologic pharmaceuticals for immune-mediated conditions such as inflammatory bowel disease, juvenile inflammatory arthritis, and even severe eczema often requires access to an infusion center for administration and carries the risk of serious side effects that must be closely monitored.

Patients and Families

When children require care from multiple subspecialists and/or require multiple other health care services, coordination of that care is time-consuming but necessary to avoid duplication of and gaps in needed services. However, such coordination is frequently absent or fragmented, leaving parents as the main link between clinicians in different organizations (Stille et al., 2007). These themes were highlighted by Ileana Barron, parent of a child who receives pediatric subspecialty care, during the committee's first webinar on patient and family perspectives.[2]

---

[2] The webinar recording can be accessed at https://www.nationalacademies.org/event/07-19-2022/the-pediatric-subspecialty-workforce-and-its-impact-on-child-health-and-well-being-webinar-1.

Along this journey, my family has seen the ways the system makes getting care easier, but we've also seen the gaps that make specialty care complicated and frustrating. And for those issues that complicate care, we can put coordination of care at the top of the list…First, unless the subspecialists share a combined clinic, communication is often difficult, even within the same hospital system. And in many cases, it relies on individual initiatives to maintain those connections. When we think that communication will be easy when clinicians have access to the same medical record system, but it often isn't, it is essential that the subspecialists talk to each other and develop a shared care plan. But doing so is often difficult, and we have found ourselves being passed back and forth between specialists many times. The second problem in coordinating care is a lack of communication effort between subspecialists and primary care clinicians. Pediatricians are rarely well informed about what subspecialists are doing. They're rarely fully included in the care plan, and parents like me and my husband often have to be the ones keeping the pediatrician up to date with the care plan. Our complicated son should be able to go to the pediatrician instead of the top specialist to handle acute exacerbations of his chronic illnesses. And although some hospitals have created specific complex care clinics that are meant to deal with these issues, the benefits of these clinics are limited to current patients of these large hospitals. Children like my son will continue getting colds that potentially become pneumonias, and gastrointestinal illnesses that would require a specific and unique care plan of care. So having a pediatrician who is part of the team and feels comfortable treating these complex children in those situations will keep families like mine from having to go to the ED [emergency department] or having to reach out to the subspecialist for one of those impossible to get sick child appointments…. For the things that make the system work more efficiently…[having] other professionals, health professionals support the specialist practices, having NPs or PAs [physician assistants] that are trained in the subspecialty field, is very important.

This sentiment was reiterated by a clinician who responded to the committee's call for perspectives:

I find families either do not access what is needed or end up duplicating evaluations/services or spend time accessing unnecessary resources because of poor communication and fragmented care (need to see a different professional for every problem even though one clinician might be able to address) which increases the stress on families and cost to the health care system.
—Developmental-Behavioral Pediatrician, Wyckoff, NJ

Care Coordination during Transitions from Pediatric to Adult Care

As discussed in Chapter 2, the transition from pediatric to adult care can be difficult. One review of 29 studies that focused on adolescents and young adults with chronic health conditions concluded that shared models of care and communication among the primary care clinician, the adolescent/young adult, and the pediatric subspecialist were associated with positive outcomes during transition (Schraeder et al., 2022). Without adequate support during this transition, adolescents and young adults with chronic illnesses face an increased risk of adverse outcomes, including medical complications, decreased treatment adherence, increased emergency department use and hospitalization, and increased health care costs (McManus et al., 2020; White et al., 2018).

Transitions of care require support, planning, and intentional actions among multiple clinicians to create a defined, purposeful transition from pediatric to adult care (Castillo and Kitsos, 2017; Got Transition, 2022). Registered nurses are well suited to act as the liaison between the pediatric and adult practices. Specifically, registered nurses can help with the management of referral documents, quality improvement processes to ensure effective communication among clinicians, and in monitoring the transition overall (Betz, 2017; Varty et al., 2020). During one of the committee's information-gathering sessions, Christian Lawson discussed his transition from pediatric to adult care:

> [The] transition from pediatrics to adult GI was a little bit of a challenge… eventually when I did transition, we were able to form this partnership between my physician and my specialist, so now they kind of work hand in hand with trying to make sure that the records are up to date on both sides…it works well, primarily if it's kind of in the same network or same area where the specialist might be.[3]

Adult subspecialists have found the transition of care for children with special health care needs to be more complex compared with assuming care of adult chronic care patients (Kobussen et al., 2021). Specifically, adult subspecialists found challenges that include increased time and resource burdens; the management of the expectations of patients and families; navigation of the discrepancies in goals of care; the complexity of coordination among services; and a need for increased efforts in coordinating discharge from the hospital (Kobussen et al., 2021). To facilitate successful transitions of care for pediatric patients, clinicians who provide care for adults have

---

[3] The webinar recording can be accessed at https://www.nationalacademies.org/event/07-19-2022/the-pediatric-subspecialty-workforce-and-its-impact-on-child-health-and-well-being-webinar-1.

expressed a desire for improved infrastructure (e.g., links to community resources, consultation support when needed) and education and training about specific diseases as well as the physical and behavioral stages of adolescent development (White et al., 2016). Given gaps in physician training around transitions of care and extensive role of care coordination associated with transitions of care, there is a vital role for interprofessional teams (particularly the inclusion of registered nurses and NPs) in supporting these transitions (Betz, 2017; Castillo and Kitsos, 2017; Lestishock et al., 2018; Lestishock, 2020; NASEM, 2021a; Sharma et al., 2014).

CHALLENGES OF CONSULTATION, REFERRAL, AND CO-MANAGEMENT

Primary care clinicians often care for many patients with chronic conditions. For example, Nasir et al. (2018) found that more than half of pediatric patients in community clinics had at least one chronic problem, and 25 percent had at least two. Primary care clinicians generally refer to subspecialists when children: (1) have problems that are rare; (2) require a technical procedure; (3) need recommendations to support a specific diagnosis or treatment; (4) do not respond to conventional therapy; or (5) display signs and symptoms that could indicate the presence of a condition that is more severe than can be typically managed within primary care.

Referral Processes

Referral from primary care clinicians to subspecialists is a multistep process, and barriers can exist within these steps. During one of the committee's information-gathering sessions, Kristin Ray, associate professor of pediatrics at the University of Pittsburgh School of Medicine, presented on pediatric referral processes; much of the following section is based on this presentation.[4] (See Chapter 2 for more information on demand for referrals.)

A 2017 report from the Institute for Healthcare Improvement provided insight into the steps that are required for optimal referral and the degree to which optimal closed-loop referrals involves multiple people (see Figure 7-1).

According to the report, primary care clinicians, specialists, patients, and schedulers are involved in nine overall steps, each of which can experience barriers that contribute to suboptimal access to pediatric subspecialty

---

[4] The webinar recording can be accessed at https://www.nationalacademies.org/event/11-09-2022/the-pediatric-subspecialty-workforce-and-its-impact-on-child-health-and-well-being-webinar-4.

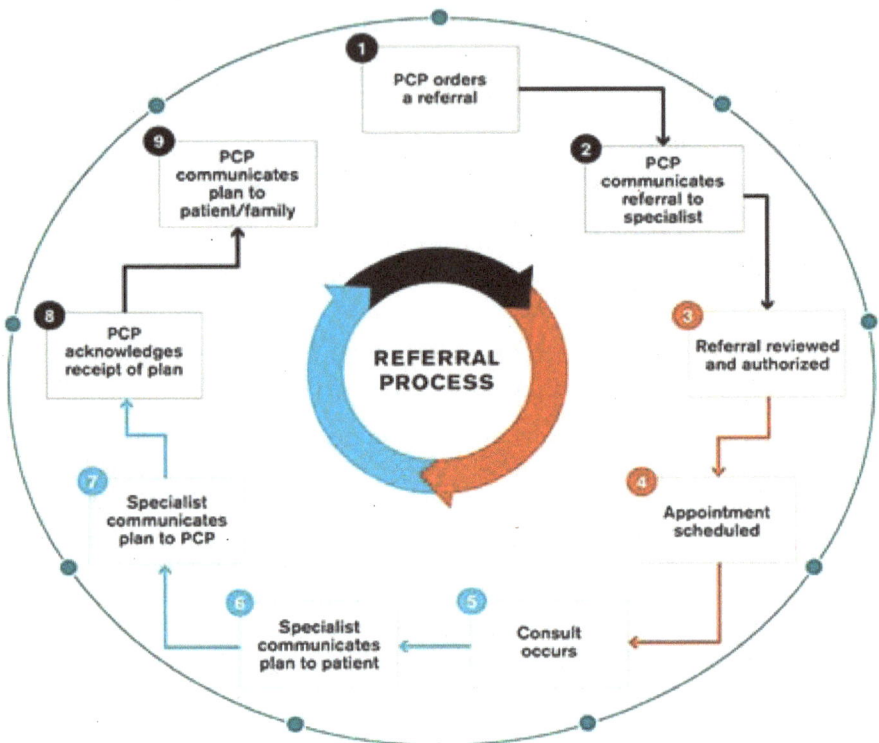

FIGURE 7-1 Closed-loop process for optimal referrals.
NOTE: Technical (hardware, software) factors are noted in blue; sociological factors (workflow, staff) are noted in orange; PCP = primary care provider
SOURCE: Institute for Healthcare Improvement and the National Patient Safety Foundation (2017). Reprinted with permission from the Institute for Healthcare Improvement, ihi.org.

care. At the initial step of referral decision, primary care clinicians may be uncertain regarding whether to refer, where to refer, and the degree of work to be completed before referral. At the next step of preconsultative communication, information may not be sent, received, or reviewed. In appointment scheduling, there may be inadequate capacity for scheduling due to demand exceeding supply, leading to an inability to schedule or to long wait times. In addition, barriers are present internally to the scheduling process; long phone trees or unattended voice mailboxes can lead to unscheduled or suboptimally scheduled appointments. Within the consultative visit, there may be geographic or time barriers, language and literacy barriers, or other equity issues that interfere with an optimal visit. At the postconsultative communication step, there may be inadequate communication processes among patients, specialists, and primary care clinicians that lead to confusion, inadequate care, or care redundancies.

Many referrals are never completed due to these barriers. A study of one year of referrals from primary care clinicians to medical and surgical subspecialists was found that only 51 percent of referrals resulted in a completed visit within 3 months of referral (Bohnhoff, 2019). Out of the remainder of referrals, a third were never scheduled, and an additional sixth were scheduled, but not attended. According to the 2020–2021 National Survey of Children's Health,[5] 26 percent of families in need of subspecialty care encountered difficulty in obtaining specialty care (NSCH, n.d.).[6] This percentage increased to 32 percent for families with a primary household language other than English, 32 percent for children receiving public insurance, and 40 percent for children who are uninsured, thereby contributing to inequities in access and use (NSCH, n.d.). (See Chapter 2 for more on the influences on children's access to subspecialty care.)

Training for Consultation and Referral

Truly integrated care will require enhanced training in some areas, particularly subspecialty referral and appropriate consultation (Ray et al., 2016). The American Board of Pediatrics has identified "provide consultation to other health care providers caring for children" and "refer patients who require consultation" as essential, entrustable professional activities[7] for graduating pediatric residents (ABP, 2023; Hamburger et al., 2015). However, among pediatric residents from 2015 to 2018, nearly one-third (31 percent) of graduating residents did not achieve "entrustment with unsupervised practice" for providing consultations and 18 percent did not achieve this benchmark for making referrals (Schumacher et al., 2020).

Training medical residents on how to interact effectively with consultants can improve collaborative care (Adekolujo et al., 2019). For example, Freed et al. (2020) suggested that focusing education on essential condition-specific management strategies for commonly referred oncology conditions enhances primary care management of these diagnoses. The Children's National Hospital Syncope Education Project is an example of enhanced training for residents in the referral process wherein pediatric residents on

---

[5] In the National Survey of Children's Health, specialist doctors were defined as "doctors like surgeons, heart doctors, allergy doctors, skin doctors, and others who specialize in one area of health care" (NSCH, n.d.). See Indicator 4.5 for more information.

[6] This percentage was calculated using Indicator 4.5a. The denominator of this measure is based on the response to the question which asks whether the child received a specialist care.

[7] Entrustable professional activities for pediatrics are "observable, routine activities that a general pediatrician should be able to perform safely and effectively to meet the needs of their patients" (ABP, 2023).

rotation in cardiology completed a "workshop focusing on red-flag criteria for cardiology referral and practiced with standardized parents" (Stave et al., 2022). The project resulted in "significant improvements in self-efficacy and parents' rating of their communication" (Stave et al., 2022, pg.2). When the curriculum was expanded to focus on advanced communication skills, Stave et al. (2022) found that residents' communication skills improved immediately postintervention for subspecialty referral. The authors suggest that this curriculum can be broadened to include other patient scenarios.

Expansion of the Role of Primary Care

The appropriate scope of pediatric primary care has been debated in the United States for decades (Leslie et al., 2000; NASEM, 2021b). Recent trends in the expansion of the role of primary care include integration with behavioral health, specifically, and with community providers to address social and structural determinants of health more generally (AACAP, 2023; Arbour et al., 2021; CMS, 2022b; Gillespie et al., 2022). Collaboration and co-management with subspecialists are a natural fit with these trends; however, this expansion of scope has not been met with a concurrent expansion of resources (Price et al., 2020), making it difficult for most primary care clinicians to embrace co-management to the degree they might otherwise. See Box 7-2 for clinician perspectives on resource challenges at the primary–specialty care interface.

Expanding the scope of primary care clinicians is particularly relevant in rural areas. During one of the committee's public webinars, Robert Hostoffer, clinical professor at the Ohio University Heritage College of Osteopathic Medicine at Athens, and associate professor at Case Western Reserve University in Cleveland), provided his perspectives on rural pediatric scope of practice, stating: "[for rural pediatricians], their scope of practice is large...a lot of time is spent on things that they can't get a hold of a subspecialist for. I think their scope of practice has expanded."[8]

PROMISING PRIMARY–SPECIALTY CARE MODELS

Appropriate primary care management and referral to subspecialists are important factors that affect demand for subspecialty care. Many diagnoses for which patients are referred may be addressable to some extent in primary care, and many specialist-induced follow-up visits for a referred health problem could be done in primary care settings. Reserving care by primary

---

[8] The webinar recording can be accessed at https://www.nationalacademies.org/event/09-06-2022/the-pediatric-subspecialty-workforce-and-its-impact-on-child-health-and-well-being-webinar-2.

> **BOX 7-2**
> **Clinician Perspectives—Resource Challenges at the Primary–Specialty Care Interface**
>
> "There would be less need for subspecialists if primary care docs were paid enough to be able to spend a reasonable amount of time with patients so they could care for the more common subspecialty problems, like constipation."
> **– Attending Physician in Pediatric Gastroenterology, San Francisco, CA**
>
> "With the shortage of pediatric subspecialists, especially in my subspecialty, and insurance pressures (reimbursement levels and policies) it is much more difficult to be able to spend the time needed to do a comprehensive evaluation, collaborate with other specialists, and spend the time needed to provide excellent care for complex patients whose issues cross a variety of disciplines."
> **– Developmental-Behavioral Pediatrician, Wyckoff, NJ**
>
> *These quotes were collected from the committee's online call for trainee, clinician, and family perspectives.*

care clinicians for pediatric patients with common chronic conditions, such as asthma, attention deficit hyperactivity disorder (ADHD), and obesity, or preparing them to provide some part of the care they might otherwise refer to a subspecialist would allow subspecialists to focus on the children with more severe and/or complex care needs and the technical work that primary care cannot address. However, the data analyses in Chapter 3, as well as older studies (e.g., Forrest et al., 1999), provide evidence that many common diagnoses in medical subspecialists' practices may be conditions or health problems that can and should be routinely managed in primary care settings, suggesting a potential inefficiency in the use of referrals to pediatric medical subspecialists. Factors needed to facilitate optimal management and referral include education and mutual dialogue between primary care and subspecialty pediatric clinicians; prereferral management and treatment guidelines; new models of care; and payment models that acknowledge the time requirements and value of collaboration (Children's National, 2023; Cornell et al., 2015; Feyissa et al., 2015; Harahsheh et al., 2021; NASEM, 2021b; Rubin et al., 2014; Seattle Children's, 2023).

To achieve seamless integration of primary care and subspecialty care, innovations in workforce, processes, technology, payment, and setting of care are needed, with a consideration of equity within each of these elements. Several evidence-based models show promise to increase access to pediatric subspecialty care and support the judicious use of all members of interprofessional pediatric care teams. Viewed broadly as innovations in pediatric care delivery, provider education, and interprofessional care, the committee categorized each innovation into a typology and summarized their supporting evidence below. The typology consists of the following:

1. Integrating primary care and subspecialty care;
2. Using telemedicine and telehealth (broadly defined);
3. Facilitating access through nursing; and
4. Appropriately financing the primary–specialty care interface.

Integrating Primary Care and Subspecialty Care

Promising models that integrate primary care and subspecialty care include models for co-management and co-location of primary care clinicians and subspecialists, educational activities to encourage expanded primary care clinician scope of practice, and the determination of appropriate management and referral guidelines.

Models of Co-Management

Co-managed care is a type of team-based care that is planned, delivered, and evaluated by two or more clinicians (Fevissa et al., 2015). The pediatric subspecialist can have different levels of responsibility in the co-management model. For example, the subspecialist could be a co-manager with shared care and share long-term management with a primary care clinician for a patient's referred health problem, or the subspecialist could be a co-manager with principal care and assume total responsibility for the long-term management of a referred health problem, while the primary care clinician cares for all other health conditions and concerns (Forrest, 2009). In exceptional cases where a child has a condition primarily involving a single organ system that requires intensive management, such as sickle cell disease or cancer, it may be appropriate for the subspecialist to serve as the primary manager, either for the short term (e.g., with cancer) or longer term (e.g., with sickle cell disease) (Antonelli et al., 2005; Van Cleave et al., 2016). Outcomes of co-management models have found improved communication and decreased inpatient use (de Banate et al., 2019; Cady and Belew, 2017; Casey et al., 2011; Cohen et al., 2012; McClain et al., 2014). Importantly, when co-management is arranged, making sure that primary care clinicians, subspecialists, and families agree on the specifics of the arrangement is essential so that expectations from clinicians and families are met and access to subspecialty care is maximized. According to a survey conducted on pediatricians and family practitioners in New Hampshire, there was a widespread endorsement of the co-management model, particularly for conditions that were seldom encountered (McClain et al., 2014).

Several models promote co-management within the context of available local and regional resources for local primary care clinicians and subspecialists at referral centers (Cooley et al., 2013; Crego et al., 2020; Feyissa et al., 2015; Rubin et al., 2014). The implementation of co-management models can enhance the ability of primary care clinicians to treat prevalent pediatric conditions in the medical home, while allocating subspecialty resources for more urgent or complex care. Feyissa et al. (2015) found that co-management significantly improved the likelihood of pediatric concussion patients receiving primary care follow-up. A similar co-management model has also been used to address mild to moderate depression and anxiety (Rubin et al., 2014).

Two NP-led co-management models, TeleFamilies (using an advanced practice registered nurse [APRN] coordinator embedded within an established medical home) and PRoSPer (using a registered nurse/social worker care coordinator team embedded within a specialty care system), were developed for children with medical complexity in Minnesota and funded by research grants (Cady et al., 2015). These models used a nurse to undertake care coordination between primary care providers, subspecialists, and families of children with medical complexity, serving as a "one-stop shop" for care coordination among multiple services. A study of the TeleFamilies model indicated that patients and families highly value relationships and access to single individuals in care coordination and the APRN's extended scope of practice lessened the handoffs necessary during care coordination, resulting in a faster resolution time and decreased risk of interruptions or delays in care (Looman et al., 2015). The PRoSPer model's success was contingent on building relationships with families and primary care partners, helping the specialty care coordination team to communicate questions, concerns, and education on care management (Cady et al., 2015; Cady and Belew, 2017).

Co-Location of Primary and Subspecialty Care

Co-location, where clinicians work together in the same physical space, is another potential element of integration (Richman et al., 2018). Co-location allows clinicians to more easily communicate and coordinate care and offers opportunities for "warm handoffs"[9] between clinicians (Blount, 2003; Bonciani et al., 2018; Platt et al., 2018; Richman et al., 2018).

---

[9] A warm handoff is "a handoff that is conducted in person, between two members of the health care team, in front of the patient (and family if present)" (AHRQ, 2023).

Integrated Behavioral Health and Primary Care

Most evidence around the effectiveness of co-location comes from integrated behavioral health care, where behavioral health and primary care are provided in the same location (Bower et al., 2001; National Council for Mental Wellbeing, 2021; SAMHSA, 2023; Yonek et al., 2020). Co-location of primary care and specialty behavioral health services is a new strategic priority of the U.S. Department of Health and Human Services to address the urgent need for improved access to behavioral health care (HHS, 2022). The model uses mental health clinicians (primarily child psychologists, psychology trainees, and master's-level social workers, as well as child psychiatrists and psychiatry trainees) who provide services at the same site as primary care; the model is generally supported by primary care clinicians because onsite specialty mental health services help to overcome access barriers (Collins et al., 2010; Platt et al., 2018; Strosahl, 2005).

According to a scoping review, integrated care programs have been found to increase the likelihood of families attending an initial appointment, complying with recommended treatment, and receiving specialty mental health care when needed, as compared with referrals to usual specialty care (Platt et al., 2018). The review also suggested that having the integrated care provider co-employed in both the primary care and specialty settings facilitated referrals to specialty care when necessary (Briggs et al., 2012; Levy et al., 2017; Platt et al., 2018; Subotsky and Brown, 1990; Ward-Zimmerman and Cannata, 2012). Implementation of co-location models varied, with team-based models (including psychology, social work, and psychiatry) receiving higher rates of referrals to the behavioral health clinician compared with a sole co-located provider (Germán et al., 2017).

Generalist Embedded in Specialty Clinics (Reverse Co-Location)

Multidisciplinary clinics for complex or rare conditions located within academic medical centers often become the medical home for children with these conditions. In many cases, these clinics benefit from the presence of a general pediatrician who can work with families to address aspects of the conditions that may not be easily addressed by a single subspecialty (Simon et al., 2017). For example, a general pediatrician embedded within a clinic treating children with myelomeningocele may address preventive, developmental, educational, and community resource needs of children in the clinic, filling an important gap in their care while allowing subspecialists to focus on their area of strength. There is some evidence for this model in adult behavioral health, known as "reverse co-location," where a primary care clinician is stationed part- or full-time in a mental health specialty setting to monitor the physical health of patients (Collins et al., 2010) with evidence of decreased emergency department visits (Boardman, 2006).

A variation on this model involves a general pediatrician embedded in the same physical spaces with subspecialists, but without their direct involvement, to evaluate uncomplicated potential referrals and escalate them to subspecialty care as needed, also called "access clinics." Matt Di Guglielmo, director of the Division of General Academic Pediatrics at Nemours Children's Hospital, described the access clinics at Nemours Children's Health in his presentation at one of the committee's public webinars.[10] Given that wait times for specific pediatric subspecialties ranged from weeks to months, Nemours developed access clinics to improve 5-day access for new pediatric patients by embedding a general pediatrician, assisted by a nurse navigator into subspecialty clinics (Di Guglielmo et al., 2013, 2016). This model was initially implemented in three clinics: ADHD, headache, and gastroenterology. The ADHD clinic was staffed by psychologists, and the headache and gastroenterology clinics were staffed by general pediatricians who were not formally trained in those subspecialties. The generalists were given additional, specific training (in an ongoing manner), and the clinics were in the same physical space as the relevant subspecialists, enabling real-time consultation. Complementary strategies included physician priority telephone lines that were available for clinicians to call in and speak to a subspecialist within 5 minutes, and having a number of slots in the subspecialist's schedule that would only open several days prior to the appointment.

Initial barriers included the reluctance of some general pediatricians to refer to another general pediatrician, but positive experiences led to greater use of the clinics. The clinics were successful in reducing wait times for new patient appointments. In these early clinics, wait times for a new patient visit in gastroenterology decreased from an average of 25 days to 1 day; similarly, wait times for headache/ADHD decreased from an average of 77 days to 1 or 2 days. Some clinics were phased out and others have been added. Nemours currently has these types of clinics in a variety of other subspecialty areas and is experiencing similar reductions in wait times. For example, the wait for a new patient visit in dermatology is now 1 week (compared with 4 months previously) and 1 month for behavioral and developmental health care (compared to with months previously). Additionally, clinicians, patients, and families reported high levels of satisfaction.

---

[10] The webinar recording can be accessed at https://www.nationalacademies.org/event/11-09-2022/the-pediatric-subspecialty-workforce-and-its-impact-on-child-health-and-well-being-webinar-4.

Subspecialist Office Hours within the Primary Care Practice

For relatively common conditions requiring some degree of subspecialty input but not fully integrated care, subspecialists may be available for limited hours (e.g., 1 day a week) within a primary care clinic. This model may be particularly helpful for children with difficulty accessing the specialty care system because of distance or transportation difficulties.

Educational Activities to Encourage Expanded Primary Care Clinician Scope of Practice

Extending primary care clinician capacity to manage conditions that are commonly referred to subspecialists can be valuable for patients and enhance primary care clinicians' satisfaction. While the American Board of Pediatrics defines numerous areas in which pediatricians should generally be able to provide a complete consultation (e.g., common behavioral and developmental concerns, acute and chronic health conditions, and mental health conditions), there are also areas in which general pediatricians should usually seek additional consultation such as critical care issues; complex or serious mental health conditions (e.g., suicidal or homicidal behavior, mental health conditions not responding to usual therapies); and complex or rare health conditions requiring medical or surgical subspecialty expertise (ABP, 2021).

Multiple-provider primary care practices often support the development of concentrations among individual clinicians who become the practice's expert in caring for patients with common conditions that have specialty care needs (Cohen et al., 2018). Examples include behavioral health, pulmonary medicine for children with asthma, and gastroenterology for children with abdominal pain. This approach may avoid low-level or unneeded referrals to pediatric subspecialists, though it may require clinicians to attend trainings (e.g., mini-fellowships ranging from a few days to a few months) or to engage in onsite subspecialist observation to gain needed knowledge and skills. Primary care clinicians who acquire this type of expertise may benefit from referrals to subspecialists for only the most complex cases, as there is acknowledgement of the primary care clinician's capability to manage many conditions, increasing the perceived urgency of these subspecialist referrals (Canin and Wunsch, 2008). The REACH model for patient-centered mental health care in primary care, which supports clinicians in developing skills to diagnose and treat a spectrum of pediatric mental health conditions, is one example of how condition-focused education can expand the capacity of primary care to the most needed subspecialty care (Green et al., 2019; The REACH Institute, 2022). Ongoing education on these conditions as part of maintenance of certification can ensure that clinicians' knowledge evolves with dynamic subspecialty practice.

Referral and Management Guidelines

Even prior to a patient evaluation in subspecialty care, guidelines and recommendations for initial evaluation and management in the primary care setting reduce subspecialty demand by eliminating unnecessary referrals. For example, children who are seen in subspecialty care frequently lack complete or appropriate initial work-up and can face delays in care while awaiting results after the initial subspecialist visit (Ip et al., 2022). Vernacchio et al. (2012) suggested that frequently visited subspecialties and commonly referred diagnoses such as acne (Strauss et al., 2007), asthma (NHLBI, 2007), chronic abdominal pain (Di Lorenzo et al., 2005), and ADHD (AAP, 2000, 2001) should be targeted for enhanced primary care management. Referral guidelines include criteria for when and how to refer these types of conditions to subspecialists and can help reduce unnecessary referrals, thereby improving access (Cornell et al., 2015). Referral guidelines also support primary care clinicians in the ongoing management of patients who need and are awaiting subspecialty care, help to address discrepancies in opinion, and build buy-in and receptivity for subspecialty care by patients and families (Children's National, 2023; Cornell et al., 2015; Kwok et al., 2018; Seattle Children's, 2023). Referral guidelines that include communication about referral may also improve show rates because, historically, when there is less good communication, referrals are not completed (Zuckerman et al., 2011). See Box 7-3 for clinician perspectives on the need for guidance on subspecialty care referrals.

Primary care and subspecialty clinicians do not necessarily find all guidelines for every condition to be useful (Ip et al., 2022). As a result, involvement of representatives from both primary care and specialty care is a critical aspect of successful referral guideline development and dissemination. Active dissemination can be promoted by directing clinicians to relevant referral guidelines (Cornell et al., 2015). The use of technology-enabled referral support also improves the interface between primary care and specialty clinicians; electronic messaging between clinicians where there is a planned referral needs to include initial management and referral guidelines (Ray and Kahn, 2020). Clinical decision support tools may offer automated recommendations based on specialists' practice patterns, further tailoring an initial work-up, and evaluation in primary care prior to specialist care (Ip et al., 2022).

> **BOX 7-3**
> **Clinician Perspectives—Challenges at the**
> **Primary–Specialty Care Interface**
>
> "Pediatric subspecialty care is important, yet we have also become so ingrained in the specific needs of a patient that the general care of the patient is often overlooked or downplayed. General pediatricians defer almost everything to the subspecialists, and it's rather frustrating that there is an expectation that for every symptom, there must be a referral."
> **– Professor of Pediatrics, Atlanta, GA**
>
> "General practitioners are not able to provide basic and secondary level of care to these patients due to lack of time and training on their part. There are no established guidelines or references for a [primary care clinician] who may want to assist with specialty management. The tendency is to refer for even minor issues."
> **– Attending Physician, California**
>
> "Subspecialization can be helpful, but it can give the false impression that only the highly specialized can/should handle a problem. This can be bad especially in the rural setting."
> **– Clinician**
>
> *These quotes were collected from the committee's online call for trainee, clinician, and family perspectives.*

Using Telemedicine and Telehealth

A variety of technological approaches can extend subspecialists' reach and improve the primary–subspecialty care interface. The terms "telehealth" and "telemedicine" have been used interchangeably. However, according to the Office of the National Coordinator for Health Information Technology, "while telemedicine refers specifically to remote clinical services, telehealth can refer to remote non-clinical services, such as providing training, administrative meetings, and continuing medical education, in addition to clinical services" (ONC, 2019). Even before the COVID-19 pandemic, telehealth technologies were recognized as an important mechanism for increasing access to pediatric subspecialty care and reducing urban/rural disparities (Marcin et al., 2016; Ray et al., 2017).

The American Academy of Pediatrics (AAP) endorses the use of telehealth as an essential strategy to reduce health care disparities, and many state Medicaid programs now cover this care model for pediatric care, with coverage that rapidly expanded during the COVID-19 pandemic (Price et al., 2020; Rudich et al., 2022). However, challenges regarding the use of telehealth in providing pediatric care management persist, including the inability for patients to access broadband services in rural areas, limited access to smartphone technology, patients and families with limited English proficiency, privacy for patients in their homes with other family members present, licensing across state lines, reimbursement, and education and training barriers (Buchi et al., 2022; Curfman et al., 2021; Preminger, 2022). Additionally, the impact of increased telehealth use on the workforce depends on whether patients use telehealth as a substitute for in-person visits or as a way to see their clinician more often; it will also depend on whether increased use of telehealth affects provider productivity or the decision to enter fields with higher levels of telehealth use (IHS Markit Ltd., 2021). Patients and families that use telehealth value transparent and reliable scheduling, continuity with trusted providers, clear directions on telemedicine use, and preserving family choice regarding method of care delivery (Ray et al., 2017).

Different types of telehealth and telemedicine, such as live interactive patient visits, store-and-forward patient visits[11] (also known as electronic visits, or e-visits), telementoring, and electronic consultations (e-consults), are distinct and synergistic in their ability to improve collaborative care (Giavina-Bianchi et al., 2020). For example, patients and subspecialists can connect in real-time through live, interactive patient visits or e-visits. E-visits are built robustly in teledermatology, in which patients can send pictures to a dermatologist and receive treatment advice in return (Faucon, 2022; Sud and Anjankar, 2022; Tensen et al., 2016). Live, interactive visits and e-visits can address geographic and time barriers that may limit attendance at scheduled visits (Olayiwola et al., 2019). Technology can also be used to connect primary care clinicians and subspecialists through telementoring that occurs in real-time or through asynchronous electronic consultations (e-consults).

e-Consults

Electronic consults (or e-consults) are defined as "directed communication between providers over a secure electronic medium that involves sharing of patient-specific information and discussing clarification or guidance regarding clinical care" and have been touted as a mechanism to improve access to subspecialty care, in addition to improved collaborations among clinicians. One Milbank report declared e-consults a "triple win for

---

[11] Store-and-forward telehealth is a type of asynchronous telemedicine service that allows patients to submit clinical information for evaluation without an in-person visit.

patients, clinicians, and payers" (Thielke and King, 2020). Clinician-to-clinician e-consults have been successful when there is clinical uncertainty and concern for timely access to care (Kwok et al., 2018; Ray and Kahn, 2020). Effective use of these types of technologies assists the primary care clinicians in managing the family experience during referral along with expectations of subspecialty care (Ray et al., 2016; Ray and Kahn, 2020).

E-consults can help to deliver care and save costs through reduced subspecialist use and improved care coordination. A growing body of literature highlights e-consults' contributions to reductions in wait times and improvements in patient satisfaction across multiple settings (Abu Libdeh et al., 2022; Bhanot et al., 2021; Patel et al., 2020; Porto et al., 2021; Vimalananda et al., 2020). Furthermore, e-consults can potentially address multiple barriers in the first half of the referral process by addressing uncertainties about referrals, facilitating preconsultative communication between primary care clinicians and specialists, and addressing the supply and demand imbalance by reducing the demand for in-person subspecialty visits. Some e-consult infrastructure systems pay specialists for their consultation, but they often do not pay primary care clinicians for their increased labor and care coordination (which would not be needed in traditional models if the subspecialist communicated directly with the patient) (Thompson et al., 2021; Vimalananda et al., 2015).

In his presentation to this committee during a public webinar, Alexander Li, deputy chief medical officer of L.A. Care, highlighted several challenges to the successful implementation of e-consults, including the need for reimbursement for both primary care clinicians and subspecialists, the time required to assist patients with the technology, and the lack of infrastructure in smaller practices.[12] Resources and payment models are needed to remedy these challenges given that prior studies have found that e-consults (when combined with evidence-based care pathways) can allow more care to be delivered in primary care and therefore reduce demand on subspecialists and improve access (Porto et al., 2021).

In guidance issued in January 2023, the Centers for Medicare and Medicaid Services (CMS) clarified that interpersonal consultation services is "a distinct, coverable service in the Medicaid program and in the Children's Health Insurance Program, for which payment can be made directly to the consulting provider" (CMS, 2023e). This policy superseded previous policy under which additional payment for the consulting provider went to the treating provider, who then passed on that reimbursement to the consulting provider. While CMS encourages states to base fees for consulting services

---

[12] The webinar recording can be accessed at https://www.nationalacademies.org/event/11-09-2022/the-pediatric-subspecialty-workforce-and-its-impact-on-child-health-and-well-being-webinar-4.

off Medicare rates for the same services, it confirms that states hold flexibility in determining payment rates for consultation services. As of July 12, 2023, no states had approved state plan amendments to cover e-consult services under this rule.[13] See later in this section for more on telehealth/telemedicine coverage.

The Coordinating Optimal Referral Experiences Model

In his presentation to this committee during a public webinar, Scott Shipman, CyncHealth Endowed Chair of Population Health at Creighton University, described the Coordinating Optimal Referral Experiences (CORE) Model.[14] The CORE Model was developed for primary care in general, including pediatrics. In this model, primary care physicians determine whether to refer patients directly to a specialist or use an e-consult while continuing to manage that patient's care. The primary care physician can share the information asynchronously so that the specialist can determine if the case is too complex for an e-consult and instead requires a traditional referral. The Project CORE Network began in 2014 when the Association of American Medical Colleges was awarded a Healthcare Innovation Award from the Center for Medicare & Medicaid Innovation Center. Most of the initial sites expanded the model to their children's hospitals and pediatric patients over time. Limited evaluations of the CORE model have demonstrated high levels of patient and provider satisfaction in adult care, as well as improvements in timely access to specialty expertise, and reductions over time in referral rates and volumes from primary care providers with above average use of eConsults, when compared to their peers (Ackerman et al., 2020; Deeds et al., 2019; Gilman et al., 2020). The degree to which this is generalizable to the use of eConsults for pediatric patients is unclear, though early trends from children's hospitals are favorable. Providers overwhelmingly believed that the program affects patients positively, and 80 to 85 percent of primary care clinicians voluntarily used e-consults (CHA, 2021; McCulloch et al., 2023). By the third year of the project, 86 percent of e-consults were resolved without a subsequent specialist visit.

However, e-consult volumes, and the degree to which they replace referrals, differs by specialty. Generally, specialties that place more emphasis on laboratory results and the non-procedural specialties tend to have higher levels of penetration for e-consults, reflected in both child and adult data.

---

[13] The most updated list of Medicaid State Plan Amendments can be found at https://www.medicaid.gov/medicaid/medicaid-state-plan-amendments/index.html (accessed July 12, 2023).

[14] The webinar recording can be accessed at https://www.nationalacademies.org/event/11-09-2022/the-pediatric-subspecialty-workforce-and-its-impact-on-child-health-and-well-being-webinar-4.

Non-procedural specialties, particularly those to whom referral are commonly triggered by abnormal lab or imaging results, have been shown to have the highest use of e-consults in both adult and pediatric populations.[15] The effectiveness of e-consults in changing care depends not only on the penetration of using e-consults in place of referrals, but also the volume of consultations.

Using e-Consults for Precision Scheduling

In his presentation to this committee during a public webinar, Hal Yee Jr., chief deputy director, Clinical Affairs and chief medical officer, Los Angeles County Department of Health Services, highlighted using e-consults for precision scheduling.[16] Precision scheduling is an attempt to move toward a "right time" model of care. It is defined as scheduling an appointment within the time frame recommended after dialogue between the primary care clinician and specialist about the patient's needs and available specialist access after using an e-consult to define the situation. The "right time" should not be too late, but also not too early. Precision scheduling aims to optimize use of specialty capacity in both face-to-face and real-time video. Patients who are scheduled "on-time" are within the precision scheduling definition; "late" scheduling (not within the precision scheduling time) may occur when patients are not available for a visit, lack transportation, or have personal preferences.

Telephone Consultation

A "lower tech" approach to improve access to real-time consultations for primary care clinicians is the use of a standing telephone call line. A key example is the availability of behavioral health consultation with child psychiatrists and mental health specialists. The Massachusetts Child Psychiatry Access Project (MCPAP), now replicated in most states, was created in the mid-2000s, and includes initial consultation via a hotline, outpatient mental health consultation within 2 weeks if clinically indicated, care coordination, and primary care clinician continuing education (Sarvet et al., 2010; Connor et al., 2006). The consultation team includes a care coordinator, psychotherapist, and child psychiatrist. The care coordinator provides information about community mental health services for children and routes clinical questions to the available child psychiatrist or psychotherapist. If

---

[15] Data provided by Scott Shipman in his presentation to the committee, November 9, 2022.
[16] The webinar recording can be accessed at https://www.nationalacademies.org/event/11-09-2022/the-pediatric-subspecialty-workforce-and-its-impact-on-child-health-and-well-being-webinar-4.

the question is related to differential diagnosis or medication, the call is directly sent to the child psychiatrist. The overarching goal is to provide consultation while the patient is still with the primary care clinician.

Statewide implementation was made possible through funding included in the Massachusetts state budget to cover all operational expenses (Sarvet et al., 2010; Van Cleave et al., 2018). One analysis of calls from primary care clinicians to MCPAP from October 1, 2010, to July 31, 2011, showed that reasons for use among frequent users included timely and tailored guidance to the child, the ability to arrange therapy referrals, and the ability to provide a plan at point of care for families, including keeping mental health care in their primary care setting, when preferred (Van Cleave et al., 2018). Findings from other states also suggest that statewide implementation is feasible (Cotton et al., 2021; Hilt et al., 2013; Sullivan et al., 2021). According to Stein et al. (2019), "children from states with statewide child psychiatric telephone access programs are significantly more likely to receive mental health services than children residing in states without such programs."

As programs expand to other states, however, there are concerns about sustainability and that traditional insurance mechanisms are not designed to reimburse child psychiatrists' time spent on pediatrician consultation, indicating the need for state or other sources of funding (Sullivan et al., 2021). Nevertheless, variations of the MCPAP model have been replicated in 38 states, the District of Columbia, and British Columbia. In October 2014, the National Network of Child Psychiatry Access Programs, Inc., a Massachusetts nonprofit organization, was created to provide technical assistance to support the development of the model in other states (NNCPAP, 2022). Future research is needed to examine use at the child and clinician levels by sociodemographic characteristics and clinical characteristics (e.g., type of psychiatric diagnosis, clinical severity, psychosocial complexity); use by type of intervention component; the extent to which real-time consultation (while the patient is in a primary care setting) is met; and the relationships among use of the intervention, provision of evidence-based mental health care, and clinical outcomes.

Telementoring

An important example of remote integration of primary and subspecialty care is Project Extension for Community Healthcare Outcomes (ECHO). The 2021 National Academies report on high-quality care described this example of telemonitoring:

> Project ECHO connects governments, academic medical centers, nongovernmental organizations, and centers of excellence around the world to

> "telementor" clinicians for the purpose of training, enabling collaborative problem solving and co-management of cases, and ultimately improving quality of care in underserved communities (UNM, 2022a). Originally designed by the University of New Mexico for the treatment of hepatitis C, today Project ECHO operates in 45 countries (UNM, 2022b) and has been used to disseminate clinical training on cancer screening, addiction management, perinatal care, COVID-19 treatment, and many other primary care domains (Archbald-Pannone et al., 2020; Coulson and Galvin, 2020; Francis et al., 2020; Komaromy et al., 2016; Nethan et al., 2020). With its hub-and-spoke model, Project ECHO enables regular, bidirectional knowledge sharing and collaboration between geographically isolated care team members; fostering new local partnerships; or facilitating the development of new services where they were previously unavailable or insufficient. Project ECHO has been successful, with outcomes including increased knowledge and self-efficacy among clinicians, decreased feelings of professional isolation, increased safety and improved treatment outcomes for patients, and greater ability to enact practice transformation projects (McDonnell et al., 2020). (NASEM, 2021b)

Many pediatric programs have adopted the ECHO model. ECHO has been found to be both feasible and acceptable to conduct virtual education of interprofessional health care providers in managing children with medical complexity. Indeed, AAP has created and launched more than 100 ECHO programs in over 20 topics, including childhood anxiety, childhood obesity, and spina bifida (AAP, 2023), and most recently, pain management (Lalloo et al., 2023). AAP has acted as an ECHO Superhub to train organizations in the model and to support peer and expert learning communities. Recently, the ECHO model has helped support pediatricians in learning about COVID-19 (Bernstein et al., 2022).

Telehealth Coverage

The 2020 AAP Policy Statement on Financing the Medical Home emphasizes the importance of paying for telehealth, urging that:

> Appropriate non–face-to-face encounters via telephone and video and those on digital platforms, such as the Internet, e-mail, electronic health record portals, and other secure encrypted communication, that provide meaningful care should be paid for adequately to facilitate optimal function of the medical home and to improve patient and family satisfaction. These interactions may occur between the patient and family and the medical home or between the medical home and specialty care providers (Price et al., 2020).

This position has been reaffirmed in other policy statements (Brown et al., 2021; Carlson et al., 2022; Curfman et al., 2021).

Many commercial health plans broadened coverage for telehealth in response to COVID-19 and cover at least some form of telehealth service. As of May 2023, 43 states, the District of Columbia, and the Virgin Islands have a private payer law that addresses telehealth reimbursement, with 24 states requiring payment parity for at least one specialty (CCHP, 2023a; HHS, 2023). States have flexibility to cover telehealth services under Medicaid. Unless specifically required by regulation or policy, states can cover such services without submitting a state plan amendment if they reimburse telehealth in the same way and amount as face-to-face services. If states want to reimburse telehealth services differently from face to face, they must submit and receive approval for a state plan amendment if that is not already specified in the state plan (CMS, 2023b). States also have flexibility in setting payment policy for telehealth services in Medicaid, though reimbursement "must satisfy federal requirements of efficiency, economy, and quality of care" (CMS, 2023a). Even before the pandemic, most states covered telehealth for at least some services (CCHP, 2020; Chu et al., 2021).

Most states require managed care organizations that serve Medicaid beneficiaries to follow state fee-for-service telehealth rules, and some allow managed care organizations to adopt more expansive policies than the state fee-for-service requirements. According to research conducted between January and March 2023, all 50 states and Washington, DC, provide reimbursement for some form of live video in Medicaid fee-for-service,[17] 28 states allow store-and-forward telehealth services in Medicaid,[18] 34 allow remote patient monitoring,[19] and 36 states and Washington, DC, reimburse for audio-only telephone in some capacity (CCHP, 2023b). Most states also allowed a patient's home (versus provider office) to serve as the originating site and covered other sites such as schools (CCHP, 2023b; Chu et al., 2021). According to Hinton et al. (2022b): "In 2021, all responding states indicated that they ensured payment parity between telehealth and in-person delivery of [fee-for service] services (as of July 1, 2021), which may have been under emergency policy; most states reported no changes in FY2022 or FY2023 to parity requirements. A small number of states reported that in FY2022 or FY2023 they established telehealth payment parity on a permanent basis." As of June 2023, 21 states have implemented payment parity

---

[17] Puerto Rico and the Virgin Islands do not indicate reimbursement for live video in their Medicaid programs (CCHP, 2023a).

[18] Three states (Illinois, North Carolina, and Ohio) solely reimburse store-and-forward as a part of Communications Technology Based Services (CTBS), which is limited to specific codes and reimbursement amounts (CCHP, 2023a).

[19] Four of the states reimburse only for specific remote patient-monitoring CTBS codes, including California, Massachusetts, Hawaii, and West Virginia (CCHP, 2023a).

policies, 8 states have these policies with certain caveats, and 21 states have no payment parity (Augenstein and Marks Smith, 2023) (see Figure 7-2). Moreover, an important barrier to primary care-subspecialty collaboration in care is that payment for a telehealth visit is only made to one provider, rendering joint primary care-subspecialty visits infeasible. See later in this section for more on telehealth coverage during the COVID-19 pandemic.

Cross-State Telehealth Policy

State licensing issues arise when the patient and the provider are in different states. States have the authority to regulate the practice of physicians and other health care professionals within their state boundary. Because telehealth generally takes place at the patient's home and not in the clinical setting, most states require that out-of-state providers be licensed in the state of the patient's residence (Curfman et al, 2021). States may pay for Medicaid services provided to a beneficiary who is out of state under certain circumstances, including emergencies, services being more readily available in another state, or if it is general practice for beneficiaries in a locality to use medical resources in another state (42 CFR § 431.52). However, states vary in their policies, and there may be substantial administrative burden in accessing out-of-state providers (GAO 2019; MACPAC, 2020; Manetto et al., 2020). (See Chapter 2 for more information on out-of-state access barriers for in-person visits.) In October 2021, CMS issued guidance to states on care provided by out-of-state providers to children with medical complexity who are covered by Medicaid (CMS, 2021). The guidance included best practices for facilitating care from out-of-state providers, including (among others) coverage of telehealth services from out-of-state providers and payment to support services provided to out-of-state providers. See later in this section for more on cross-state licensing rules during the COVID-19 pandemic.

The Interstate Medical Licensure Compact is an "agreement among participating U.S. states to work together to significantly streamline the licensing process for physicians who want to practice in multiple states. It offers a voluntary, expedited pathway to licensure for physicians who qualify" (IMLCC, 2022). The expansion of this compact could help to break down regulatory barriers to accessing subspecialty care for children in states with few pediatric subspecialists via telehealth.

Telehealth during the COVID-19 Pandemic

Patients' reluctance to visit traditional health care settings early in the COVID-19 pandemic prompted health care systems to rapidly adopt telehealth for clinical care and for patients to engage providers via telehealth

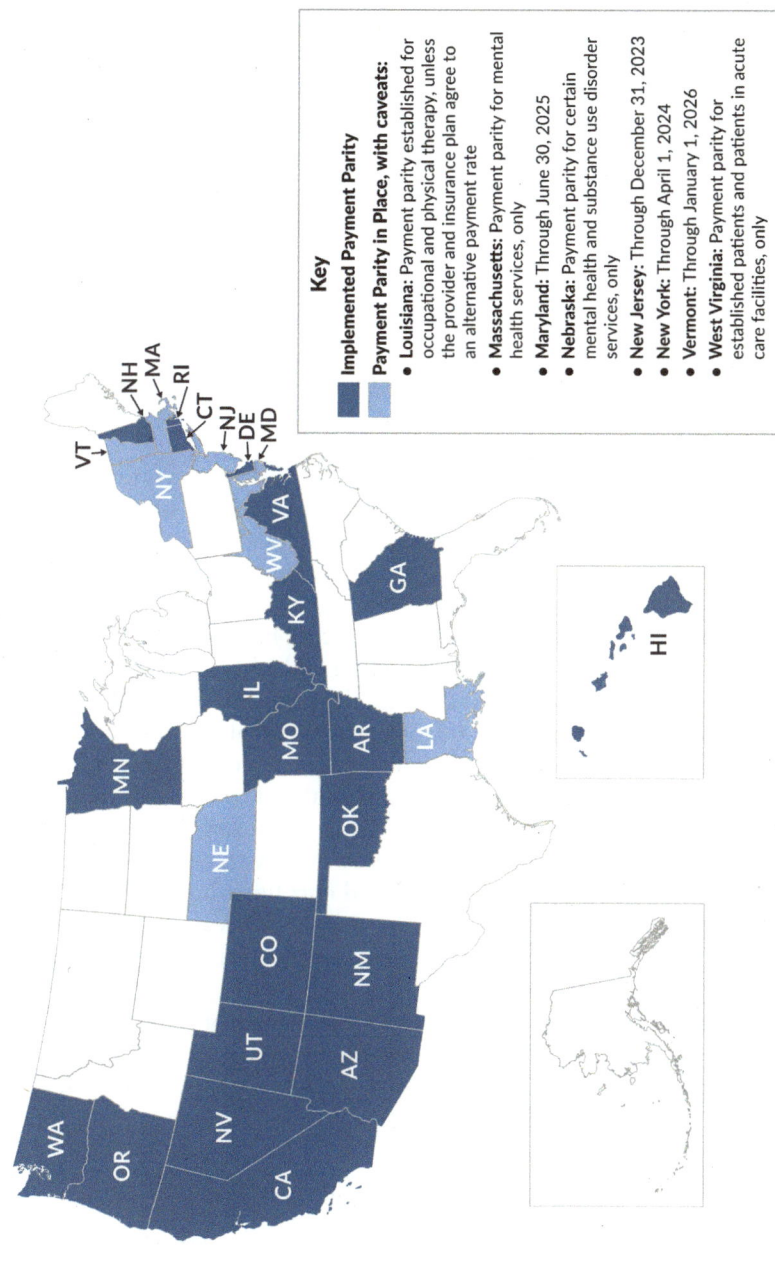

FIGURE 7-2 Map of States with Laws Requiring Insurers to Implement Payment Parity (as of June 2023).
SOURCE: Adapted from Augenstein and Marks Smith, 2023. Reprinted with permission from Manatt, Phelps & Phillips, LLP.

modalities at an accelerated rate. The early stages of the pandemic were associated with a major and very rapid shift from in-person appointments to telehealth encounters (Curfman et al., 2021). One study that examined telehealth use among patients requiring pediatric subspecialty management before and after the COVID-19 pandemic at a single academic health system found that the nature and scale of pandemic effects were complex and varied by pediatric subspecialty type, social demographics, and established patient status (Cahan et al., 2022). Consistent with other studies, established patients were more likely to complete telehealth appointments and newer patients were less likely to use the technology (Cahan et al., 2022; Nguyen et al., 2022). While in-person office visits declined for all subspecialties in 2020, the completion of telehealth visits was lower in pulmonology, oncology, and cardiology compared with endocrinology and neurology. These patterns may correspond with different subspecialty practice requirements, such as the need for a physical exam or imaging study (Cahan et al., 2022; Ray et al., 2015).

During the pandemic, states enacted a range of modifications to their Medicaid telehealth policies to expand access to and use of these services (Augenstein and Marks Smith, 2023; Cahan et al., 2022). These changes included waiving restrictions on distant and originating sites, modalities, and provider–patient relationships as well as issuing guidance focused on expanded telehealth access for specific services. For example, at least 13 states issued guidance for telehealth well-child and early and periodic screening, diagnostic, and treatment visits during the pandemic (AAP, 2021). Now that the infrastructure for telehealth practice is in place in many settings and patients have familiarity with remote clinical services, much care will likely continue to be delivered via telehealth, subject to continued favorable regulatory and reimbursement policies. While all states implemented Section 1135 waivers to allow out-of-state providers with equivalent licensing in another state to provide care to Medicaid enrollees during the pandemic (Guth and Hinton, 2020), many states have let those waivers lapse, though this varies by state (CCHP, 2023c). For example, Arizona allows out-of-state licensed health care providers without registration for certain criteria with no expiration date; Colorado allows occasional out-of-state provider telehealth services; Michigan and Minnesota allow out-of-state ability with no exception; and New Mexico can do so with registration (FSMB, 2023; University of Chicago, 2022).

Facilitating Access through Nursing

Since the *Patient Protection and Affordable Care Act of 2010* (ACA), greater emphasis has been placed on team care and optimization of each team member's contribution to care and care outcomes. The report *Assessing*

Progress on the Institute of Medicine Report The Future of Nursing noted, "in new collaborative models of practice, it is imperative that all health professionals practice to the full extent of their education and training to optimize the efficiency and quality of services for patients" (IOM, 2016, pg. 48). Subsequent National Academies reports reinforce the necessity of the health care team, with each member working to their fullest capabilities as well as identifying models of care that have potential application for improving pediatric care delivery (NASEM, 2021a,b). Nurses in both primary and subspecialty care settings can assume responsibilities that allow them to increase the availability of subspecialty care clinicians to meet the most critical or complex pediatric health care needs.

The Role of Nurse Practitioners

Models of care that include NPs often result from workforce needs and are informed by state regulatory structures. In common models, NPs have roles as (1) an adjunct to a resident or fellow, (2) a substitute for residents, (3) a supplement in an attending physician-only model, and/or (4) an independent clinician in a free-standing practice (Gigli et al., 2021; Wall et al., 2014; Winter et al., 2021). Pediatric NPs increase access to care for vulnerable populations, including children who have chronic health care needs, who live in rural and underserved areas, or are from low-income families (Buerhaus, 2018; Martyn et al., 2013). Furthermore, NPs are poised to improve individual- and population-level health inequities through their care delivery and partnership with communities (NASEM, 2021a). Additionally, initial studies of advanced practice providers as primary care clinicians for patients with complex care needs have found no increase in use and costs (Morgan et al., 2019). This sentiment was reiterated by a clinician who responded to the committee's call for perspectives:

> One way to increase the availability of subspecialty [care] for patients is to increase the use of pediatric nurse practitioners. In our area almost all pediatric subspecialties employ pediatric nurse practitioners. A significant number of my graduates elect to take positions in subspecialties. Most who make that choice stay in that subspecialty and are experts in the area.
>
> – Pediatric nurse practitioner, Cleveland, OH

Despite the opportunities for NPs to increase access to high-quality pediatric care, barriers exist that limit their practice. One example is state-based, scope-of-practice regulations, namely state laws that delineate the amount of physician supervision or collaboration an NP must have to practice in a state. Currently, 27 states and the District of Columbia allow NPs

TABLE 7-1 Specific Exemplars of Implementation of Nurse-Led Care Responsibilities

Patient Population	Care Setting	Nurse-Led Care Responsibilities
Children with obesity	Primary care	Education, health promotion and facilitation of social determinants of heatlh needs (Cheng et al., 2021); intervention delivery (Seburg et al., 2015)
Adolescents with complex health needs (e.g., spina bifida, type 1 diabetes mellitus)	Ambulatory care	Support to teach self-management of chronic disease, facilitate transitions of care to adult clinicians, care coordination (Campbell et al., 2016)
		Monitor the acquisition of self-management knowledge and skills, including core self-management skills (e.g., knowledge of spina bifida, bladder management, skin care) and peripheral self-management skills (e.g., emergency resources in the community, medication refills, and equipment maintenance and replacement) (Betz et al., 2016)
	Transition to adult care	Care coordination; building and maintaining trust with families of young people as they transition into adult services (O'Connell et al., 2019)
Children in need of referral to subspecialty care	Primary care/ outpatient	Triaging of patient referrals (Hong et al., 2015)
Children discharged from hospital after acute-care stay	Acute to primary care transition	Nurse home visits to provide education and health promotion interventions (Pickler et al., 2016); nurse-led telephone counseling intervention to provide pain management education, symptom management, and reduced readmissions (Özalp et al., 2016)
Children discharged from hospital	Acute care	Discharge planning, education, and referral for outpatient services (Breneol et al., 2018; Khair and Chaplin, 2017)

full practice authority to "evaluate patients; diagnose, order, and interpret diagnostic tests; and initiate and manage treatments, including prescribing medications and controlled substances, under the exclusive licensure authority of the state board of nursing" (AANP, 2022). The remaining states impose requirements for collaborative or supervisory practice that are associated with smaller NP workforces, lower ability for patients to access care, and no evidence of improved care quality (Buerhaus, 2018; Kuo et al., 2013; Reagan and Salsberry, 2013). Within individual provider practices, hospitals, and health systems, NPs must also be granted privileges to practice. There is growing evidence that institutions restrict NP practice through the privileging process, even within states that allow full practice authority, without evidence to demonstrate these institutional restrictions improve safety or quality (Bowman et al., 2022; Freund et al., 2015; Pittman et al., 2020). Additionally, within interprofessional teams in all practice settings, local practices create a culture that contributes to NPs' work environment. The work environment includes (1) professional visibility, (2) NP–administration relations, (3) NP–physician relations, and (4) independent practice and support (Poghosyan et al., 2013b). The NP work environment contributes to patient and organizational outcomes, and lower quality NP work environments restrict NP practice and limit patient access to NP-provided care (Frogner et al., 2020; Poghosyan and Aiken, 2015; Poghosyan et al., 2013a, 2015; Scanlon et al., 2018). Furthermore, NPs are paid less than physicians for providing the same care. Medicare reimburses NPs at 85 percent of the physician rate, and private payers also pay NPs less than physicians (CMS, 2022a). These variations and limitations hamper NPs' ability to contribute to high-quality, cost-effective pediatric care delivery (NASEM, 2021a). Elimination of unnecessary restrictions to NP practice can increase the types and amount of high-quality health care services that can be provided by NPs to those with complex health and social needs, thereby improving access to care and health equity (NASEM, 2021a).

Financing Innovations to Support Primary–Specialty Care Collaboration

Payment in pediatrics traditionally has been made on a fee-for-service basis, in which providers are paid for each specific service provided. Starting several decades ago, payers began moving to risk-based payment models (i.e., capitation payments) in which providers receive a set amount per month to care for patients on their panel. Often capitated payments were made to primary care providers, with specialists continuing to be paid on a fee-for-service basis (Alguire, 2023; Berenson et al., 2016; NASEM, 2021b; Volpp et al., 2018). These models created incentives for primary care to refer cases and sometimes hindered collaborative care. In some cases, multispecialty groups that combined primary care and specialty care jointly entered risk contracts, creating incentives for joint, efficient patient management, but these arrangements did not account for most patient care and often did not include pediatric care (Mechanic and Zinner, 2016). There is some evidence that children in capitated plans have greater use of urgent care and well-child and acute care delivered by the primary care provider, with lower odds of visits to emergency departments and specialty care (Canares et al., 2020).

In more recent years, payers have explored value-based payment (VBP) models, which generally tie payment to quality or health outcome (and sometimes cost or efficiency) goals (MACPAC, 2023). VBPs range from bonus systems tied to performance for an individual provider to payment at a population level. Within Medicaid, states have been using VBP in a variety of forms, including population-based payment models (CMS, 2020; Houston and Brykman, 2022); however, while children may be included in VBP models, most of these models are not specifically designed to serve pediatric populations (Bachman et al., 2017; Brykman et al., 2021; Counts et al., 2021; Heller et al., 2017). Commentators have noted several challenges in the potential use of VBP for children with special health care needs, including "low prevalence of specific special health care need conditions, how to factor in a life course perspective, in which investments in children's health pay off over a long period of time, the marginal savings that may or may not accrue, the increased risk of family financial hardship, and the potential to exacerbate existing inequities across race, class, ethnicity, functional status, and other social determinants of health" (Bachman et al., 2017, pg. S96). Other challenges noted include measurement issues (lack of measures appropriate to subspecialty care or data systems in place to systematically collect data) (Bachman et al., 2017); complexity of pediatric patients who receive subspecialty care and the need to consider individual and family-specific circumstances (Kevill et al., 2019); and potential mismatch between outcomes in VBP and family or patient preferences for care (Anderson et al., 2017; Garg et al., 2019). Still, others believe that VBP holds promise to align payment with medical needs of children with complex needs and could be a promising avenue to advance high quality care for children.

The federal government has provided several funding streams and technical assistance to support population-based payment models under Medicaid. For example, Delivery System Reform Incentive Payments (DSRIPs) were Medicaid supplemental payments to provider-led initiatives to support state delivery system goals. Most frequently, payments were made to hospitals or health systems, though they sometimes included community partners; DSRIPs tied supplemental payments to milestones (e.g., provider training, telemedicine capacity building, chronic care management systems, establishment of medical homes, patient navigation programs, or integrating physical and behavioral health) or outcomes (e.g., lowering errors, complications, or readmissions, patient satisfaction, accreditation by the National Committee for Quality Assurance) (Gates et al., 2014). When DSRIP funds ended in 2020, states turned to new ways to continue these efforts, such as directed payments under Medicaid managed care (Hinton et al., 2022a). The State Innovation Model (SIM) initiative, which ran from 2013 to 2019, was another Medicaid effort to provide federal funds to support state delivery system reform through multipayer efforts. SIM funds generally supported a shift to VBP as well as infrastructure development (e.g., shared electronic health information and development of team-based care) and included awards to both develop models and pilot test models (CMS, 2023c; Kissam et al., 2019). Most SIM programs focused on patient-centered medical homes and care linkages between primary care and care in other settings. SIM programs also used a range of payment incentives to support specific aims (KFF, 2015). The federal government has also supported the development of accountable care organizations (ACOs) in Medicaid, which uses VBP tied to population health outcomes for the population served by a provider, though there are not targeted additional federal funds tied to ACO development or implementation (CHCS, 2018).

Among the broad range of VBP and population health payment models, few focus specifically on children. ACO models are typically broad population-based models and therefore include children along with adults, and some include pediatric-specific outcome measures or adjustments to measures (Brykman et al., 2021). Notably for the pediatric primary–specialty care interface, current ACO models for children focus mainly on primary care, and often still "carve out" subspecialty care into a fee-for-service model. Moreover, they do not acknowledge the importance or benefits of collaborative primary–subspecialty care in either outcome measures or payment structures (Fogler et al., 2022; Perrin et al., 2017). State efforts to support patient-centered medical homes within Medicaid include children and may include child-focused components, such as outcomes tied to pediatric specific outcome measures (e.g., immunization or developmental screening) or episode-of-care payment programs (in which payment is made for conditions or procedures over a period of time) that include pediatric conditions (Brykman et al., 2021). CMS has supported pediatric-focused efforts through the Innovation Accelerator Program, which provided technical assistance to states to support implementation of VBP in maternal and infant health, and the Integrated Care for Kids (InCK) model, which provides grants to six states to support integration of care for children across health and social services (CMS, 2023b,d).[20] Because relatively few VBP programs are targeted to pediatrics and because valuable pediatric outcomes (e.g., developmental milestones, high school graduation, employment) often occur over a much longer time period than adult outcomes, there is limited evidence of the effect they have on children's health or health care spending, including use of subspecialty care. A report based

---

[20] During an information-gathering session, the Committee heard from Steven Kairys (New Jersey InCK model) and Charlene Wong (North Caroline InCK model) about their respective state models. The webinar recording can be accessed at https://www.nationalacademies.org/event/11-09-2022/the-pediatric-subspecialty-workforce-and-its-impact-on-child-health-and-well-being-webinar-4.

on expert interviews concluded that while VBP offers opportunities for investment in children's health, ongoing barriers to implementation include difficulty realizing short-term, direct savings from population-based investments in children's health; challenges in coordinating with sectors outside of health care; and limited existing outcomes and quality measures to reflect the range of pediatric care needs (Brykman et al., 2021).

INVESTING IN PEDIATRIC PRIMARY CARE TO IMPROVE THE PRIMARY–SPECIALTY CARE INTERFACE

Many of the innovations discussed in this chapter have the potential to increase efficiency and coordination at the pediatric primary–specialty care interface, improving communication, coordination, and access to care, while supporting patients and families. However, these models have the potential to increase the burden on primary care clinicians. The increased scope of practice and judicious use of appropriate subspecialty referrals by primary care clinicians will require investment in primary care, including payment change and support to develop and implement new models, as well as education and training for new models for both primary care clinicians and pediatric subspecialties. Decades of evidence show that a strong foundation of primary care yields better health outcomes overall, greater equity in health care access and outcomes, and lower per capita health costs (FitzGerald et al., 2022; Shi, 2012; Starfield et al., 2005). The committee recognizes the importance of high-quality primary care as a foundation for high-quality subspecialty care. While the committee did examine some new models of subspecialist-primary care clinician interaction for patient care, the 2021 National Academies report *Implementing High-Quality Primary Care: Rebuilding the Foundation of Health Care* specifically addresses strategies to improve primary care broadly and this current committee considered their work to build upon the previous study (NASEM, 2021b). The 2021 report developed an implementation plan for high-quality primary care in the United States (NASEM, 2021b); the implementation of many of the 2021 report's recommendations will support the innovative care and delivery models discussed in this chapter. Additionally, while this chapter's recommendations are focused on improving the delivery of subspecialty care through innovations at the primary–specialty care interface, many recommendations will also help to support primary care clinicians. The committee also recognizes a study currently in progress at the National Academies, which is charged to address "innovations that can be implemented in the health care system to improve the health and wellbeing of children and youth," including workforce development and team-based care.[21]

KEY FINDINGS AND CONCLUSIONS

Key Findings

<u>Finding #7-1</u>: Care coordination is critical for high-quality pediatric subspecialty care.

<u>Finding #7-2</u>: There are inconsistent and ill-defined expectations within the U.S. health care system and among providers regarding the scope of practice for pediatric subspecialists and primary care clinicians.

<u>Finding #7-3</u>: Pediatric subspecialists and pediatric primary care clinicians are not optimally trained about their role and responsibilities in the referral process.

<u>Finding #7-4</u>: Many of the common and lower complexity diagnoses referred to subspecialists are conditions that could be managed by primary care clinicians either alone (with appropriate resources and training) or through co-management with the subspecialist.

<u>Finding #7-5</u>: Both pediatric subspecialists and primary care clinicians (e.g., general pediatricians, family medicine physicians, APRNs, PAs) face suboptimal systems that negatively impact efficiency. Factors that contribute to this inefficiency include misaligned financial and non-financial incentives (e.g., regulation); barriers to the use of innovative consultation and referral interventions; non-clinical demands on clinicians' time; and lack of education and training in team-based care, in making referrals, and in the use and equitable compensation of modalities such as telehealth and e-consults.

<u>Finding #7-6</u>: Many innovative, collaborative primary–subspecialty care models exist to improve children's access to care and outcomes.

<u>Finding #7-7</u>: Beneficial policies developed during the COVID-19 pandemic to promote telehealth and access to care across state lines are threatened as the public health emergency ends.

---

[21] For more information, see https://www.nationalacademies.org/our-work/improving-the-health-and-wellbeing-of-children-and-youth-through-health-care-system-transformation (accessed July 7, 2023).

<u>Finding #7-8</u>: Current payment models neither measure nor incentivize increasing primary care scope nor primary care–subspecialty collaboration.

<u>Finding #7-9</u>: The issues of state licensing and payment for services across state lines is a barrier for the expansion of some effective models of care.

Conclusions

<u>Conclusion #7-1</u>: *Current care models will not be able to meet future needs just by expanding the overall size of the subspecialty workforce. Alternative approaches are needed among pediatric subspecialists and primary care clinicians, as well as allied health providers, to use their training and expertise efficiently and effectively.*

<u>Conclusion #7-2</u>: *The use of new technologies and methods of care delivery can increase patient access, improve care coordination, and allow subspecialists the time to provide inpatient and outpatient care that is best for children in a manner that is feasible, fulfilling, and financially sustainable.*

<u>Conclusion #7-3</u>: *Inconsistent and inadequate reimbursement for some models of care (e.g., telehealth, team-based care, e-consults), coupled with the lack of support for the increased scope of primary care clinicians, serves as a barrier to the use of more efficient and effective models.*

<u>Conclusion #7-4</u>: *The provision of subspecialty care to children across U.S. rural and urban areas will require removal of regulatory barriers to the delivery of pediatric subspecialty care, both in-person and virtual, to ensure timely and equitable access to care for all children who need pediatric subspecialty care.*

RECOMMENDATIONS

Pediatric subspecialists need to focus on their essential role in the care of children with complex, severe, and rare disorders or those requiring technical procedures, while collaborating with primary care clinicians. However, in general, both groups of clinicians are not optimally trained about their role and responsibilities in the referral process. Many children with common and lower-complexity or -severity diagnoses referred to subspecialists could be managed by primary care clinicians either alone (with appropriate time, financial resources, and training), or through active, collaborative co-management with the subspecialist. In addition, the COVID-19 pandemic has shown how rapidly technology such as telehealth can be implemented and widely adopted. The use of new technologies and methods of care can increase patient access, improve care coordination, strengthen the role of the primary care clinician, and allow subspecialists the time to provide inpatient and outpatient care in a manner that is feasible, fulfilling, and financially sustainable and best for children. However, barriers in payment and regulation prevent the full implementation and scaling of current evidence-based models of team-based care. Finally, innovative models of care are needed to reset the relationship between pediatric subspecialists and primary care clinicians, making them greater *partners* in the care of children. Enhanced communication at the primary–subspecialty care interface is essential within these models. Therefore, to achieve a goal of **promoting collaboration and effective use of services between pediatric primary care clinicians and subspecialty physicians,** the committee provides the following recommendations:

RECOMMENDATION 7-1 The American Academy of Pediatrics, the Council of Pediatric Subspecialties, and other pediatric professional societies should collaboratively develop, disseminate, and implement testing, management, and referral guidelines for health conditions commonly managed by subspecialists. This should include when to consult, when to co-manage, and what the appropriate follow-up roles are for both the primary care clinician and the subspecialist.

RECOMMENDATION 7-2 Public and private health insurance payers should adequately reimburse evidence-based care delivery models that improve interprofessional, integrated, team-based care to enhance access to pediatric subspecialty care. These models include but are not limited to
- E-consults (with payment for both the referring and the receiving clinician);
- Telehealth visits (both within and across state lines); and
- Integrated care teams that support mental and physical primary and specialty health care clinicians and include advanced practice providers, social workers, and care coordinators.

RECOMMENDATION 7-3 CMS (in conjunction with state Medicaid agencies), private foundations, and health systems should sponsor the development, implementation, and evaluation of innovations (including new models of care delivery and reimbursement) in the primary–specialty care interface and the pediatric subspecialty referral and care coordination processes.

REFERENCES

AACAP (American Academy of Child and Adolescent Psychiatry). Committee on Collaborative and Integrated Care and AACAP Committee on Quality Issues. 2023. Clinical update: Collaborative mental health care for children and adolescents in pediatric primary care. *Journal of the American Academy of Child & Adolescent Psychiatry* 62(2):91-119.

AANP (American Association of Nurse Practitioners). 2022. *State practice environment.* https://www.aanp.org/advocacy/state/state-practice-environment (accessed May 4, 2023).

AAP (American Academy of Pediatrics). 2000. Clinical practice guideline: Diagnosis and evaluation of the child with attention-deficit/hyperactivity disorder. American Academy of Pediatrics. *Pediatrics* 105(5):1158-1170.

AAP. 2001. Clinical practice guideline: Treatment of the school-aged child with attention-deficit/hyperactivity disorder. *Pediatrics* 108(4):1033-1044.

AAP. 2021. *State notices on telehealth policy in response to COVID-19 (as of March 9, 2021).* https://downloads.aap.org/DOCCSA/State-Telehealth-Notices.pdf (accessed May 2, 2023).

AAP. 2023. Pediatric ECHOs. https://www.aap.org/en/practice-management/project-echo/pediatric-echos/ (accessed July 12, 2023).

ABP (American Board of Pediatrics). 2021. *Entrustable professional activities: EPA 1 for general pediatrics.* https://www.abp.org/sites/abp/files/pdf/combined_gp_epas.pdf (accessed December 21, 2022).

ABP. 2023. *Entrustable professional activities for general pediatrics* https://www.abp.org/content/entrustable-professional-activities-general-pediatrics (accessed April 30, 2023).

Abu Libdeh, A., J. Flanigan, and K. Heinan. 2022. Experience with pediatric neurology e-consults from a specialist perspective at an academic center. *Journal of Child Neurology* 37(5):373-379.

Ackerman, S. L., N. Gleason, and S. A. Shipman. 2020. Comparing patients' experiences with electronic and traditional consultation: Results from a multisite survey. *Journal of General Internal Medicine* 35(4):1135-1142.

Adekolujo, O. S., S. E. Roskos, and O. O. Adekolujo. 2019. Teaching medical residents to collaborate with specialist consultants. *International Journal of Medical Education* 10:172-173.

AHRQ (Agency for Healthcare Research and Quality). 2023. *Warm handoffs: A guide for clinicians.* https://www.ahrq.gov/sites/default/files/wysiwyg/professionals/quality-patient-safety/patient-family-engagement/pfeprimarycare/warm-handoff-guide-for-clinicians.pdf (accessed May 8, 2023).

Alguire, P. C. 2023. *Understanding capitation.* https://www.acponline.org/about-acp/about-internal-medicine/career-paths/residency-career-counseling/resident-career-counseling-guidance-and-tips/understanding-capitation (accessed April 19, 2023).

Anderson, B., J. Beckett, N. Wells, and M. Comeau. 2017. The eye of the beholder: A discussion of value and quality from the perspective of families of children and youth with special health care needs. *Pediatrics* 139(Suppl 2):S99-S108.

Antonelli, R. C., C. J. Stille, and L. C. Freeman. 2005. Enhancing collaboration between primary and subspeciality care providers for children and youth with special health care needs.

Arbour, M. C., B. Floyd, S. Morton, P. Hampton, J. M. Sims, S. Doyle, S. Atwood, and R. Sege. 2021. Cross-sector approach expands screening and addresses health-related social needs in primary care. *Pediatrics* 148(5):e2021050152.

Archbald-Pannone, L. R., D. A. Harris, K. Albero, R. L. Steele, A. F. Pannone, and J. B. Mutter. 2020. COVID-19 collaborative model for an academic hospital and long-term care facilities. *Journal of the American Medical Directors Association* 21(7):939-942.

Asarnow, J. R., M. Rozenman, J. Wiblin, and L. Zeltzer. 2015. Integrated medical-behavioral care compared with usual primary care for child and adolescent behavioral health: A meta-analysis. *JAMA Pediatrics* 169(10):929-937.

Augenstein, J., and J. Marks Smith. 2023. *Executive summary: Tracking telehealth changes state-by-state in response to COVID-19*. https://www.manatt.com/insights/newsletters/covid-19-update/executive-summary-tracking-telehealth-changes-stat (accessed July 12, 2023).

Bachman, S. S., M. Comeau, and T. F. Long. 2017. Statement of the problem: Health reform, value-based purchasing, alternative payment strategies, and children and youth with special health care needs. *Pediatrics* 139(Supplement_2):S89-S98.

Berenson, R. A., D. Upadhyay, S. F. Delbanco, and R. Murray. 2016. *Payment methods: How they work*. Washington, DC: Urban Institute.

Bernstein, H. H., T. Calabrese, P. Corcoran, L. E. Flint, and F. M. Munoz. 2022. The power of connections: AAP COVID-19 ECHO accelerates responses during a public health emergency. *Journal of Public Health Management and Practice* 28(1):E1-E8.

Betz, C. L. 2017. SPN position statement: Transition of pediatric patients into adult care. *Journal of Pediatric Nursing* 35:160-164.

Betz, C. L., K. A. Smith, A. Van Speybroeck, F. V. Hernandez, and R. A. Jacobs. 2016. Movin' on up: An innovative nurse-led interdisciplinary health care transition program. *Journal of Pediatric Health Care* 30(4):323-338.

Bhanot, N., G. Dimitriou, L. McAninch, C. Rossi, D. Thompson, and S. Manzi. 2021. Perspectives of health care providers in an integrated health care delivery network on inpatient electronic consultation (e-consult) use during the COVID-19 pandemic. *Journal of Patient Experience* 8:23743735211007696.

Blount, A. 2003. Integrated primary care: Organizing the evidence. *Families, Systems, & Health* 21:121-133.

Boardman, J. B. 2006. Health access and integration for adults with serious and persistent mental illness. *Families, Systems, & Health* 24:3-18.

Bohnhoff, J. C., J. M. Taormina, L. Ferrante, D. Wolfson, and K. N. Ray. 2019. Unscheduled referrals and unattended appointments after pediatric subspecialty referral. *Pediatrics* 144(6).

Bonciani, M., W. Schäfer, S. Barsanti, S. Heinemann, and P. P. Groenewegen. 2018. The benefits of co-location in primary care practices: The perspectives of general practitioners and patients in 34 countries. *BMC Health Services Research* 18(1):132.

Bower, P., E. Garralda, T. Kramer, R. Harrington, and B. Sibbald. 2001. The treatment of child and adolescent mental health problems in primary care: A systematic review. *Family Practice* 18(4):373-382.

Bowman, A. F., M. B. Goreth, A. B. Armstrong, and K. H. Gigli. 2022. Hospital regulation of pediatric-focused nurse practitioners: A multistate survey. *Journal for Nurse Practitioners* 18(5):558-562.e551.

Breneol, S., A. Hatty, A. Bishop, and J. A. Curran. 2018. Nurse-led discharge in pediatric care: A scoping review. *Journal of Pediatric Nursing* 41:60-68.

Briggs, R. D., E. M. Stettler, E. J. Silver, R. D. Schrag, M. Nayak, S. Chinitz, and A. D. Racine. 2012. Social-emotional screening for infants and toddlers in primary care. *Pediatrics* 129(2):e377-e384.

Brown, K. M., A. D. Ackerman, T. K. Ruttan, S. K. Snow, Committee on Pediatric Emergency Medicine, American College of Emergency Physicians Pediatric Emergency Medicine Committee, Emergency Nurses Association Pediatric Committee 2018–2019, G. P. Conners, J. Callahan, T. Gross, M. Joseph, L. Lee, E. Mack, J. Marin, S. Mazor, R. Paul, N. Timm, A. M. Dietrich, K. H. Alade, C. S. Amato, Z. Atanelov, M. Auerbach, I. A. Barata, L. S. Benjamin, K. T. Berg, C. Chang, J. Chow, C. E. Chumpitazi, I. A. Claudius, J. Easter, A. Foster, S. M. Fox, M. Gausche-Hill, M. J. Gerardi, J. M. Goodloe, M. Heniff, J. L. Homme, P. T. Ishimine, S. D. John, M. M. Joseph, S. H.-F. Lam, S. L. Lawson, M. O. Lee, J. Li, S. D. Lin, D. I. Martini, L. B. Mellick, D. Mendez, E. M. Petrack, L. Rice, E. A. Rose, M. Saidinejad, G. Santillanes, J. N. Simpson, S. M. Sivasankar, D. Slubowski, A. Sorrentino, M. J. Stoner, C. D. Sulton, J. H. Valente, S. Vora, J. J. Wall, D. Wallin, T. A. Walls, M. Waseem, D. P. Woolridge, C. Brandt, K. M. Kult, J. J. Milici, N. A. Nelson, M. A. Redlo, M. R. Curtis Cooper, K. Logee, D. E. Bryant, and K. Cline. 2021. Access to optimal emergency care for children. *Pediatrics* 147(5):e2021050787.

Brykman, K., R. Houston, M. Bailey. 2021. *Value-based payment to support children's health and wellness: Shifting the focus from short-term to life course impact.* https://www.bluecrossmafoundation.org/sites/g/files/csphws2101/files/2021-09/Value-Based%20Pmt_Childrens-Health_FINAL.pdf (accessed April 19, 2023).

Buchi, A. B., D. M. Langlois, and R. Northway. 2022. Use of telehealth in pediatrics. *Primary Care* 49(4):585-596.

Buerhaus, P. 2018. *Nurse practitioners: A solution to America's primary care crisis.* https://www.aei.org/research-products/report/nurse-practitioners-a-solution-to-americas-primary-care-crisis (accessed April 30, 2023).

Burkhart, K., K. Asogwa, N. Muzaffar, and M. Gabriel. 2020. Pediatric integrated care models: A systematic review. *Clinical Pediatrics* 59(2):148-153.

Cady, R. G., and J. L. Belew. 2017. Parent perspective on care coordination services for their child with medical complexity. *Children* 4(6): https://doi.org/10.3390/children4060045.

Cady, R., W. Looman, L. Lindeke, B. LaPlante, B. Lundeen, A. Seeley, and M. Kautto. 2015. Pediatric care coordination: Lessons learned and future priorities. *Online Journal of Issues in Nursing* 20(3).

Cahan, E. M., J. Maturi, P. Bailey, S. Fernandes, A. Addala, S. Kibrom, J. R. Krissberg, S. M. Smith, S. Shah, and E. Wang. 2022. The impact of telehealth adoption during COVID-19 pandemic on patterns of pediatric subspecialty care utilization. *Academic Pediatrics* 22(8):1375-1383.

Campbell, F., K. Biggs, S. K. Aldiss, P. M. O'Neill, M. Clowes, J. McDonagh, A. While, and F. Gibson. 2016. Transition of care for adolescents from paediatric services to adult health services. *Cochrane Database of Systematic Reviews*(4).

Canares, T. L., A. Friedman, J. Rodean, R. R. Burns, D. Berkowitz, M. Hall, E. Alpern, and A. Montalbano. 2020. Pediatric outpatient utilization by differing Medicaid payment models in the United States. *BMC Health Services Research* 20(1):532.

Canin, L., and B. Wunsch. 2008. *Fuller scope of practice for primary care providers: A strategy to improve access to specialty care in the safety net.* https://www.academia.edu/6326002/Fuller_Scope_of_Practice_for_Primary_Care_Providers_A_Strategy_to_Improve_Access_to_Specialty_Care_in_the_Safety_Net_Prepared_for_the_Specialty_Care_Access_Initiative_A_Partnership_of_Kaiser_Permanente_Community_Benefits_California_Association_of_Public_Hospitals_and_Health_Systems_and_Californ_ (accessed April 27, 2023).

Carlson, K. M., S. K. Berman, J. Price, and the Committee on Child Health Financing. 2022. Guiding principles for managed care arrangements for the health of newborns, infants, children, adolescents and young adults. *Pediatrics* 150(2):e2022058396.

Casey, P. H., R. E. Lyle, T. M. Bird, J. M. Robbins, D. Z. Kuo, C. Brown, A. Lal, A. Tanios, and K. Burns. 2011. Effect of hospital-based comprehensive care clinic on health costs for Medicaid-insured medically complex children. *Archives of Pediatrics & Adolescent Medicine* 165(5):392-398.

Castillo, C., and E. Kitsos. 2017. Transitions from pediatric to adult care. *Global Pediatric Health* 4:2333794X17744946.

CCHP (Center for Connected Health Policy). 2020. *State telehealth Medicaid fee-for-service policy: A historical analysis of telehealth: 2013–2019.* https://www.cchpca.org/2021/04/Historical-State-Telehealth-Medicaid-Fee-For-Service-Policy-Report-FINAL.pdf (accessed April 12, 2023).

CCHP. 2023a. *State telehealth laws and reimbursement policies report, Spring 2023.* https://www.cchpca.org/resources/state-telehealth-laws-and-reimbursement-policies-report-spring-2023/ (accessed July 11, 2023).

CCHP. 2023b. *Policy trend maps.* https://www.cchpca.org/policy-trends (accessed May 4, 2023).

CCHP. 2023c. *Cross-state licensing.* https://www.cchpca.org/topic/cross-state-licensing-covid-19/ (accessed April 19, 2023).

CHA (Children's Hospital Association). 2021. *Improving communication between primary care providers and specialists.* https://www.childrenshospitals.org/news/childrens-hospitals-today/2021/02/improving-communication-between-primary-care-providers-and-specialists#.YiZ_TXrMKUk (accessed April 14, 2023).

CHCS (Center for Health Care Strategies). 2018. *Medicaid accountable care organizations: State update.* https://www.chcs.org/media/ACO-Fact-Sheet-02-27-2018-1.pdf (accessed April 19, 2023).

Cheng, H., C. George, M. Dunham, L. Whitehead, and E. Denney-Wilson. 2021. Nurse-led interventions in the prevention and treatment of overweight and obesity in infants, children and adolescents: A scoping review. *International Journal of Nursing Studies* 121:104008.

Children's National. 2023. *Referral guidelines.* https://childrensnational.org/healthcare-providers/refer-a-patient/referral-guidelines (accessed April 14, 2023).

Chu, R. C., C. Peters, N. De Lew, and B. D. Sommers. 2021. *State Medicaid telehealth policies before and during the COVID-19 public health emergency.* https://aspe.hhs.gov/sites/default/files/2021-07/medicaid-telehealth-brief.pdf (accessed April 14, 2023).

CMS (Centers for Medicare & Medicaid Services). 2020. *Re: Value-based care opportunities in Medicaid.* https://www.medicaid.gov/Federal-Policy-Guidance/Downloads/smd20004.pdf (accessed April 19, 2023).

CMS. 2021. *Guidance on coordinating care provided by out-of-state providers for children with medically complex conditions.* https://www.medicaid.gov/federal-policy-guidance/downloads/cib102021.pdf (accessed April 18, 2023).

CMS. 2022a. *Advanced practice registered nurses, anesthesiologist assistants, and physician assistants.* https://www.cms.gov/Outreach-and-Education/Medicare-Learning-Network-MLN/MLNProducts/MLN-Publications-Items/CMS1244981 (accessed December 29, 2022).

CMS. 2022b. *Integrated Care for Kids (InCK) model.* https://innovation.cms.gov/innovation-models/integrated-care-for-kids-model (accessed April 19, 2023).

CMS. 2022c. *Re: Health homes for children with medically complex conditions.* https://www.medicaid.gov/federal-policy-guidance/downloads/smd22004.pdf

CMS. 2023a. *Reimbursement for telehealth and provider and facility guidelines.* https://www.medicaid.gov/medicaid/benefits/telehealth/reimbursement-for-telehealth-and-provider-and-facility-guidelines/index.html (accessed April 12, 2023).

CMS. 2023b. *Telehealth.* https://www.medicaid.gov/medicaid/benefits/telehealth/index.html (accessed April 12, 2023).

CMS. 2023c. *State innovation models initiative: General information.* https://innovation.cms.gov/innovation-models/state-innovations (accessed April 19, 2023).

CMS. 2023d. *Maternal & infant health initiative value-based payment.* https://www.medicaid.gov/resources-for-states/innovation-accelerator-program/functional-areas/value-based-payment/maternal-infant-health-initiative-value-based-payment/index.html (accessed April 19, 2023).

CMS. 2023e. *Re: Coverage and payment of interprofessional consultation in Medicaid and the Children's Health Insurance Program (CHIP)* https://www.medicaid.gov/federal-policy-guidance/downloads/sho23001.pdf (accessed May 4, 2023).

Cohen, E., A. Lacombe-Duncan, K. Spalding, J. MacInnis, D. Nicholas, U. G. Narayanan, M. Gordon, I. Margolis, and J. N. Friedman. 2012. Integrated complex care coordination for children with medical complexity: A mixed-methods evaluation of tertiary care-community collaboration. *BMC Health Services Research* 12(1):1-11.

Cohen, E., C. J. Wang, and B. Zuckerman. 2018. Specialized care without the subspecialist: A value opportunity for secondary care. *Children* 5(6):69.

Collins, C., D. L. Hewson, and R. Munger. 2010. *Evolving models of behavioral health integration in primary care.* Millbank Fund Report. New York: New York Milbank Memorial Fund.

Connor, D. F., T. J. McLaughlin, M. Jeffers-Terry, W. H. O'Brien, C. J. Stille, L. M. Young, and R. C. Antonelli. 2006. Targeted child psychiatric services: A new model of pediatric primary clinician—child psychiatry collaborative care. *Clinical Pediatrics* 45(5):423-434.

Cooley, W. C., A. R. Kemper, G. and the Medical Home Workgroup of the National Coordinating Center for the Regional, and C. Newborn Screening Service. 2013. An approach to family-centered coordinated co-management for individuals with conditions identified through newborn screening. *Genetics in Medicine* 15(3):174-177.

Cornell, E., L. Chandhok, and K. Rubin. 2015. Implementation of referral guidelines at the interface between pediatric primary and subspecialty care. *Healthcare* 3(2):74-79.

Cotton, A., M. A. Riddle, S. P. Reinblatt, and A. F. Bettencourt. 2021. Characteristics of providers using a child psychiatry access program. *Psychiatric Services* 72(10):1213-1217.

Coulson, C. C., and S. Galvin. 2020. Navigating perinatal care in western North Carolina: Access for patients and providers. *North Carolina Medical Journal* 81(1):41-44.

Counts, N. Z., K. B. Mistry, and C. A. Wong. 2021. The need for new cost measures in pediatric value-based payment. *Pediatrics* 147(2).

Crego, N., C. Douglas, E. Bonnabeau, M. Earls, K. Eason, E. Merwin, G. Rains, P. Tanabe, and N. Shah. 2020. Sickle-cell disease co-management, health care utilization, and hydroxyurea use. *Journal of the American Board of Family Medicine* 33(1):91-105.

Curfman, A., S. D. McSwain, J. Chuo, B. Yeager-McSwain, D. A. Schinasi, J. Marcin, N. Herendeen, S. L. Chung, K. Rheuban, and C. A. Olson. 2021. Pediatric telehealth in the COVID-19 pandemic era and beyond. *Pediatrics* 148(3).

de Banate, M. A., J. Maypole, and M. Sadof. 2019. Care coordination for children with medical complexity. *Current Opinion in Pediatrics* 31(4):575-582.

Deeds, S. A., K. J. Dowdell, L. D. Chew, and S. L. Ackerman. 2019. Implementing an opt-in econsult program at seven academic medical centers: A qualitative analysis of primary care provider experiences. *Journal of General Internal Medicine* 34(8):1427-1433.

Di Guglielmo, M. D., J. S. Greenspan, and D. J. Abatemarco. 2016. Pediatrician preferences, local resources, and economic factors influence referral to a subspecialty access clinic. *Primary Health Care Research & Development* 17(6):628-635.

Di Guglielmo, M. D., J. Plesnick, J. S. Greenspan, and I. Sharif. 2013. A new model to decrease time-to-appointment wait for gastroenterology evaluation. *Pediatrics* 131(5):e1632-e1638.

Di Lorenzo, C., R. B. Colletti, H. P. Lehmann, J. T. Boyle, W. T. Gerson, J. S. Hyams, R. H. Squires, Jr., L. S. Walker, and P. T. Kanda. 2005. Chronic abdominal pain in children: A technical report of the American Academy of Pediatrics and the North American Society for Pediatric Gastroenterology, Hepatology and Nutrition. *Journal of Pediatric Gastroenterology and Nutrition* 40(3):249-261.

Eichner, J. M., J. M. Betts, M. B. Chitkara, J. A. Jewell, P. S. Lye, L. J. Mirkinson, C. Brown, K. Heiss, L. Lostocco, R. A. Salerno, J. M. Percelay, S. N. Alexander, B. H. Johnson, M. Abraham, E. Ahmann, E. Crocker, N. DiVenere, G. MacKean, W. E. Schwab, and T. Shelton. 2012. Patient- and family-centered care and the pediatrician's role. *Pediatrics* 129(2):394-404.

Faucon, C., D. Gribi, D. S. Courvoisier, P. Senet, O. Itani, A. Barbaud, A. M. Magnier, C. Frances, J. Chastang, and F. Chasset. 2022. Performance accuracy, advantages and limitations of a store-and-forward teledermatology platform developed for general practitioners: A retrospective study of 298 cases. *Annales de Dermatologie et de Venereologie* 149(4):245-250.

Feyissa, E. A., E. Cornell, L. Chandhok, D. Wang, C. Ionita, J. Schwab, R. Kostyun, F. Wilion, and K. Rubin. 2015. Impact of co-management at the primary-subspecialty care interface on follow-up and referral patterns for patients with concussion. *Clinical Pediatrics* 54(10):969-975.

FitzGerald, M., M. Z. Gunja, and R. Tikkanen. 2022. *Primary care in high-income countries: How the United States compares.* https://www.commonwealthfund.org/publications/issue-briefs/2022/mar/primary-care-high-income-countries-how-united-states-compares (accessed May 11, 2023).

Fogler, S., M. O'Connell, J. Quinton, C. Ritter, B. Waldersen, and P. Rawal. 2022. Pathways for specialty care coordination and integration in population-based models: CMS. https://www.cms.gov/blog/pathways-specialty-care-coordination-and-integration-population-based-models (accessed April 24, 2023).

Forrest, C. B. 2009. A typology of specialists' clinical roles. *Archives of Internal Medicine* 169(11):1062-1068.

Forrest, C. B., G. B. Glade, A. E. Baker, A. B. Bocian, M. Kang, and B. Starfield. 1999. The pediatric primary-specialty care interface: How pediatricians refer children and adolescents to specialty care. *Archives of Pediatrics & Adolescent Medicine* 153(7):705-714.

Francis, E., K. Shifler Bowers, G. Buchberger, S. Ryan, W. Milchak, and J. Kraschnewski. 2020. Reducing alcohol and opioid use among youth in rural counties: An innovative training protocol for primary health care providers and school personnel. *JMIR Research Protocols* 9(11):e21015.

Freed, J. A., A. J. Hale, D. Rangachari, and D. N. Ricotta. 2020. Twelve tips for teaching oncology to non-oncologists. *Medical Teacher* 42(9):987-992.

Freund, T., C. Everett, P. Griffiths, C. Hudon, L. Naccarella, and M. Laurant. 2015. Skill mix, roles and remuneration in the primary care workforce: Who are the healthcare professionals in the primary care teams across the world? *International Journal of Nursing Studies* 52(3):727-743.

Frogner, B. K., E. P. Fraher, J. Spetz, P. Pittman, J. Moore, A. J. Beck, D. Armstrong, and P. I. Buerhaus. 2020. Modernizing scope-of-practice regulations—time to prioritize patients. *New England Journal of Medicine* 382(7):591-593.

FSMB (Federation of State Medical Boards). 2023. *U.S. States and territories modifying requirements for telehealth in response to COVID-19.* https://www.fsmb.org/siteassets/advocacy/pdf/states-waiving-licensure-requirements-for-telehealth-in-response-to-covid-19.pdf (accessed April 19, 2023).

GAO (U.S. Government Accountability Office). 2019. CMS oversight should ensure state implementation of screening and enrollment requirements. Report no. GAO-20-8. Washington, DC: GAO. https://www.gao.gov/products/GAO-20-8 (accessed July 12, 2023).

Garg, A., C. J. Homer, and P. H. Dworkin. 2019. Addressing social determinants of health: Challenges and opportunities in a value-based model. *Pediatrics* 143(4).

Gates, A., R. Rudowitz, and J. Guyer. 2014. *An overview of Delivery System Reform Incentive Payment (DSRIP) waivers.* https://www.kff.org/report-section/an-overview-of-delivery-system-reform-incentive-payment-waivers-issue-brief/ (accessed April 19, 2023).

Germán, M., M. L. Rinke, B. A. Gurney, R. S. Gross, D. E. Bloomfield, L. A. Haliczer, S. Colman, A. D. Racine, and R. D. Briggs. 2017. Comparing two models of integrated behavioral health programs in pediatric primary care. *Child and Adolescent Psychiatric Clinics* 26(4):815-828.

Giavina-Bianchi, M., A. P. Santos, and E. Cordioli. 2020. Teledermatology reduces dermatology referrals and improves access to specialists. *EClinicalMedicine* 29-30:100641.

Gigli, K. H., B. S. Davis, G. R. Martsolf, and J. M. Kahn. 2021. Advanced practice provider-inclusive staffing models and patient outcomes in pediatric critical care. *Medical Care* 59(7):597-603.

Gillespie, C., J. A. Wilhite, K. Hanley, K. Hardowar, L. Altshuler, H. Fisher, B. Porter, A. Wallach, and S. Zabar. 2022. Addressing social determinants of health in primary care: A quasi-experimental study using unannounced standardised patients to evaluate the impact of audit/feedback on physicians' rates of identifying and responding to social needs. *BMJ Quality & Safety* PMID: 35623722.

Gilman, B., D. B. Whicher, Randall, N. McCall, S. Dale, L. Felland, R. Schmitz, J. Schurrer, L. Forrow Vollmer, M. Flick, J. Derzon, and R. Lakhani. 2020. *Evaluation of the Health Care Innovation Award, Round 2: Final report.* Mathematica.

Got Transition. 2022. *Six Core Elements of Health Care Transition.* https://www.gottransition.org/six-core-elements/ (accessed December 29, 2022).

Green, C. M., J. M. Foy, M. F. Earls, A. Lavin, G. L. Askew, R. Baum, E. Berger-Jenkins, T. B. Gambon, A. A. Nasir, and L. S. Wissow. 2019. Achieving the pediatric mental health competencies. *Pediatrics* 144(5).

Guth, M., and E. Hinton. 2020. *State efforts to expand Medicaid coverage & access to telehealth in response to COVID-19.* https://www.kff.org/coronavirus-covid-19/issue-brief/state-efforts-to-expand-medicaid-coverage-access-to-telehealth-in-response-to-covid-19/ (accessed April 14, 2023).

Hamburger, E. K., J. L. Lane, D. Agrawal, C. Boogaard, J. L. Hanson, J. Weisz, and M. Ottolini. 2015. The referral and consultation entrustable professional activity: Defining the components in order to develop a curriculum for pediatric residents. *Academic Pediatrics* 15(1):5-8.

Harahsheh, A. S., E. K. Hamburger, L. Saleh, L. M. Crawford, E. Sepe, A. Dubelman, L. Baram, K. M. Kadow, C. Driskill, K. Prestidge, J. E. Bost, and D. Berkowitz. 2021. Promoting judicious primary care referral of patients with chest pain to cardiology: A quality improvement initiative. *Medical Decision Making* 41(5):559-572.

Heller, R. E., III, B. D. Coley, S. F. Simoneaux, D. J. Podberesky, M. Hernanz-Schulman, R. L. Robertson, and L. F. Donnelly. 2017. Quality measures and pediatric radiology: Suggestions for the transition to value-based payment. *Pediatric Radiology* 47(7):776-782.

HHS (U.S. Department of Health and Human Services). 2022. *HHS roadmap for behavioral health integration.* https://www.hhs.gov/about/news/2022/12/02/hhs-roadmap-for-behavioral-health-integration-fact-sheet.html (accessed March 30, 2023).

HHS. 2023. *Private insurance coverage for telehealth.* https://telehealth.hhs.gov/providers/billing-and-reimbursement/private-insurance-coverage-for-telehealth (accessed May 4, 2023).

Hilt, R. J., M. A. Romaire, M. G. McDonell, J. M. Sears, A. Krupski, J. N. Thompson, J. Myers, and E. W. Trupin. 2013. The partnership access line: Evaluating a child psychiatry consult program in Washington state. *JAMA Pediatrics* 167(2):162-168.

Hinton, E., L. Stolyar, M. Guth, and M. Nardone. 2022a. *State delivery system and payment strategies aimed at improving outcomes and lowering costs in Medicaid.* https://www.kff.org/medicaid/issue-brief/state-delivery-system-and-payment-strategies-aimed-at-improving-outcomes-and-lowering-costs-in-medicaid/ (accessed April 19, 2023).

Hinton, E., M. Guth, J. Raphael, S. Haldar, and R. Rudowitz. 2022b. *How the pandemic continues to shape Medicaid priorities: Results from an annual Medicaid budget survey for state fiscal years 2022 and 2023.* https://files.kff.org/attachment/REPORT-How-the-Pandemic-Continues-to-Shape-Medicaid-Priorities-Results-from-an-Annual-Medicaid-Budget-Survey-for-State-Fiscal-Years-2022-and-2023.pdf (accessed May 8, 2023).

Hong, P., K. Ritchie, C. Beaton-Campbell, L. Cavanagh, J. Belyea, and G. Corsten. 2015. The effectiveness of nurse-led outpatient referral triage decision making in pediatric otolaryngology. *International Journal of Pediatric Otorhinolaryngology* 79(4):576-578.

Houston, R., A. Smithey, and K. Brykman. 2022. *Medicaid population-based payment: The current landscape, early insights, and considerations for policymakers.* https://www.chcs.org/media/Medicaid-Population-Based-Payment-Current-Landscape-Early-Insights-and-Considerations-for-Policymakers_111622.pdf (accessed April 19, 2023).

Huang, X., and M. B. Rosenthal. 2014. Transforming specialty practice—the patient-centered medical neighborhood. *New England Journal of Medicine* 370(15):1376-1379.

Institute for Healthcare Improvement, and the National Patient Safety Foundation. 2017. *The nine steps of the closed-loop EHR referral process. Closing the loop: A guide to safer ambulatory referrals in the EHR era.* Cambridge, Massachusetts: Institute for Healthcare Improvement.

IHS Markit Ltd. 2021. *The complexities of physician supply and demand: Projections from 2019 to 2034.* Washington, DC: Association of American Medical Colleges.

IMLCC (Interstate Medical Licensure Compact). 2022. *A faster pathway to physician licensure.* https://www.imlcc.org/a-faster-pathway-to-physician-licensure (accessed December 22, 2022).

IOM (Institute of Medicine). 2001. *Crossing the quality chasm: A new health system for the 21st century.* Washington, DC: National Academy Press.

Ip, W., P. Prahalad, J. Palma, and J. H. Chen. 2022. A data-driven algorithm to recommend initial clinical workup for outpatient specialty referral: Algorithm development and validation using electronic health record data and expert surveys. *JMIR Medical Informatics* 10(3):e30104.

Katkin, J. P., S. J. Kressly, A. R. Edwards, J. M. Perrin, C. A. Kraft, J. E. Richerson, J. S. Tieder, L. Wall, Task Force on Pediatric Practice Change. 2017. Guiding principles for team-based pediatric care. *Pediatrics* 140(2).

Kevill, K. A., A. Bazzy-Asaad, and S. Pati. 2019. Opportunities on the road to value-based payment for children with chronic respiratory disease. *Pediatric Pulmonology* 54(2):105-116.

KFF (Kaiser Family Foundation). 2015. *The State Innovation Models (SIM) program: A look at Round 2 grantees.* https://www.kff.org/medicaid/fact-sheet/the-state-innovation-models-sim-program-a-look-at-round-2-grantees (accessed April 19, 2023).

Khair, K., and S. Chaplin. 2017. What is a nurse-led service? A discussion paper. *Journal of Haemophilia Practice* 4(1):4-13.

Kirschner, N., and M. Greenlee. 2010. The patient-centered medical home neighbor: The interface of the patient-centered medical home with specialty/subspecialty practices. Philadelphia, PA: American College of Physicians.

Kissam, S. M., H. Beil, C. Cousart, L. M. Greenwald, and J. T. Lloyd. 2019. States encouraging value-based payment: Lessons from CMS's State Innovation Models Initiative. *Milbank Quarterly* 97(2):506-542.

Kobussen, T. A., G. Hansen, and T. R. Holt. 2021. Comparing subspecialty and intensive care providers perspectives on pediatric complex chronic patients: A survey study. *International Journal of Care Coordination* 24(3-4):133-141.

Komaromy, M., D. Duhigg, A. Metcalf, C. Carlson, S. Kalishman, L. Hayes, T. Burke, K. Thornton, and S. Arora. 2016. Project ECHO (Extension for Community Healthcare Outcomes): A new model for educating primary care providers about treatment of substance use disorders. *Substance Abuse* 37(1):20-24.

Kuo, D. Z., M. Comeau, J. M. Perrin, C. Coleman, P. White, C. Lerner, and C. J. Stille. 2022. Moving from spending to investment: A research agenda for improving health care financing for children and youth with special health care needs. *Academic Pediatrics* 22(2, Suppl):S47-S53.

Kuo, Y. F., F. L. Loresto, Jr., L. R. Rounds, and J. S. Goodwin. 2013. States with the least restrictive regulations experienced the largest increase in patients seen by nurse practitioners. *Health Affairs* 32(7):1236-1243.

Kwok, J., J. N. Olayiwola, M. Knox, E. J. Murphy, and D. S. Tuot. 2018. Electronic consultation system demonstrates educational benefit for primary care providers. *Journal of Telemedicine and Telecare* 24(7):465-472.

Lalloo, C., V. Mohabir, F. Campbell, N. Sun, S. Klein, J. Tyrrell, G. Mesaroli, S. Ataollahi-Eshqoor, J. Osei-Twum, and J. Stinson. 2023. Pediatric Project ECHO for pain: Implementation and mixed methods evaluation of a virtual medical education program to support interprofessional pain management in children and youth. *BMC Medical Education* 23(1):71.

Landon, B. E. 2014. Structuring payments to patient-centered medical homes. *JAMA* 312(16):1633-1634.

Lax, Y., E. Bathory, and S. Braganza. 2021. Pediatric primary care and subspecialist providers' comfort, attitudes and practices screening and referring for social determinants of health. *BMC Health Services Research* 21(1):956.

Leslie, L., P. Rappo, H. Abelson, R. R. Jenkins, S. R. Sewall, R. W. Chesney, H. J. Mulvey, J. L. Simon, and E. R. Alden. 2000. Final report of the FOPE II pediatric generalists of the future workgroup. *Pediatrics* 106(5):1199-1223.

Lestishock, L. 2020. NAPNAP position statement on supporting the transition from pediatric to adult focused health care. *Journal of Pediatric Health Care* 34(4):390-394.

Lestishock, L., A. M. Daley, and P. White. 2018. Pediatric nurse practitioners' perspectives on health care transition from pediatric to adult care. *Journal of Pediatric Health Care* 32(3):263-272.

Levy, S. L., E. Hill, K. Mattern, K. McKay, R. C. Sheldrick, and E. C. Perrin. 2017. Colocated mental health/developmental care. *Clinical Pediatrics* 56(11):1023-1031.

Looman, W. S., M. Antolick, R. G. Cady, S. A. Lunos, A. E. Garwick, and S. M. Finkelstein. 2015. Effects of a telehealth care coordination intervention on perceptions of health care by caregivers of children with medical complexity: A randomized controlled trial. *Journal of Pediatric Health Care* 29(4):352-363.

MACPAC (Medicaid and CHIP Payment and Access Commission). 2020. *Medicaid payment policy for out-of-state hospital services.* https://www.macpac.gov/wp-content/uploads/2020/01/Medicaid-Payment-Policy-for-Out-of-State-Hospital-Services.pdf (accessed July 12, 2023).

MACPAC. 2023. *Value-based payment.* https://www.macpac.gov/subtopic/value-based-purchasing/ (accessed April 19, 2023).

Manetto, N., Greenberg, J., and C. Reddy. 2020. *Policies to enhance care of out-of-state pediatric Medicaid beneficiaries.* In Health Affairs Blog. https://www.healthaffairs.org/content/forefront/policies-enhance-care-out-of-state-pediatric-medicaid-beneficiaries (accessed July 12, 2023).

Marcin, J. P., U. Shaikh, and R. H. Steinhorn. 2016. Addressing health disparities in rural communities using telehealth. *Pediatric Research* 79(1):169-176.

Martyn, K. K., J. Martin, S. M. Gutknecht, and H. E. Faleer. 2013. The pediatric nurse practitioner workforce: Meeting the health care needs of children. *Journal of Pediatric Health Care* 27(5):400-405.

McClain, M. R., W. C. Cooley, T. Keirns, and A. Smith. 2014. A survey of the preferences of primary care physicians regarding the comanagement with specialists of children with rare or complex conditions. *Clinical Pediatrics* 53(6):566-570.

McCulloch, M. R., J. F. Thomas, M. A. Thompson, and K. D. Carel. 2023. Outpatient electronic consultations in pediatric allergy and immunology. *Annals of Allergy, Asthma & Immunology* 130(1):115-117.

McDonnell, M. M., N. C. Elder, R. Stock, M. Wolf, A. Steeves-Reece, and T. Graham. 2020. Project ECHO integrated within the Oregon Rural Practice-Based Research Network (ORPN). *Journal of the American Board of Family Medicine* 33(5):789-795.

McLeigh, J. D., L. Malthaner, C. Winebrenner, and K. E. Stone. 2022. Paediatric integrated care in the primary care setting: A scoping review of populations served, models used and outcomes measured. *Child: Care, Health and Development* 48(5):869-879.

McManus, M., P. White, A. Schmidt, M. Barr, C. Langer, K. Barger, and A. Ware. 2020. Health care gap affects 20% of United States population: Transition from pediatric to adult health care. *Health Policy OPEN* 1:100007.

Mechanic, R. E., and D. Zinner. 2016. Risk contracting and operational capabilities in large medical groups during national healthcare reform. *American Journal of Managed Care* 22(6):441-446.

Medical Home Initiatives for Children with Special Needs Project Advisory Committee. 2002. The medical home. *Pediatrics* 110(1 Pt 1):184-186.

Meyers, D. J., A. T. Chien, K. H. Nguyen, Z. Li, S. J. Singer, and M. B. Rosenthal. 2019. Association of team-based primary care with health care utilization and costs among chronically ill patients. *JAMA Internal Medicine* 179(1):54-61.

Mitchell, P., M. Wynia, R. Golden, B. McNellis, S. Okun, C. E. Webb, V. Rohrbach, and I. Von Kohorn. 2012. *Core principles & values of effective team-based health care.* https://nam.edu/wp-content/uploads/2015/06/VSRT-Team-Based-Care-Principles-Values.pdf (accessed April 28, 2023).

Morgan, P. A., V. A. Smith, T. S. Berkowitz, D. Edelman, C. H. Van Houtven, S. L. H. Woolson, C. C. Hendrix, Christine M. Everett, B. S. White, and G. L. Jackson. 2019. Impact of physicians, nurse practitioners, and physician assistants on utilization and costs for complex patients. *Health Affairs* 38(6):1028-1036.

NASEM (National Academies of Sciences, Engineering, and Medicine). 2016. *Assessing progress on the Institute of Medicine report* The Future of Nursing. Edited by S. H. Altman, A. S. Butler and L. Shern. Washington, DC: The National Academies Press.

NASEM. 2021a. *The future of nursing 2020–2030: Charting a path to achieve health equity.* Edited by M. K. Wakefield, D. R. Williams, S. Le Menestrel, and J. L. Flaubert. Washington, DC: The National Academies Press.

NASEM. 2021b. *Implementing high-quality primary care: Rebuilding the foundation of health care.* Edited by L. McCauley, R. L. Phillips, Jr., M. Meisnere, and S. K. Robinson. Washington, DC: The National Academies Press.

Nasir, A., L. Nasir, A. Tarrell, D. Finken, A. Lacroix, S. Pinniniti, S. Pitner, and M. McCarthy. 2018. Complexity in pediatric primary care. *Primary Health Care Research & Development* 20:e59.

National Council for Mental Wellbeing. 2021. *The four quadrant clinical integration model.* https://www.thenationalcouncil.org/resources/the-four-quadrant-clinical-integration-model/ (accessed July 7, 2023).

Nethan, S. T., R. Hariprasad, R. Babu, V. Kumar, S. Sharma, and R. Mehrotra. 2020. Project ECHO: A potential best-practice tool for training healthcare providers in oral cancer screening and tobacco cessation. *Journal of Cancer Education* 35(5):965-971.

Nguyen, O. T., A. K. Watson, K. Motwani, C. Warpinski, K. McDilda, C. Leon, N. Khanna, R. W. Nall, and K. Turner. 2022. Patient-level factors associated with utilization of telemedicine services from a free clinic during COVID-19. *Telemedicine and e-Health* 28(4):526-534.

NHLBI (National Heart, Lung, and Blood Institute). 2007. *Expert panel report 3: Guidelines for the diagnosis and management of asthma.* https://www.ncbi.nlm.nih.gov/books/NBK7232/pdf/Bookshelf_NBK7232.pdf (accessed April 27, 2023).

NNCPAP (National Network of Child Psychiatry Access Programs). 2022. *National Network of Child Psychiatry Access Programs.* https://www.nncpap.org (accessed December 22, 2022).

NSCH (National Survey of Children's Health). n.d. *Health Resources and Services Administration, Maternal and Child Health Bureau.* https://www.childhealthdata.org/browse/survey/results?q=9392&r=1 (accessed July 11, 2023).

O'Connell, A., and J. Petty. 2019. Preparing young people with complex needs and their families for transition to adult services. *Nursing Children and Young People* 31(1):25-31.

Olayiwola, J. N., A. Potapov, A. Gordon, J. Jurado, C. Magana, M. Knox, and D. Tuot. 2019. Electronic consultation impact from the primary care clinician perspective: Outcomes from a national sample. *Journal of Telemedicine and Telecare* 25(8):493-498.

ONC (Office of the National Coordinator for Health Information Technology). 2019. *Frequently asked questions.* https://www.healthit.gov/faq/what-telehealth-how-telehealth-different-telemedicine (accessed July 12, 2023).

Özalp Gerçeker, G., G. Karayağız Muslu, and F. Yardimci. 2016. Children's postoperative symptoms at home through nurse-led telephone counseling and its effects on parents' anxiety: A randomized controlled trial. *Journal for Specialists in Pediatric Nursing* 21(4):189-199.

Pany, M. J., L. Chen, B. Sheridan, and R. S. Huckman. 2021. Provider teams outperform solo providers in managing chronic diseases and could improve the value of care. *Health Affairs* 40(3):435-444.

Patel, V., D. Stewart, and M. J. Horstman. 2020. E-consults: An effective way to decrease clinic wait times in rheumatology. *BMC Rheumatology* 4:54.

Perrin, J. M., E. Zimmerman, A. Hertz, T. Johnson, T. Merrill, and D. Smith. 2017. Pediatric accountable care organizations: Insight from early adopters. *Pediatrics* 139(2).

Pickler, R., S. Wade-Murphy, J. Gold, H. Tubbs-Cooley, C. M. White, A. Statile, C. Hoying, H. Sauers-Ford, S. S. Shah, and J. Simmons. 2016. A nurse transitional home visit following pediatric hospitalizations. *Journal of Nursing Administration* 46(12):642-647.

Pittman, P., B. Leach, C. Everett, X. Han, and D. McElroy. 2020. NP and PA privileging in acute care settings: Do scope of practice laws matter? *Medical Care Research and Review* 77(2):112-120.

Platt, R. E., A. E. Spencer, M. D. Burkey, C. Vidal, S. Polk, A. F. Bettencourt, S. Jain, J. Stratton, and L. S. Wissow. 2018. What's known about implementing co-located paediatric integrated care: A scoping review. *International Review of Psychiatry* 30(6):242-271.

Poghosyan, L., and L. H. Aiken. 2015. Maximizing nurse practitioners' contributions to primary care through organizational changes. *Journal of Ambulatory Care Management* 38(2):109-117.

Poghosyan, L., A. Nannini, and S. Clarke. 2013a. Organizational climate in primary care settings: Implications for nurse practitioner practice. *Journal of the American Association of Nurse Practitioners* 25(3):134-140.

Poghosyan, L., A. Nannini, S. R. Finkelstein, E. Mason, and J. A. Shaffer. 2013b. Development and psychometric testing of the nurse practitioner primary care organizational climate questionnaire. *Nursing Research* 62(5):325-334.

Poghosyan, L., J. Shang, J. Liu, H. Poghosyan, N. Liu, and B. Berkowitz. 2015. Nurse practitioners as primary care providers: Creating favorable practice environments in New York State and Massachusetts. *Health Care Management Review* 40(1):46-55.

Porto, A., K. Rubin, K. Wagner, W. Chang, G. Macri, and D. Anderson. 2021. Impact of pediatric electronic consultations in a federally qualified health center. *Telemedicine and e-Health* 27(12):1379-1384.

Preminger, T. J. 2022. Telemedicine in pediatric cardiology: Pros and cons. *Current Opinion in Pediatrics* 34(5):484-490.

Price, J., M. L. Brandt, M. L. Hudak, S. K. Berman, K. M. Carlson, A. P. Giardino, L. Hammer, K. Heggen, S. A. Pearlman, and B. G. Sood. 2020. Principles of financing the medical home for children. *Pediatrics* 145(1).

Ray, K. N., and J. M. Kahn. 2020. Connected subspecialty care: Applying telehealth strategies to specific referral barriers. *Academic Pediatrics* 20(1):16-22.

Ray, K. N., J. R. Demirci, D. L. Bogen, A. Mehrotra, and E. Miller. 2015. Optimizing telehealth strategies for subspecialty care: Recommendations from rural pediatricians. *Telemedicine Journal and e-Health* 21(8):622-629.

Ray, K. N., L. E. Ashcraft, J. M. Kahn, A. Mehrotra, and E. Miller. 2016. Family perspectives on high-quality pediatric subspecialty referrals. *Academic Pediatrics* 16(6):594-600.

Ray, K. N., L. E. Ashcraft, A. Mehrotra, E. Miller, and J. M. Kahn. 2017. Family perspectives on telemedicine for pediatric subspecialty care. *Telemedicine Journal and e-Health* 23(10):852-862.

REACH Institute. 2022. *The REACH Institute.* https://thereachinstitute.org/ (accessed December 27, 2022).

Reagan, P. B., and P. J. Salsberry. 2013. The effects of state-level scope-of-practice regulations on the number and growth of nurse practitioners. *Nursing Outlook* 61(6):392-399.

Reiss-Brennan, B., K. D. Brunisholz, C. Dredge, P. Briot, K. Grazier, A. Wilcox, L. Savitz, and B. James. 2016. Association of integrated team-based care with health care quality, utilization, and cost. *JAMA* 316(8):826-834.

Richardson, L., E. McCauley, and W. Katon. 2009. Collaborative care for adolescent depression: A pilot study. *General Hospital Psychiatry* 31(1):36-45.

Richman, E. L., B. Lombardi, L. Zerden, and R. Randolph. 2018. *Where is behavioral health integration occurring? Mapping national co-location trends using national provider identifier data.* Ann Arbor, MI: University of Michigan Behavioral Health Workforce Research Center.

Rubin, K., E. Cornell, E. Feyissa, S. Macary, L. Chandhok, and L. Honigfeld. 2014. *Working together to meet children's health needs: Primary and specialty care co-management.* Farmington, CT: Child Health and Development Institute of Connecticut.

Rudich, J., A. B. Conmy, R. C. Chu, C. Peters, N. De Lew, and B. D. Sommers. 2022. *State Medicaid telehealth policies before and during the COVID-19 public health emergency: 2022 update.* Washington, DC: ASPE Office of Health Policy.

SAMHSA (Substance Abuse and Mental Health Services). 2023. *Integrated models for behavioral health and primary care.* https://www.samhsa.gov/resource/ebp/integrated-models-behavioral-health-primary-care (accessed January 3, 2023).

Sarvet, B., J. Gold, J. Q. Bostic, B. J. Masek, J. B. Prince, M. Jeffers-Terry, C. F. Moore, B. Molbert, and J. H. Straus. 2010. Improving access to mental health care for children: The Massachusetts Child Psychiatry Access Project. *Pediatrics* 126(6):1191-1200.

Scanlon, A., M. Murphy, K. Tori, and L. Poghosyan. 2018. A national study of Australian nurse practitioners' organizational practice environment. *Journal for Nurse Practitioners* 14(5):414-418.e413.

Schraeder, K., B. Allemang, A. N. Felske, C. M. Scott, K. A. McBrien, G. Dimitropoulos, and S. Samuel. 2022. Community based primary care for adolescents and young adults transitioning from pediatric specialty care: Results from a scoping review. *Journal of Primary Care & Community Health* 13:21501319221084890.

Schumacher, D. J., D. C. West, A. Schwartz, S. T. Li, L. Millstein, E. C. Griego, T. Turner, B. E. Herman, R. Englander, J. Hemond, V. Hudson, L. Newhall, K. McNeal Trice, J. Baughn, E. Giudice, H. Famiglietti, J. Tolentino, K. Gifford, and C. Carraccio. 2020. Longitudinal assessment of resident performance using entrustable professional activities. *JAMA Network Open* 3(1):e1919316.

Seattle Children's. 2023. *Referral information by clinic*. https://www.seattlechildrens.org/healthcare-professionals/access-services/ambulatory-services/clinic-referrals/clinic-referral-information (accessed April 14, 2023).

Seburg, E. M., B. A. Olson-Bullis, D. M. Bredeson, M. G. Hayes, and N. E. Sherwood. 2015. A review of primary care-based childhood obesity prevention and treatment interventions. *Current Obesity Reports* 4(2):157-173.

Sharma, N., K. O'Hare, R. C. Antonelli, and G. S. Sawicki. 2014. Transition care: Future directions in education, health policy, and outcomes research. *Academic Pediatrics* 14(2):120-127.

Shi, L. 2012. The impact of primary care: A focused review. *Scientifica (Cairo)* 2012:432892.

Simon, T. D., K. B. Whitlock, W. Haaland, D. R. Wright, C. Zhou, J. Neff, W. Howard, B. Cartin, and R. Mangione-Smith. 2017. Effectiveness of a comprehensive case management service for children with medical complexity. *Pediatrics* 140(6).

Starfield, B. 1998. *Primary care: Balancing health needs, services, and technology*. New York: Oxford University Press.

Starfield, B., L. Shi, and J. Macinko. 2005. Contribution of primary care to health systems and health. *Milbank Q* 83(3):457-502.

Stave, E. A., L. Greenberg, E. Hamburger, M. Ottolini, D. Agrawal, K. Lewis, J. R. Barber, J. E. Bost, and A. S. Harahsheh. 2022. An educational intervention to facilitate appropriate subspecialty referrals: A study assessing resident communication skills. *BMC Medical Education* 22(1):533.

Stein, B. D., A. Kofner, W. B. Vogt, and H. Yu. 2019. A national examination of child psychiatric telephone consultation programs' impact on children's mental health care utilization. *Journal of the American Academy of Child & Adolescent Psychiatry* 58(10):1016-1019.

Stille, C. J., T. J. McLaughlin, W. A. Primack, K. M. Mazor, and R. C. Wasserman. 2006. Determinants and impact of generalist–specialist communication about pediatric outpatient referrals. *Pediatrics* 118(4):1341-1349.

Stille, C. J., W. A. Primack, T. J. McLaughlin, and R. C. Wasserman. 2007. Parents as information intermediaries between primary care and specialty physicians. *Pediatrics* 120(6):1238-1246.

Stille, C. J., L. Honigfeld, L. A. Heitlinger, D. Z. Kuo, and E. J. Werner. 2017. The pediatric primary care-specialist interface: A call for action. *Journal of Pediatrics* 187:303-308.

Strauss, J. S., D. P. Krowchuk, J. J. Leyden, A. W. Lucky, A. R. Shalita, E. C. Siegfried, D. M. Thiboutot, A. S. Van Voorhees, K. A. Beutner, and C. K. Sieck. 2007. Guidelines of care for acne vulgaris management. *Journal of the American Academy of Dermatology* 56(4):651-663.

Strosahl, K. 2005. Training behavioral health and primary care providers for integrated care: A core competencies approach. In *Behavioral Integrative Care: Treatments That Work in the Primary Care Setting*, edited by W. O'Donohue, M. Byrd, N. Cummings, and D. Henderson. New York: Brunner-Routledge. pp. 15-52.

Subotsky, F., and R. M. Brown. 1990. Working alongside the general practitioner: A child psychiatric clinic in the general practice setting. *Child: Care, Health and Development* 16(3):189-196.

Sud, E., and A. Anjankar. 2022. Applications of telemedicine in dermatology. *Cureus* 14(8):e27740.

Sullivan, K., P. George, and K. Horowitz. 2021. Addressing national workforce shortages by funding child psychiatry access programs. *Pediatrics* 147(1).

Tensen, E., J. P. van der Heijden, M. W. Jaspers, and L. Witkamp. 2016. Two decades of teledermatology: Current status and integration in national healthcare systems. *Current Dermatology Reports* 5:96-104.

Thielke, A., and V. King. 2020. *Electronic consultations (eConsults): A triple win for patients, clinicians, and payers.* https://www.milbank.org/publications/electronic-consultations-a-triple-win-for-patients-clinicians-and-payers (accessed April 30, 2023).

Thompson, M. A., A. L. Fuhlbrigge, D. W. Pearson, D. R. Saxon, L. A. Oberst-Walsh, and J. F. Thomas. 2021. Building eConsult (electronic consults) capability at an academic medical center to improve efficiencies in delivering specialty care. *Journal of Primary Care and Community Health* 12:21501327211005303.

University of Chicago. 2022. *Table of state licensure requirements during the COVID-19 PHE.* https://compliance.bsd.uchicago.edu/Documents/Table%20of%20State%20Licensure%20Requirements.pdf (accessed April 19, 2023).

UNM (University of New Mexico). 2022a. *About Project ECHO.* https://hsc.unm.edu/echo/about-us/ (accessed December 29, 2022).

UNM. 2022b. *Our work.* https://hsc.unm.edu/echo/partner-portal/ (accessed December 29, 2022).

Van Cleave, J., M. J. Okumura, N. Swigonski, K. G. O'Connor, M. Mann, and J. L. Lail. 2016. Medical homes for children with special health care needs: Primary care or subspecialty service? *Academic Pediatrics* 16(4):366-372.

Van Cleave, J., C. Holifield, and J. M. Perrin. 2018. Primary care providers' use of a child psychiatry telephone support program. *Academic Pediatrics* 18(3):266-272.

Varty, M., B. Speller-Brown, L. Phillips, and K. P. Kelly. 2020. Youths' experiences of transition from pediatric to adult care: An updated qualitative metasynthesis. *Journal of Pediatric Nursing* 55:201-210.

Vernacchio, L., J. M. Muto, G. Young, and W. Risko. 2012. Ambulatory subspecialty visits in a large pediatric primary care network. *Health Services Research* 47(4):1755-1769.

Vimalananda, V. G., G. Gupte, S. M. Seraj, J. Orlander, D. Berlowitz, B. G. Fincke, and S. R. Simon. 2015. Electronic consultations (e-consults) to improve access to specialty care: A systematic review and narrative synthesis. *Journal of Telemedicine and Telecare* 21(6):323-330.

Vimalananda, V. G., J. D. Orlander, M. K. Afable, B. G. Fincke, A. K. Solch, S. T. Rinne, E. J. Kim, S. L. Cutrona, D. D. Thomas, J. L. Strymish, and S. R. Simon. 2020. Electronic consultations (e-consults) and their outcomes: A systematic review. *Journal of the American Medical Informatics Association* 27(3):471-479.

Volpp, K. G., A. Navathe, E. O. Lee, M. Mugishii, A. B. Troxel, K. Caldarella, A. Hodlofski, S. Bernheim, E. Drye, J. Yoshimoto, K. Takata, M. B. Stollar, and E. Emanuel. 2018. Redesigning provider payment: Opportunities and challenges from the Hawaii experience. *Healthcare* 6(3):168-174.

Wall, S., D. Scudamore, J. Chin, M. Rannie, S. Tong, J. Reese, and K. Wilson. 2014. The evolving role of the pediatric nurse practitioner in hospital medicine. *Journal of Hospital Medicine* 9(4):261-265.

Ward-Zimmerman, B., and E. Cannata. 2012. Partnering with pediatric primary care: Lessons learned through collaborative colocation. *Professional Psychology: Research and Practice* 43(6):596.

White, P., C. Cuomo, H. C. Johnson-Hooper, and T. M. McManus. 2016. *Adult provider willingness to accept young adults into their practice: Results from three integrated delivery systems.* Poster presented at the 17th Annual Chronic Illness and Disability Conference, Houston, TX, October 27–28, 2016.

White, P. H., W. C. Cooley, Transitions Clinical Report Authoring Group, American Academy of Pediatrics, American Academy of Family Physicians, American College of Physicians, A. D. A. Boudreau, M. Cyr, B. E. Davis, D. E. Dreyfus, E. Forlenza, A. Friedland, C. Greenlee, M. Mann, M. McManus, A. I. Meleis, and L. Pickler. 2018. Supporting the health care transition from adolescence to adulthood in the medical home. *Pediatrics* 142(5):e20182587.

Will, K. K., M. L. Johnson, and G. Lamb. 2019. Team-based care and patient satisfaction in the hospital setting: A systematic review. *Journal of Patient-Centered Research and Reviews* 6(2):158-171.

Willard-Grace, R., D. Hessler, E. Rogers, K. Dubé, T. Bodenheimer, and K. Grumbach. 2014. Team structure and culture are associated with lower burnout in primary care. *Journal of the American Board of Family Medicine* 27(2):229-238.

Winter, S. G., E. Matsuda, L. M. Stephan, and S. A. Chapman. 2021. Enablers, barriers, and contributions of pediatric nurse practitioners to ambulatory specialty care. *Journal of Pediatric Health Care* 35(2):226-230.

Yonek, J., C. M. Lee, A. Harrison, C. Mangurian, and M. Tolou-Shams. 2020. Key components of effective pediatric integrated mental health care models: A systematic review. *JAMA Pediatrics* 174(5):487-498.

Zuckerman, K. E., K. Nelson, T. K. Bryant, K. Hobrecker, J. M. Perrin, and K. Donelan. 2011. Specialty referral communication and completion in the community health center setting. *Academic Pediatrics* 11(4):288-296.

8

Financing Children's Health Care

In 2019, children represented just under one-quarter of the U.S. population, yet only approximately 9 percent of total health care spending (Ortaliza et al., 2021). Expenditures for children's health care services tend to be disproportionately distributed, with a relatively small share of children accounting for a majority of costs. Children with special health care needs are more likely to have persistently high health care costs than other children, indicating an ongoing need for intense services (Leininger at al., 2015; Liptak et al., 2006). In addition, spending on health care during childhood has been documented to improve health into adulthood and even subsequent generations, and investments in child health can be considered a long-term, multigenerational investment (East et al., 2023; Miller and Wherry, 2018; Wherry et al., 2018). Data from the 2019 National Ambulatory Medical Care Survey reported that while private insurance was the primary expected source of payment for most pediatric office-based physician visits (56 percent), Medicaid was the primary expected source of payment for 39 percent of pediatric office-based physicians' visits (Ashman et al., 2023). Additionally, Weiss et al. (2022) found that nearly half of pediatric hospital stays were from children with Medicaid coverage in 2019, with approximately 61 percent of hospitalized infants (less than 1 year of age) covered by Medicaid.

Financing of children's subspecialty care directly affects payments to health care institutions and providers, which impacts provider salary, practice decisions, and, ultimately, provider supply. In this way, financing of child health care affects access to pediatric subspecialty physician care. Financing and payment for specific services, providers, or practice models also affect access, as lack of coverage or limited reimbursement may limit benefits, scope of practice, or innovations in care delivery. Therefore, while this chapter discusses the financing of children's health care broadly, the focus is on the issues that are particularly challenging for pediatric subspecialty physicians.

FINANCING AND COVERAGE OF CHILDREN'S SUBSPECIALTY CARE

Specialty health care services for children in the United States are financed through a combination of private and public funds. Private funds include commercial health insurance that is primarily obtained through the parents' employers and usually paid as an employment benefit. Other private funds include payments made directly by individuals, either for insurance or for services. Public financing is primarily through Medicaid or the Children's Health Insurance Program (CHIP).[1] Medicaid/CHIP funds are a combination of federal and state (and sometimes local) funds, and the federal government matches states' spending, based on the Federal Medical Assistance Percentage (FMAP). The FMAP is based on a formula set in federal statute that accounts for a state's per-capita income, relative to that of other states, with lower income states receiving a higher FMAP, and ranges from a minimum of 50 percent to a high of 77 percent in Mississippi in FY2024 (HHS, 2022). The federal government pays different FMAPs for some services, such as family planning or administrative services, or for specific populations (e.g., ACA expansion populations under the *Patient Protection and Affordable Care Act [ACA]*[2] or children covered through CHIP) (MACPAC, 2023a,b). Increased FMAPs have been used by the federal government to provide incentives for states to expand Medicaid eligibility or benefits, to offset state spending and provide fiscal relief during economic downturns, and to finance federal initiatives or priorities that flow through Medicaid (MACPAC, 2023b; Rudowitz et al., 2020). Because Medicaid is an entitlement program, spending is open-ended, which means that the federal government must match allowable state expenditures and states must pay for covered services provided to covered individuals. While the federal government is allowed to accrue a deficit to cover entitlement spending, states generally must balance their budgets each year and cannot run a deficit on Medicaid spending (Rueben and Randall, 2017).

---

[1] The Children's Health Insurance Program was enacted in 1997 as a block grant program to reduce the number of uninsured children. To be eligible for CHIP, the child must not be eligible for Medicaid and not otherwise insured (CMS, 2023a).

[2] The Patient Protection and Affordable Care Act of 2010, Public Law 111-148; 42 USC 18022 (March 23, 2010).

In 2021, the most recent full year for which data are available, half (52 percent) of all children (aged 0–18 years) were covered through private, employer-based insurance; approximately one-third (36 percent) through Medicaid/CHIP; 5 percent through other private insurance (e.g., ACA Marketplace coverage); and 2.5 percent through other public coverage (KFF, 2022a).[3] In 2021, only 5 percent of children were uninsured (see Figure 8-1). Pediatric insurance coverage varies by state, reflecting both private coverage rates and variation in Medicaid eligibility levels for children. There are racial/ethnic differences across types of coverage, with more than half of Black, Hispanic, American Indian/Alaska Native, and Native Hawaiian/Other Pacific Islander children covered by Medicaid and CHIP (Artiga, 2022). Children with special health care needs represent a distinct subgroup that includes many children who require specialty care; 44 percent of this subgroup is covered by Medicaid, including 8 percent who have both Medicaid and private coverage (Williams and Musumeci, 2021).

Out-of-pocket payments made by families for cost sharing and uncovered services represent financing for a portion of children's health care in the United States. In 2016–2017, more than 13 percent of parents reported that they made annual out-of-pocket health care expenses at or above $1,000 for their children's care (Jones et al., 2021). Over time, as a greater share of children with private coverage are covered through high-deductible health plans,[4] some families' financial burden for health care costs has increased (KFF, 2022b; Larson et al., 2021).

Health care expenditures for children are skewed toward those with higher levels of medical needs, similar to the pattern observed for adults. Within Medicaid, overall, about 10 percent of pediatric-specific spending is for outpatient specialty services (not including behavioral health services); while the distribution of spending on outpatient specialty care was fairly consistent across higher and lower spending groups, spending levels for this service increased from $8 per member per month for the least expensive 80 percent of children to $768 per member per month for children in the top 1 percent of spenders (Kuo et al., 2015). Other work finds that outpatient specialty care is the second highest cost category among Medicaid-covered children with complex chronic conditions (second to pharmacy spending) (Ming et al., 2022) or medical complexity (second to inpatient spending)

---

[3] Children with end-stage renal disease may qualify for Medicare coverage if their parents meet work history requirements and they need regular dialysis or have had a kidney transplant. In 2021, approximately 1,300 people under age 18 were covered by Medicare (CMS, 2023b).

[4] "A developing body of evidence suggests that high-deductible health plans discourage families from seeking high-value and/or medically necessary medical services" (Price et al., 2020). This discouragement decreases inappropriate or excessive use, but also can restrict access to appropriate care (Agarwal et al., 2017; Brot-Goldberg et al, 2017; Price et al., 2020). See Chapter 2 for more information on financial accessibility to care.

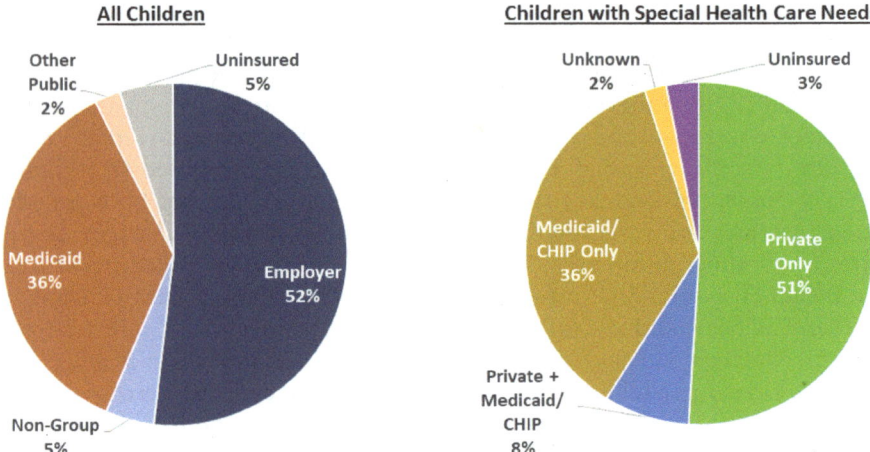

FIGURE 8-1 Health insurance coverage of all children and children with special health care needs.
¹ See https://www2.census.gov/programs-surveys/cps/techdocs/cpsmar21.pdf (accessed June 30, 2023).
NOTES: Data for all children are for 2021 and include children aged 0–19; data for children with special health care needs (CSHCN) are for 2019 and include children aged 0–17. "In this analysis, individuals are sorted into only one category of insurance coverage using the following hierarchy: Medicaid: Includes those covered by Medicaid, Medical Assistance, Children's Health Insurance Plan (CHIP), or any kind of government-assistance plan for those with low incomes or a disability, as well as those who have both Medicaid and another type of coverage, such as dual-eligibles who are also covered by Medicare. Employer: Includes those covered by employer-sponsored coverage either through their own job or as a dependent in the same household. Other public: Includes those covered under the military or Veterans Administration as well as non-elderly Medicare enrollees. Non-group: Includes individuals and families that purchased or are covered as a dependent by non-group insurance. Uninsured: Includes those without health insurance and those who have coverage under the Indian Health Service only."
SOURCES: KFF estimates for all children are based the Census Bureau's March Current Population Survey (CPS: Annual Social and Economic Supplements)¹, KFF (2022a); For CSHCN, KFF analysis of 2019 National Survey of Children's Health (Williams and Musumeci, 2021).

(Berry et al., 2014). Similar patterns exist for children covered by other types of insurance, including private insurance.

The benefits covered by private and public health insurance vary substantially, both across states and across insurers. Since 2014, under the ACA most private plans are required to provide, at a minimum, "essential health benefits" that include pediatric services, including oral and vision care.[5] However, some plans are exempt from these requirements, and private plans may still impose substantial cost sharing for these services. Private plans also may use limited provider networks as a strategy to manage costs. Medicaid benefits vary by state, although federal law requires all states to provide Early and Periodic Screening, Diagnosis, and Treatment (EPSDT) services to children enrolled in Medicaid. Under EPSDT, states must provide regular medical, vision, hearing, and dental screening as well as services necessary to correct or ameliorate health conditions, regardless of whether these services are otherwise covered under the state's Medicaid plan. Medicaid covers services not typically covered by private plans, such as non-emergency medical transportation, and long-term services as well as supports that may be required by children who have substantial health care needs. States that provide CHIP coverage through a separate (non-Medicaid) program may provide different benefits under these programs, but many states use a benefits package that is equivalent to Medicaid in separate CHIP programs.

Under both private and public health insurance, most children participate in managed care, under which financing flows to a managed care organization that in turn structures a care delivery system for enrollees. As of 2022, nearly half (49 percent) of people covered through employer-sponsored coverage were enrolled in a preferred provider organization, with nearly all of the rest enrolled in another type of managed care plan such as a health maintenance organization (12 percent), point-of-service plan (9 percent), or high-deductible plan coupled with a managed care plan (29 percent) (KFF, 2022b). As of July 2022, 41 states and the District of Columbia had contracts with Medicaid managed care organizations (Hinton et al., 2022). More than three-quarters of children covered by Medicaid (excluding CHIP) were enrolled in comprehensive managed care organizations, or health plans that cover comprehensive benefits including acute, primary, and specialty care, in 37 of the 41 states (Hinton and Raphael, 2023). Medicaid managed care plans include private for-profit, private non-profit, and public plans, but a small number of private for-profit firms (United Health Group, Centene, Molina, Aetna/CVS, and Elevance Health) account for the majority of Medicaid managed care enrollment (Klukoff et al., 2023).

---

[5] The Patient Protection and Affordable Care Act of 2010, Public Law 111-148; 42 USC 18022 (March 23, 2010).

In states that have not implemented comprehensive Medicaid managed care, children may receive services on a fee-for-service basis or may be covered by limited service plans (e.g., prepaid inpatient health plans or prepaid ambulatory health plans) or primary care case management arrangements, under which a primary care provider is paid a small, monthly amount per member per month to provide case management services in addition to regular primary care. For children covered through Medicaid managed care, states must still ensure that they receive the full scope of Medicaid services (either through the managed care plan or through wrap-around services). In some cases, Medicaid managed care plans provide additional services beyond those covered in the state Medicaid plan (e.g., social needs services). States and Medicaid managed care plans are subject to federal regulations as a condition of federal matching payments, though states and plans maintain some flexibility in setting standards for network adequacy and payment within federal rules (and subject to federal approval).

The providers that are available to serve children covered by private or public insurance depend not only on the supply of providers in an area but also on contracting and provider enrollment rules. For Medicaid, providers must enroll with each state's Medicaid program; within federal guidelines, states set standards and requirements for provider enrollment in Medicaid, which at a minimum, mirror Medicare enrollment rules (CMS, 2023c). Providers are not required to participate in Medicaid, and, as discussed elsewhere, may opt out of the program due to low payment rates or other issues. Medicaid managed care plans and private insurance plans contract with a network of providers to serve enrollees in their plans. Network adequacy—or whether health insurance networks include a sufficient number and distribution of providers to ensure access for enrollees—has been a longstanding policy issue across health care and for children's health care access (MACPAC, 2015). State Medicaid agencies are responsible for developing, publicly posting, and enforcing quantitative network adequacy standards for both adult and pediatric specialists, in addition to other provider types.[6] Metrics can include time and distance standards, provider-to-enrollee ratio, and wait time standards; states set their own standards and there are no federal minimums (Schneider and Corcoran, 2022). Some studies have examined network adequacy in the context of ACA Marketplace plans, with research on initial plan offerings in 2014, finding that such plans were more likely to have narrow networks (defined as <10% of available providers in an area being included in the insurance network) for pediatric versus adult specialists (Wong et al., 2017). More recent work has found that narrow networks in the ACA Marketplace have proliferated over time, leading to new proposed federal requirements for network adequacy

---

[6] *Network Adequacy Standards* § 438.68 (2020).

standards in this market (Pollitz, 2022). Recently proposed federal regulations governing Medicaid managed care would establish new standards for network adequacy and align these more closely with federal rules governing ACA Marketplace plans (Schneider, 2023).

PAYMENT RATES FOR CHILDREN'S SUBSPECIALTY CARE

Payment rates for children's health care services are largely determined by health plans (in negotiation with providers) or set by state Medicaid programs. In private coverage and Medicaid managed care plans, payment rates take a broad range of forms, including traditional fee-for-service (under which providers are paid per individual service), bundled payments (in which payment is made for an episode of care or for a set of services that are often delivered together), payment models that place providers at risk (e.g., as monthly capitation payments), or pay-for-performance models (in which providers may be paid a bonus or face a penalty depending on whether they meet quality or outcome measures), among others (OECD, 2016). In more recent years, payers have also explored value-based payment models; see Chapter 7 for more information. Private commercial plans set payment rates based on negotiation or proprietary methods. Commercial payment rates are determined by a range of factors, including market forces, competition, and contracting rules. In many cases, commercial insurers pay providers using a method similar to Medicare, though providers in some areas may negotiate "multipliers" to increase rates or have sufficient market power to demand other methods (CBO, 2022). Medicaid rates are similarly determined by market factors but also are governed by additional factors, including state budgets and federal regulations.

Overall, states have substantial flexibility to determine fee schedules that govern fee-for-service Medicaid payment rates (and in some cases, as described below, Medicaid managed care rates), with federal requirements stipulating that payment levels be "consistent with efficiency, economy, and quality of care and sufficient to enlist enough providers so that services under the plan are available to beneficiaries at least to the extent that those services are available to the general population" (42 CFR § 447.204).[7] Outside of this provision, known as the "equal access" provision, the federal government has over time issued some additional regulation or requirements for Medicaid payment. Under the Boren Amendment, enacted in 1980 and repealed in 1997, the federal government regulated Medicaid

---

[7] CMS Requirements for Medicaid Program—Methods for Assuring Access to Covered Medicaid Services, 42 CFR § 447.204 (2016) Under federal law, federally qualified health centers, which focus on providing primary and preventive care, are paid on a prospective payment system (PPS) that reimburses clinics a set amount per visit (MACPAC, 2017a).

payments for institutional providers such as nursing homes and hospitals; as part of the *Balanced Budget Act of 1997* that repealed the Boren Amendment, state agencies are required to use a public process to determine payment rates for institutional providers (MACPAC, 2023c; Miller, 2007). In 2015, CMS issued regulations governing Medicaid's equal access provision, including requirements that states develop access monitoring review plans (AMRP), among other requirements, and that CMS approve any payment changes that could affect access (CMS, 2015). However, the 2015 rule explicitly excluded Medicaid managed care and demonstration programs, and it did not set federal standards for payment or access (CMS, 2015; Rosenbaum, 2015). States and stakeholders have questioned the utility of the AMRP process, and in 2019, CMS proposed to rescind the 2015 rule (CMS, 2019). While the recission was never finalized, in late spring 2023, CMS issued a notice of proposed rulemaking on *Ensuring Access to Medicaid Services* that acknowledged the limits to the 2015 rule (CMS, 2023d). CMS proposed requirements to "increase the transparency of FFS provider payment rates, update and standardize the requirements for states to submit documentation about proposed payment rate reductions or restructurings, and improve the public comment process for changes to payment rates" (CMS, 2023e). These new rules would require states to post Medicaid fee-for-service payment rates to a publicly accessible website, conduct analysis comparing Medicaid fee-for-service rates to Medicare, and provide documentation for any rate changes that meet certain thresholds of reduction relative to existing rates or Medicare rates (among other provisions) (Manatt Health, 2023).

Multiple legal cases have attempted to use the judicial system as a mechanism to require states to increase Medicaid payment rates, holding that low state payment levels were a failure to adhere to the equal access provision (Berman, 2018; Perkins, 2015; Staman, 2011). However, these cases have failed for a variety of reasons, including the question of whether the plaintiffs (typically providers) have standing or a cause of action to pursue the case. The recent Supreme Court case *Health & Hospital Corporation of Marion County, Indiana v. Talevski* could have further limited the use of the courts to enforce the equal access provision, as it decided "whether Medicaid beneficiaries can seek relief in federal court when they believe their rights are being violated by state officials" (Rudowitz and Sobel, 2022). In June 2023, the Supreme Court issued a 7-2 decision that reaffirmed the private right of action under Medicaid.[8] However, the decision noted that not all federal laws create individual rights, and previous Supreme Court decisions have held that the Medicaid statute does not provide a private right of action for providers and beneficiaries to challenge

---

[8] *Health and Hosp. Corp. of Marion Cnty. v. Talevski*, No. 21-806 (U.S. Jun. 8, 2023).

payment rates in federal court, making the use of the court as a potential avenue for providers and enrollees to pursue enforcement of the equal access provision uncertain (Rosenbaum et al., 2023).

According to a review by the Medicaid and CHIP Payment and Access Commission (MACPAC):

> State Medicaid programs that pay physicians on a direct, [fee-for-service] basis typically pay physicians and other clinicians using a fee schedule that establishes base payment rates for every covered service, as with Medicare and commercial payers. State Medicaid programs generally use one of three methods for establishing base payment rates (fee schedules): the resource-based relative value scale (RBRVS), a percentage of Medicare's fee, or a state-developed fee schedule using local factors. (MACPAC, 2017b, 2022a)

The review found that 23 states used RBRVS, 15 set fees based on a percent of Medicare fees, and 12 used a fee schedule based on either market assessment or internal processes (MACPAC, 2017b). States also include a variety of adjustments to their fee schedules (e.g., adjustments to reflect geographic cost differences (e.g., urban versus rural) or adjustments to account for site of care (e.g., office versus hospital based); 25 states make upward adjustments for pediatric services. These adjustments, and the mechanisms that they are made by, vary by states. For example, certain primary care and preventive medicine services are compensated at a higher rate for individuals who are 17 or younger in California; rates for child patients are roughly 9 percent higher than those for adult patients. In Michigan, adjustments may be made for providers who care for children with special health care needs; the payment adjustment method determined by the Medical Services Administration is the lesser of the difference between the fee-for-service Medicaid fee screens and the average commercial rate, or the difference between the fee-for-service Medicaid fee screens and the physician's customary charge. States also use a range of incentive payments within fee-for-service, including supplemental payments for academic medical centers (26 states). The review did not include specific information on other adjustments or payment policies for pediatric specialty care.

Payments through Medicaid managed care plans may be bound by state contracting requirements or payment floors. A 2017 survey of Medicaid managed care plans found that 51 percent of plans set physician rates based on state Medicaid fee schedule, 5 percent based on Medicare fee schedule, and the rest negotiated (38 percent) or set in some other way (6 percent) (Garfield et al., 2018). As of July 1, 2021, 16 states have a directed minimum fee schedule for providers (physicians or other professional services) covered by Medicaid managed care (Gifford et al., 2021). Certain payments under Medicaid managed care (e.g., state directed payments) are subject to federal regulations and approval. In late spring 2023, CMS issued a proposed rule that would require states to submit an annual analysis that compares Medicaid managed care plan payment rates to Medicare for a limited number of services; the proposed rule also includes several provisions governing use of state-directed payments in Medicaid managed care (CMS, 2023d).

Adequacy of Payment Rates across Payers

A review by the Congressional Budget Office (CBO) concluded that, compared with public payers, commercial insurers face more upward pressure on prices and therefore pay higher rates and increase rates more quickly. The review also found that the ratio between commercial rates and Medicare rates for physician services was higher for specialty care (in which commercial insurance paid 144 percent of Medicare) than primary care (in which commercial insurance paid 117 percent of Medicare), though ratios varied widely by state and even metropolitan area within a state. While CBO did not include conclusions about whether rates were "adequate," it did note that there is limited evidence of "cost shifting," or higher commercial rates to providers to offset lower prices paid by public payers (CBO, 2022). Other work has reached a similar conclusion, though most research focuses on hospital cost shifting (Coughlin et al., 2021).

In comparison, there is a great deal of discussion about whether Medicaid rates are too low to cover providers' and health systems' costs and thereby contribute to cost-shifting from public to private payers or result in financial shortfalls for providers whose patient panels include a large share of Medicaid enrollees (e.g., pediatric primary care clinicians and subspecialists). While the preponderance of evidence, summarized below, shows that Medicaid payment rates are below other payers, there are some data challenges in directly comparing rates. Many private fee schedules are proprietary (including those used by Medicaid managed care plans) and are not currently publicly available. In addition, analysis of Medicaid fee schedules may not reflect actual payment (because final payment rates reflect a variety of adjustments); a Government Accountability Office study (2014a) that compared fee schedules to payments reported in claims data showed that "fee schedule rates [used in other analyses]...were rarely used in practice" due to adjustments. In some cases, actual payments were lower, reflecting adjustments downward for non-physician providers, though the study also found that payments were frequently higher, reflecting other adjustments including higher payments for services for children. Comparative analysis of fee schedules is also time-consuming and thus typically restricted to a subset of services or procedures, leading to limited insight into services specific to pediatrics in general or pediatric specialty care in particular. Analysis of claims data can address some of these limitations, but are subject to other challenges, such as inclusion of out-of-pocket payments in assessment of payment for patients covered by private insurance or Medicare or inability to directly compare reimbursement at a service-versus-visit level.

Bearing these limitations in mind, recent studies that compare Medicaid and commercial payment based on claims data find that Medicaid payment is lower, with Medicaid fee-for-service payment lower than Medicaid managed care. A Government Accountability Office (2014b) review of 26 evaluation and management services showed that Medicaid fee-for-service and managed care were generally 27 to 65 percent lower than private insurance. In all but two states included in the analysis, Medicaid managed care payments were at or above Medicaid fee-for-service payments. The report further found that differences in evaluation and management services varied by site of care, with differences being largest in emergency care and smallest in office settings. A 2017 report of differences in payments for child visits to office-based physicians (based on the Medical Expenditure Panel Survey) concluded that the median Medicaid payment per visit was approximately 65 percent of the median payment for private insurance (the mean difference was larger, mainly due to some very high payment for some private visits) (Muhuri and Machlin, 2017). The study also found that differences were consistent across Census regions and consistent across specialties included, with differences for orthopedics being much higher than other specialties. Notably, the private payment rates included out-of-pocket payments (which were applicable in 58 percent of private visits), and the authors noted an inability to adjust for service intensity.

Comparisons of Medicaid and Medicare fee schedules similarly find Medicaid rates generally to be below Medicare, with some variation across states, specialties, or services. Few studies specifically examine services common in pediatric specialty care. The most recent analysis of Medicaid fee-for-service to Medicare fee ratios published by The Urban Institute found that the 2019 national average Medicaid-to-Medicare fee index was lower for primary care (0.67) than for obstetric care (0.80) or for other services (0.78), and only five states (i.e., Alaska, Delaware, Montana, Nebraska, and North Dakota) had average Medicaid fees equal to or higher than Medicare (Zuckerman et al., 2021). The service categories included in the analysis included limited services[9] common to pediatric subspecialty care. Other studies that have examined orthopedic surgery (Lalezari et al., 2018), general surgery (Mabry et al., 2016), cochlear implants (Conduff

---

[9] Other services include endoscopy, dilation and curettage, hysterectomy, cataract removal, tympanostomy, head computerized axial tomography, chest X-ray, pathology, ophthalmologic services, echocardiogram, pregnant uterus echography, and echocardiography (Zuckerman et al., 2021; supplemental materials).

and Coelho, 2017), and musculoskeletal radiology (Santiago et al., 2020) find that while there is most commonly a shortfall between Medicaid rates relative to Medicare, this conclusion does not hold in all states and all services. In other words, while many outcomes show Medicaid payments below Medicare, there was wide variation in the scale of the shortfall, and in some cases Medicaid rates were above Medicare.

COMPENSATION FOR PEDIATRIC MEDICAL SUBSPECIALTY PHYSICIANS

The following sections address the factors that contribute to physician compensation, including payment to physicians, payments to pediatric departments and hospitals, and administrative costs.

Payments to Physicians and the Resource-Based Relative Value Scale

Physician compensation is a factor of the financing system that structures the flow of funds within the health care system, payment rates, and structure of salary or compensation. As mentioned above, provider payment generally may be on a fee-for-service basis (in which providers are paid for each service they provide), a capitated or bundled basis (in which providers are paid a set amount for a population or package of services), a flat salary, an incentive basis (in which providers are paid or penalized according to certain quality goals or other outcomes), or through a combination of approaches.

Based on data from the maintenance of certification surveys for 2018–2022, most commonly pediatric subspecialists (32 percent) indicate that their primary work setting is an academic setting affiliated with a medical school or university, with the remainder working in a nongovernmental hospital or clinic (22 percent), multispecialty group practice (20 percent), or another setting (ABP, 2023).[10] In addition, 57 percent of pediatric subspecialists hold a full-time academic position. Salaries for physicians in most academic settings (and private practices within large health care systems) are based on expected clinical productivity, and salaries for faculty members are often determined relative to national benchmarks (developed using data submitted by departments and schools across the country) (Schnapp et al., 2020; Weidemann et al., 2022). Traditionally, faculty compensation is determined using a formula for base salary, with additional rewards for

---

[10] Calculated on the ABP dashboard by choosing "overall specialty status" under "select to crosstab results" and by choosing the 15 ABP-certified subspecialties under "GP/subspecialty certification filter."

productivity, seniority, and leadership/administration. As noted in Chapter 5, pediatricians are among the lowest paid specialists, even among primary care specialties (Doximity and Curative, 2023), and pediatricians have significantly lower incentive bonuses as compared with other specialists (Martin, 2021). Incentive bonuses for pediatricians were relatively low, averaging $26,000; only psychiatrists reported a lower average bonus. See Chapter 5 for more information on salaries for pediatric subspecialists. See Box 8-1 for clinician perspectives on payment.

Faculty clinical productivity, which goes into both base salary as well as bonus payments, is often measured by work relative value units (RVUs). Developed in the early 1990s to set physician payment rates in Medicare,

---

BOX 8-1
Clinician Perspectives—Payment

"Because this is not a procedure-based specialty, it is poorly paid and largely undervalued by hospitals and department chairs."
– Pediatric Nephrologist, Bethesda, MD

"Current issues include low rates of reimbursement despite long hours, an excess of non-reimbursable time spent following up on labs and imaging studies and calling patients to discuss these, and the documentation burden that can be crippling."
– Attending Physician, Boston, MA

"As junior faculty, I have been surprised by the volume of unpaid work that is part of academia (resident lectures, calls from community providers, etc.) despite a fairly low salary."
– Pediatric Infectious Diseases Physician

"Complex pediatric hospital care is provided at many, many hospitals that do not have direct access to pediatric subspecialists; these hospitals do not hire more subspecialists because they are unable to recoup their salaries by providing complex consultative services. We therefore receive phone calls from all over the state asking for consultation. Only rarely do we receive any compensation for this care; when we do it is generally a very small amount that is much less than we would earn providing face-to-face care."
– Pediatric Infectious Diseases Physician, North Carolina

These quotes were collected from the committee's online call for trainee, clinician, and family perspectives.

the RVU system is "set nationally for a discrete piece of physician work and attempt to equilibrate aspects of care across specialties" (Schnapp et al., 2020). RVUs consist of three components: physician work RVUs; practice expense RVUs; and professional liability insurance RVUs:

1. Physician work RVUs (wRVU): Account for the time, technical effort and skill, medical decision making, and mental stress required to provide a certain service;
2. Practice expense RVUs: account for the non-physician labor, equipment, and building space; and
3. Professional liability insurance RVUs: factor in the costs of malpractice premiums (Weidemann et al., 2022).

Although RVUs themselves are not monetary values, they can be multiplied by a conversion factor (dollars per RVU) to determine the amount of payment for a service (Weidemann et al., 2022). The Centers for Medicare & Medicaid Services (CMS) and most private payers have used the RVU system for physician payment since 1992 (Weidemann et al., 2022). As outlined in the 2021 National Academies of Sciences, Engineering, and Medicine (National Academies) report, *Implementing High-Quality Primary Care*, the resource-based relative value scale, and the process for updating it, have "contributed to the differences in compensation across specialties, the distribution of physicians across specialties, inefficient distortions in use, and inadequate beneficiary access to undervalued services" (NASEM, 2021, pg 291; MedPAC, 2018). In general, the system leads to lower payment for not only primary care, but also specialty care outside of surgical or procedural services. The report further asserts that because changes to Medicare's fee schedule must be budget neutral, evaluation and management codes "have become passively devalued in the PFS [physician fee schedule] as their relative prices fall as a result of other service prices (including new technologies) increasing" (NASEM, 2021, pg.291). The National Academies report identified a variety of other factors contributing to this devaluation, including overestimation of work time for some procedures; lack of reevaluation of RVUs for these services; difficulty in the estimation of time, skill, and effort for evaluation and management services, among others. As a result, PFS is "oriented toward discrete, often procedural, technical services" (NASEM, 2021). Recent efforts to change misvalued codes resulted in significant upward revision for office visits (CMS, 2020). However, CMS efforts are hindered by "the lack of current, accurate, and objective data on clinician work time and practice expenses" (NASEM, 2021; GAO, 2015; Mulcahy et al., 2020; Wynn et al., 2015; Zuckerman et al., 2016). The multispecialty Relative Value Scale Update Committee, which includes members from 26 specialties, provides input to CMS for determining the physician fee schedule for RVUs. However, despite the inclusion of only one pediatric representative on this committee, the determination of RVUs for all pediatric services is made primarily based on this input (Moore et al., 2008). Although the Relative Value Scale Update Committee provides recommendations, CMS makes all final decisions about payments and can accept or modify these recommendations, though CMS has historically deferred to nearly all the Relative Value Scale Update Committee's recommendations (AMA, 2023; GAO, 2015; NASEM, 2021).

Current challenges with existing fee schedules are particularly problematic for pediatric subspecialty care. Because the RVU system is Medicare-driven, CMS acknowledges that it "underrepresent[s] or undervalue[s] some components of pediatric work" (AAP, 2008). As a result, the RVU system may overvalue services to adults (Massoumi et al., 2021; Weidemann et al., 2022). RVUs may undervalue the physician work input for pediatric care: Because children are accompanied by their parents, creating a triadic relationship, and may take more time to gain cooperation in the health care process than adult counterparts, services and procedures for children require more face-to-face time, more education, more information-giving and counseling, more emotional support, and more communication with child care facilities, schools, or absent parents, which can increase post-service time for an encounter (AAP, 2008; Lakshminrusimha et al., 2023). Furthermore, practice expenses for pediatric services may be higher than for adult care due to the need for more direct hands-on time by clinical staff, more case management, higher telephone call volume, and other factors (e.g., cost of supplies in multiple sizes for inpatient pediatric units). A study of pediatric nephrology payments noted that increases in fees for pediatric codes for dialysis were lower than those for adult dialysis, even though management of children on dialysis may be more time-consuming (Weidemann et al., 2022).

Furthermore, the weighting of the RVU system to procedure-based specialties persists in pediatric care, leading to differences in payment not only across pediatric subspecialties, but also between pediatric and adult specialists. An analysis of the application of the RVU system to pediatric nephrology noted that technological advances have generally increased efficiency for procedure-based practice (i.e., allowing more procedures in less time); they have decreased efficiency for non–procedure-based practice through the need for extensive documentation in the electronic record; and these documentation requirements are particularly burdensome for pediatric care (Weidemann et al., 2022). In addition, compared with adult specialists in the same field, pediatric specialists may have fewer procedures and thus lower RVU expectations, which partially accounts for salary levels. Recent analysis of productivity benchmarks for pediatric subspecialists found that the median productivity per 1.0 clinical full-time equivalent is lower for many non-ICU pediatric medical subspecialists compared to their adult counterparts (Lakshminrusimha et al., 2023). Lower patient volumes, particularly for subspecialists who are not practicing in freestanding large children's hospitals, also contributes to lower RVUs, as clinicians must be on call and cover services in between a predominantly outpatient schedule (Lakshminrusimha et al., 2023). Lower RVUs also affect RVU-based bonus payments available to providers. A study of pediatric rheumatology found that the RVU expectation for pediatric rheumatologists was about 70 percent of that for adult rheumatologists (Singer and Onel, 2019). The incentives in the RVU system and conclusion that the care of complex patients is "inadequately captured in the RVU model" (Weyand and Freed, 2020) also impact patient care by creating incentives for referrals, fewer "curbside" consultations, or focus on ongoing monitoring for patients whose acute issues have been resolved. See Box 8-2 for trainee and clinician perspectives on RVUs.

BOX 8-2
Fellow and Clinician Perspectives—RVUs

"Barrier: Inadequate RVU [relative value unit] credit for highly skilled services with shrinking representation. Beyond the realm of my personal experience, in nephrology in particular, the billing/coding structure of CMS is ill-suited to provide productivity credit through the RVU system to accurately capture the nature of our work. For hospitalized [end stage renal disease] patients requiring dialysis, the dialysis RVUs undervalue the daily work required. For critically ill infants, toddlers, and preschool children requiring dialysis, the inability for a pediatric nephrologist to bill for critical care time despite the patient population requiring an incredibly high level of technical expertise, training, attention, and detail seriously undermines the value of the care we provide for children. Our field will continue to be unable to attract an adequate number of trainees into the subspecialty as long as the value of our services continues to be so minimized."
– Mid-Career Pediatric Nephrologist

"There needs to be less of a financial emphasis on performing procedures and more on the thought process and the quality of care provided."
– Second Year Pediatric Endocrinology Fellow, Denver, CO

These quotes were collected from the committee's online call for trainee, clinician, and family perspectives.

Payments to Pediatric Departments and Hospitals

Provider reimbursement is also a factor of the flow of funds within a department and institution. Department chairs have a significant role in setting salaries and incentives for clinical faculty as well as allocating the amount of time to be spent on research, patient care, education, and administration. In turn, department budgets are a function of professional fees collected, hospital agreements for time spent in administrative and operational functions, and other funds that flow to the department from the larger institution. (Departments within academic institutions also have other revenue sources, e.g., grants and teaching agreements.) Departments are part of the larger institution, which may also collect supplemental payments. These are not tied to a specific service, such as those targeted to graduate medical education (see Chapter 5 for more information about graduate medical education payments) or payments to support safety net providers.

Analysis of Medicaid payment rates shows that, like provider payment rates, base payments to hospitals are often below hospital costs of providing services to Medicaid beneficiaries, leading to what is known as the "Medicaid shortfall" (MACPAC, 2022b). While other payers may also pay below costs, a recent analysis found that underpayment to children's hospitals (defined as payment below calculated costs) was more frequent for Medicaid compared with private payers (VonAchen et al., 2021). Medicaid disproportionate share (DSH) payments are supplemental payments intended to provide financial assistance to hospitals that serve a relatively high share of Medicaid or low-income patients, in part to offset the Medicaid shortfall (MACPAC, 2023d). DSH funds are allocated from the federal government to states, which then distribute funds to providers within broad federal guidelines. States may also make other supplemental Medicaid payments to hospitals through other mechanisms, including upper payment limits that "allow states to make up the difference between a reasonable estimate of what Medicare would pay and Medicaid payments" (in aggregate within a type and class of providers) (Rudowitz, 2020) and state directed payments (SDPs), under which a state directs a Medicaid managed care organization to pay providers certain rates or payment methodologies (MACPAC, 2022c).

Health care institutions that treat a relatively large share of patients covered by Medicaid may recoup some of the difference in reimbursement rates through supplemental payments. However, analysis finds that Medicaid DSH funds are poorly targeted, with "little meaningful relationship between DSH allotments and the number of uninsured individuals; the amounts and sources of hospitals' uncompensated care costs; and the number of hospitals with high levels of uncompensated care that also provide essential community services for low-income, uninsured, and vulnerable populations" (MACPAC, 2022b, pg. 105). MACPAC finds that, in some cases, supplemental payments may fully cover hospital costs, while in other cases, hospitals still face a shortfall relative to the cost of care for Medicaid patients (MACPAC, 2022b). Supplemental payments also typically flow to the institution and, depending on that institution's policies, may or may not flow to pediatric subspecialty departments or providers.

Given the different role of Medicaid for varied patient populations as well as how RVUs affect reimbursement in different specialties, some institutions take steps to rebalance resources across departments or support services that provide capacity but are not profitable through funds flow. "Funds flow arrangements define the financial relationships between departments, medical centers, and university entities within a coordinated academic health system" (Josephson et al., 2020, pg. 785). The clinical revenue from hospitals and medical centers represents the majority of financial support to its associated entities. The revenue generated by clinical activities is usually allocated to clinical departments to cover the costs of the centralized faculty practice plan, including faculty compensation and employee benefits (Miller et al., 2012). "System" funds may then be redistributed across entities and departments to fund the academic or other underfunded activities that are central to the organization's mission (Itri et al., 2017; Miller et al., 2012). Clinical departments that generate excess revenue may be used to support other departments that are not generating sufficient revenue to cover their own expenses. The allocation of funds among clinical departments is often negotiated among the department chair, the hospital, and the dean, and the dean may have the discretion to use the surplus generated by one department to cover the expenses of other clinical departments (Miller et al., 2012). Funds flow formulas may be based on the "shortfall" of payments per RVU needed to meet needs, calculations of FTEs needed to staff services, or some combination of both (Lakshminrusimha et al., 2022). There are a broad variety of arrangements, corporate structures, and relationships among affiliated entities. Financing within health care institutions has been described as a black box due to the seemingly randomness of typing specific revenue streams to concepts such as "knowledge" or "population health" (Miller et al., 2012).

Administrative Costs

A final aspect of reimbursement is administrative costs. Administrative burden on providers may result from a range of factors, including medical records, health insurance authorizations or referrals, care coordination, billing, or other factors. Much evidence shows that providers' administrative burden in the United States is substantial and has increased in recent years

(Casalino et al., 2009; Erickson et al., 2017; Himmelstein et al., 2014; West et al., 2018). Administrative duties may be seen as a "hassle" for providers and may also affect payment, especially if these factors lead to denied claims or take time away from other billable activities (Dunn et al., 2023). Administrative burdens are a major contributor to "burnout" or job dissatisfaction (Apaydin, 2020; Frintner et al., 2020). To the extent that these administrative duties vary by specialty or payer, they also may influence physician practice or career decisions, as discussed below. While administrative burdens may be universal, there is some evidence that certain factors that particularly affect pediatric specialists lead to heavy administrative burdens. For example, research non-specific to pediatrics finds that, within an academic medical center, administrative costs are higher for specialty care compared with primary care (Tseng et al., 2018). Other research finds that insurance denial rates are higher in Medicaid compared with other payers, leading to lower payment for these patients, lending evidence to the idea that providers with a relatively higher share of Medicaid patients may face higher administrative costs (Dunn et al., 2023). This evidence builds on previous work showing that Medicaid reimbursement delays can offset increases in Medicaid reimbursement rates to the point that "increasing these rates may be insufficient to increase physicians' participation unless accompanied by reductions in administrative burden" (Cunningham and O'Malley, 2009).

HOW FINANCING AND PAYMENT TIE TO PROVIDER SALARIES, PRACTICE DECISIONS, AND ACCESS TO CARE

Most studies that have examined the link between payment rates and provider availability have focused on Medicaid and used outcome measures such as appointment availability, insurance participation, or patient use. Several studies have examined the effect of the Medicaid primary care payment bump under ACA, which increased primary care rates to Medicare rates for 2 years in 2013 and 2014. Results are mixed, with most research finding increases in self-reported Medicaid participation (Tang et al., 2018), improvement in patient-reported difficulty finding a provider (Alexander and Schnell, 2019), and appointment availability for new patients (Candon et al., 2018; Polsky et al., 2015), but others finding no effect of the payment bump on Medicaid participation or service volume (Decker, 2018; Mulcahy et al., 2018). Other work has looked more generally at associations between Medicaid primary care payment rates and provider participation and found that states with higher average Medicaid payment rates have higher rates of appointment availability for new patients (Sharma et al., 2018) or physician participation in Medicaid (Holgash and Heberlein, 2019). Findings based on primary care may not be fully applicable to pediatric specialty care, where physicians may be less likely to opt out of Medicaid due to the higher share of patients with this coverage type as well as policies of their institutions. There is more limited research that examines payment rates and provider availability among specialists. Other studies have found an association between Medicaid rates for dental care and access to dental services (Buchmueller et al., 2015; Chalmers and Compton, 2017).

While evidence points to a link between payment rates and provider availability or insurance participation, there is less direct evidence that in turn links payment rates to overall provider supply. Studies have examined how salary expectations (which are in part driven by payment rates) relate to career decisions among physicians. (See Chapter 5 for more on the influence of earning potential on career choices.)

While there is not a robust evidence base regarding the implications of a lack of parity between Medicare and Medicaid payments, the committee's collective judgment is that the lack of parity is a major driver for the financial disincentives to pursuing a career in a pediatric subspecialty, which, in turn, contributes to access challenges for children. The general ethical rationale for parity between Medicaid and Medicare payment rates is that if Medicaid payment rates are too low, it may be difficult for health care providers to accept patients with Medicaid coverage. This limitation in access to high-quality care for children with Medicaid coverage could lead to disparities in access to care and health outcomes. As noted previously, comparisons of Medicaid and Medicare fee schedules generally find Medicaid rates to be less than Medicare, with some variation across states, specialties, or services. Given the large percentage of children on Medicaid, there are disproportionately larger adverse effects on reimbursement and compensation for pediatric care (as compared with adult care). These disparities in the compensation of health care providers can be considered unfair or unjust. Perrin et al. (2020) argued that "both the federal government and state governments haven't consistently enforced the federal requirement that Medicaid provide payments that are high enough to ensure that people with Medicaid coverage have as much access to care as people with commercial insurance" (pg. 2597). The 2021 National Academies report on high-quality primary care also discussed Medicaid payment rates in the context of access to primary care:

> As the nation's second largest payer, with disproportionate numbers of children and high-needs beneficiaries, Medicaid needs a primary care strategy that addresses the low rates state Medicaid agencies and their contractors pay for primary care, which limits children's access to it. CMS should lead this strategy, and its state partners should implement and enforce it. Reforming Medicaid to mirror Medicare's payment standards may be the most straightforward path to ensuring equitable access to high-quality

primary care for its beneficiaries. Short of that, modifying federal access-to-care standards for state Medicaid programs can catalyze state and managed care organization payment and coverage policies to prioritize high-quality primary care. Meeting federal and accrediting bodies' access standards will require states and their contracted managed care organizations to take the necessary actions, including increasing Medicaid rates for primary care and expanding primary care provider networks as needed. (NASEM, 2021)

During the committee's public webinars, Sara Rosenbaum, Harold and Jane Hirsh Professor of Health Law and Policy and founding chair of the Department of Health Policy at George Washington University's Milken Institute School of Public Health, testified about the significance of Medicaid rates for pediatric subspecialty care:

> Even though there are all these complex reasons for access problems, you cannot get anywhere in my view until you have leveled the playing field on rates…it means a reasonably competitive rate…in the case of pediatrics, it is a much deeper issue than just what any individual provider gets paid because it obviously affects the entire structural soundness of pediatric subspecialties….It makes it that much harder to attract people into subspecialties where the financial stability of the subspecialty is open to question because so many children are publicly insured, and public payers just pay much lower rates….It is a foundational issue where the subspecialties are concerned. As far as I can tell and the same is true for adult subspecialties, adults just are not as prevalent [of a] part of the [Medicaid] population and therefore impact of high Medicaid dependence is not so much in evidence…everybody knows it is more complicated than rates. But everybody also knows that you cannot get anywhere without fixing the rates. You are really doing major damage in the case of pediatrics because of the role of Medicaid….Medicaid is incomparable as a source of pediatric coverage, but the rate issue should be taken off the table and then we can go to work on the other access barriers.[11]

To address inequities in payment for pediatric subspecialty services, various mechanisms could be considered, that may differ by state. States can simply increase provider payment rates, as some states have done over time. For example, in FY2022, 16 states reported increasing payment rates for specialist physicians, and 17 states reported plans to do so in FY2023 (Hinton et al., 2022). While states that increase Medicaid payment rates will receive commensurate increased federal funds (based on the FMAP),

---

[11] The webinar recording can be accessed at https://www.nationalacademies.org/event/11-14-2022/the-pediatric-subspecialty-workforce-and-its-impact-on-child-health-and-well-being-meeting-4.

limits in state funds may restrict the ability of states to pursue this option. Further, the simplicity of this mechanism means states also may target provider payment rates for cuts as a cost-saving area during economic downturns (Smith et al., 2010). Some states have used supplemental federal funds previously to increase provider rates. For example, Gould and Honsberger (2022) reviewed how states used expanded federal funding to states' Medicaid Home and Community-Based Services (HCBS) programs (including a one-year, 10-percentage-point FMAP bump to Medicaid HCBS) so states can use the increased federal funds to address payment. Five states have outlined their intention to raise rates paid to providers (direct support professionals for children and youth) for HCBS covered through specific waivers or state plan amendments; four states plan to raise rates paid for certain services to support in-demand specialty providers; Washington State proposed directing funds to managed care organizations to increase provider payments for wraparound mental health services for youth; and West Virginia proposed a temporary 70 percent increase in reimbursement rates for services covered under the state's Children with Serious Emotional Disorder Waiver, which covers HCBS for youth with severe mental disorders (Gould and Honsberger, 2022). These mechanisms are not the only ones that could be successful in addressing inequities in payment for pediatric subspecialty services through supplemental federal funding but are listed only as examples.

During the committee's public webinars, the impact of financing of children's health on the pipeline and retention of pediatric subspecialists as well as the overall sustainability of children's health care were highlighted by multiple speakers:

> So much of this unfortunately comes down to finances....I work in a children's hospital within an adult health care system. You have to constantly, constantly fight for children here....The reimbursement and opportunity for system margin, for example, is basically disincentivized for development of programs for children with complex needs, and it ultimately leads to downward pressure on salaries for pediatricians.[12]
>
> – Stephanie Duggins Davis, Edward C. Curnen, Jr., Distinguished Professor and Chair for the Department of Pediatrics at the University of North Carolina at Chapel Hill
>
> Academic medical centers are traditionally described as having this tripartite mission that resembles a three-legged stool...with clinical care, education, and research, all given equal importance. But I recently heard

---

[12] The webinar recording can be accessed at https://www.nationalacademies.org/event/07-19-2022/the-pediatric-subspecialty-workforce-and-its-impact-on-child-health-and-well-being-webinar-1.

a different analogy, and that is [that] the reality of the academic medical centers now resembles a tricycle with clinical revenue functioning as the big wheel sort of pulling the other two along. So, we really rely on the clinical margin to fund the research and education mission. Our problem in pediatrics is that the front wheel is not very big. We are an independent children's hospital here, but when we looked at the clinical margin across the entire health system at Stanford, the Department of Pediatrics was less than 5 percent of that clinical margin—despite the fact that…we're the second biggest department. So, the front wheel is not very big and it's not very big because Medicaid and children's health insurance programs reimburse physician services in pediatrics at much lower rates than Medicare… this has really important implications for physician compensation…it has huge implications for funding the education programs…if my front wheel of my tricycle was bigger, if we had Medicaid equity, funding the research and education mission would just be much more possible.[13]

— Mary Leonard, Arline and Pete Harman Professor and Chair of the Department of Pediatrics at Stanford University; director of the Stanford Maternal and Child Health Research Institute; and physician-in-chief of Lucile Packard Children's Hospital

[Pediatrics is the] department that is thought of secondarily to all of the adult needs. It becomes the role of the department chair of pediatrics to fight that apathy toward children's health, every day in our health systems…it is something that could be solved through putting children's health first, starting with reimbursement….There is not as much margin as adult departments and surgical departments to continue allowing for research, training, and development of [physician–scientists]. What this leaves us with is a therapeutic pipeline for children that's really threatened by not having enough bright new minds going into the field and really leaves out children when it comes to early adoption of novel therapies… with more investments into our pediatric clinical care, that big wheel of the tricycle, there could be more opportunity to think about diversifying careers in ways that are going to help us deliver better care, like focusing on quality, like focusing more on research, focusing more on our diversity and our health equity…the way that we fund health care so poorly from Medicaid is leading to segregated settings of care by payer. And that needs to be brought to light and done away with.[14]

— Sallie Permar, Nancy C. Paduano Professor and Chair of Pediatrics at Weill Cornell Medicine and pediatrician-in-chief at New York-Presbyterian/ Weill Cornell Medical Center

---

[13] The webinar recording can be accessed at https://www.nationalacademies.org/event/07-19-2022/the-pediatric-subspecialty-workforce-and-its-impact-on-child-health-and-well-being-webinar-1.

[14] The webinar recording can be accessed at https://www.nationalacademies.org/event/07-19-2022/the-pediatric-subspecialty-workforce-and-its-impact-on-child-health-and-well-being-webinar-1.

I think a fair and equitable workforce will follow if we have an equitable reimbursement and finance system.[15]

– Harold Simon, Marcus Professor and Vice Chair, Department of Pediatrics, Emory University School of Medicine and Children's Healthcare of Atlanta

KEY FINDINGS AND CONCLUSIONS

Key Findings

Finding #8-1: While rates of commercial coverage are similar between children and adults, Medicaid covers 35 percent of children and a higher share of children with complex medical needs. State Medicaid agencies have discretion in setting payment rates depending on state rules. Private insurers set payment rates based on market forces, negotiation, and other proprietary factors.

Finding #8-2: Comparisons of Medicaid and Medicare fee schedules generally find Medicaid rates to be less than Medicare, with some variation across states, specialties, or services.

Finding #8-3: Efforts to increase Medicaid payment rates through litigation under the equal access provision have been unsuccessful, the federal government has issued limited regulations to enforce the equal access provision, and there has been limited oversight of state payment rates.

Finding #8-4: Research studies have established a connection between payment levels and provider participation and children's access to care.

Finding #8-5: Existing productivity-based fee schedules (i.e., RVUs) generally reward procedure-based subspecialties and undervalue the increased time needs per clinical interaction, increased pre- and post-service time, and higher practice expenses for most subspecialty care, especially pediatric subspecialty care.

Finding #8-6: There is some evidence that pediatric subspecialties generate less revenue compared with adult subspecialties, in part due to

---

[15] The webinar recording can be accessed at https://www.nationalacademies.org/event/07-19-2022/the-pediatric-subspecialty-workforce-and-its-impact-on-child-health-and-well-being-webinar-1.

insurance mix. As a result, salaries for pediatric subspecialists are often lower than for their adult medicine counterparts.

Finding #8-7: The exact methods through which pediatric subspecialists' salaries are set are subject to complex, proprietary formulas that vary by institution.

Conclusions

Conclusion #8-1: Medicaid can be a mechanism to target investments in specific types of health care services for specific populations. Low Medicaid payments represent an underinvestment by federal and state governments in children's health. States can raise Medicaid payment rates using matched state-federal funds, but limits on state finances or other pressures may prevent states from doing so.

Conclusion #8-2: The large percentage of children on Medicaid, especially those cared for by subspecialists, coupled with the low payment rates and RVUs, adversely affects reimbursement for pediatric care. This, in turn, results in lower salaries for most pediatric subspecialties compared with adult subspecialties and compared with private practice primary care (or general) pediatricians. The relatively lower salaries for pediatric subspecialties, particularly medical subspecialties, can influence the career decisions of trainees pursuing pediatrics and pediatric subspecialty training.

Conclusion #8-3: Payment rates are one of many inputs that influence access to pediatric subspecialists.

RECOMMENDATIONS

Expansions in insurance coverage over the past decades, including via CHIP, expanded Medicaid eligibility for children, and the Affordable Care Act, have successfully removed financial barriers to health care for most children. While Medicaid and CHIP provide affordable coverage for families, the low rates of reimbursement coupled with low RVUs contribute to comparatively lower salaries for pediatric subspecialists, especially medical subspecialists. As a result, as discussed in Chapter 4, lower salaries may create disincentives for individuals to pursue careers in pediatrics.

Therefore, to achieve a goal of **reducing financial and payment disincentives,** the committee provides the following recommendations:

RECOMMENDATION 8-1 To invest in children's health and address the factors that contribute to limited access to pediatric subspecialty care, Congress should allocate additional federal funding to increase payment for pediatric services.
- Within 5 years, Congress should provide federal funds to states to increase Medicaid payment rates for pediatric services to achieve or exceed parity with Medicare payment rates.

These federal funds should be provided to all states, and the federally funded payment increases should be mandatory and apply to payments in managed care. The committee recognizes that this recommendation may be difficult to implement immediately but believes that it should be phased in as soon as possible—no later than within five years. The committee also recognizes that states can, and some have, increased payments for pediatric services themselves and encourages states to use their flexibility under Medicaid to address the payment challenges facing pediatric subspecialists. Medicaid is a policy lever that states can use in both fee-for-service and managed care settings. However, many states have not done so on their own, which is why the committee believes these mandatory, federal funds are needed.

RECOMMENDATION 8-2 The Centers for Medicare & Medicaid Services should prioritize attention to pediatric services in assigning relative value units that accurately reflect the time and resource use for pediatric subspecialty care.

REFERENCES

AAP (American Academy of Pediatrics). 2008. Application of the resource-based relative value scale system to pediatrics. *Pediatrics* 122(6):1395-1400.
ABP (American Board of Pediatrics). 2023. *Results: Continuing certification (MOC) enrollment surveys for 2018 to 2022.* https://www.abp.org/dashboards/results-continuing-certification-moc-enrollment-surveys-2018-2022 (accessed July 17, 2023).
Agarwal, R., O. Mazurenko, and N. Menachemi. 2017. High-deductible health plans reduce health care cost and utilization, including use of needed preventive services. *Health Affairs* 36(10):1762-1768.
Alexander, D., and M. Schnell. 2019 (unpublished). *The impacts of physician payments on patient access, use, and health (wp-19-23).*
AMA (American Medical Association). 2023. *RVS Update Committee (RUC).* https://www.ama-assn.org/about/rvs-update-committee-ruc/rvs-update-committee-ruc (accessed July 3, 2023).
Apaydin, E. 2020. Administrative work and job role beliefs in primary care physicians: An analysis of semi-structured interviews. *SAGE Open* 10(1): https://doi.org/10.1177/2158244019899092.

Artiga, S., L. Hill, and A. Damico. 2022. *Health coverage by race and ethnicity, 2010–2021.* https://www.kff.org/racial-equity-and-health-policy/issue-brief/health-coverage-by-race-and-ethnicity/ (accessed April 21, 2023).

Ashman, J. J., L. Santo, and T. Okeyode. 2023. *Characteristics of office-based physician visits, 2019.* Hyattsville, MD: National Center for Health Statistics.

Berman, S. 2018. State Medicaid payment levels and the federal "equal access" statute. *Pediatrics* 141(1)e20173241. https://doi.org/10.1542/peds.2017-3241.

Berry, J. G., M. Hall, J. Neff, D. Goodman, E. Cohen, R. Agrawal, D. Kuo, and C. Feudtner. 2014. Children with medical complexity and Medicaid: Spending and cost savings. *Health Affairs* 33(12):2199-2206.

Brot-Goldberg, Z. C., A. Chandra, B. R. Handel, and J. T. Kolstad. 2017. What does a deductible do? The impact of cost-sharing on health care prices, quantities, and spending dynamics.* *The Quarterly Journal of Economics* 132(3):1261-1318.

Buchmueller, T. C., S. Orzol, and L. D. Shore-Sheppard. 2015. The effect of Medicaid payment rates on access to dental care among children. *American Journal of Health Economics* 1(2):194-223.

Candon, M., S. Zuckerman, D. Wissoker, B. Saloner, G. M. Kenney, K. Rhodes, and D. Polsky. 2018. Declining Medicaid fees and primary care appointment availability for new Medicaid patients. *JAMA Internal Medicine* 178(1):145-146.

Casalino, L. P., S. Nicholson, D. N. Gans, T. Hammons, D. Morra, T. Karrison, and W. Levinson. 2009. What does it cost physician practices to interact with health insurance plans? *Health Affairs* 28(Suppl 1):w533-w543.

CBO (Congressional Budget Office). 2022. *The prices that commercial health insurers and Medicare pay for hospitals' and physicians' services.* https://www.cbo.gov/system/files/2022-01/57422-medical-prices.pdf (accessed January 4, 2023).

Chalmers, N. I., and R. D. Compton. 2017. Children's access to dental care affected by reimbursement rates, dentist density, and dentist participation in Medicaid. *American Journal of Public Health* 107(10):1612-1614.

CMS (Centers for Medicare & Medicaid Services). 2015. *Final rule: Medicaid program; methods for assuring access to covered Medicaid services.* https://www.federalregister.gov/documents/2015/11/02/2015-27697/medicaid-program-methods-for-assuring-access-to-covered-medicaid-services (accessed June 30, 2023).

CMS. 2019. *Proposed rule: Medicaid Program; Methods for Assuring Access to Covered Medicaid Services-Rescission.* https://www.federalregister.gov/documents/2019/07/15/2019-14943/medicaid-program-methods-for-assuring-access-to-covered-medicaid-services-rescission (accessed June 30, 2023).

CMS. 2020. *Final rule and interim final rule: Medicare program; CY2021 payment policies under the physician fee schedule and other changes to Part B payment policies.* https://www.govinfo.gov/content/pkg/FR-2020-12-28/pdf/2020-26815.pdf (accessed January 4, 2023).

CMS. 2023a. *Program history.* https://www.medicaid.gov/about-us/program-history/index.html (accessed April 26, 2023).

CMS. 2023b. *Beneficiary enrollment.* https://data.cms.gov/summary-statistics-on-beneficiary-enrollment/medicare-and-medicaid-reports/cms-program-statistics-medicare-total-enrollment (accessed July 17, 2023).

CMS. 2023c. *Affordable Care Act Program Integrity Provisions.* https://www.medicaid.gov/medicaid/program-integrity/affordable-care-act-program-integrity-provisions/index.html (July 10, 2023).

CMS. 2023d. *Proposed rule: Medicaid Program; Ensuring Access to Medicaid Services.* https://www.govinfo.gov/content/pkg/FR-2023-05-03/pdf/2023-08959.pdf (accessed June 30, 2023).

CMS. 2023e. *Summary of Medicaid and CHIP Payment-Related Provisions: Ensuring Access to Medicaid Services (CMS 2442-P) and Medicaid and Children's Health Insurance Program (CHIP) Managed Care Access, Finance, and Quality (CMS-2439-P).* https://www.cms.gov/newsroom/fact-sheets/summary-medicaid-and-chip-payment-related-provisions-ensuring-access-medicaid-services-cms-2442-p#_ftnref1 (accessed June 30, 2023).

Conduff, J. H., and D. H. Coelho. 2017. Professional reimbursement by Medicaid for cochlear implants and related services. *Otology & Neurotology* 38(7):985-989.

Coughlin, T. A., H. Samuel-Jakubos, and R. Garfield. 2021. *Sources of payment for uncompensated care for the uninsured.* https://www.kff.org/report-section/sources-of-payment-for-uncompensated-care-for-the-uninsured-issue-brief (accessed January 4, 2023).

Cunningham, P. J., and A. S. O'Malley. 2009. Do reimbursement delays discourage Medicaid participation by physicians? *Health Affairs* 28(1):w17-w28.

Decker, S. L. 2018. No association found between the Medicaid primary care fee bump and physician-reported participation in Medicaid. *Health Affairs* 37(7):1092-1098.

Doximity and Curative. 2023. *2023 physician compensation report.* https://press.doximity.com/reports/doximity-physician-compensation-report-2023.pdf (accessed May 5, 2023).

Dunn, A., J. D. Gottlieb, A. Shapiro, D. J. Sonnenstuhl, and P. Tebaldi. 2023. *A denial a day keeps the doctor away.* https://www.nber.org/papers/w29010 (accessed June 5, 2023).

East, C. N., S. Miller, M. Page, and L. R. Wherry. 2023. Multigenerational impacts of childhood access to the safety net: Early life exposure to Medicaid and the next generation's health. *American Economic Review* 113(1):98-135.

Erickson, S. M., B. Rockwern, M. Koltov, and R. M. McLean. 2017. Putting patients first by reducing administrative tasks in health care: A position paper of the American College of Physicians. *Annals of Internal Medicine* 166(9):659-661.

Frintner, M. P., D. Kaelber, E. Kirkendall, C. Lehmann, and E. Lourie. 2020. *U.S. pediatricians' perspectives on reducing administrative tasks.* https://www.aap.org/en/research/pediatrician-life-and-career-experience-study-places/results-and-publications/us-pediatricians-perspectives-on-reducing-administrative-tasks (accessed May 5, 2023).

GAO (U.S. Government Accountability Office). 2014a. *Medicaid: Use of claims data for analysis of provider payment rates.* Washington, DC: GAO.

GAO. 2014b. *Medicaid payment comparisons of selected services under fee-for-service, managed care, and private insurance.* Washington, DC: GAO.

GAO. 2015. *Medicare physician payment rates: Better data and greater transparency could improve accuracy.* Washington, DC: GAO.

Garfield, R., E. Hinton, C. Cornachione, and C. Hall. 2018. *The Kaiser Family Foundation 2017 Survey of Medicaid Managed Care Plans.* https://files.kff.org/attachment/Topline-and-Methodology-Kaiser-Family-Foundation-2017-Survey-of-Medicaid-Managed-Care-Plans (accessed January 4, 2023).

Gifford, K., A. Lashbrook, S. Barth, M. Nardone, E. Hinton, M. Guth, L. Stolyar, and R. Rudowitz. 2021. States respond to COVID-19 challenges but also take advantage of new opportunities to address long-standing issues: Results from a 50-state Medicaid budget survey for state fiscal years 2021 and 2022. https://www.kff.org/report-section/states-respond-to-covid-19-challenges-but-also-take-advantage-of-new-opportunities-to-address-long-standing-issues-provider-rates-and-taxes/ (accessed January 4, 2023).

Gould, Z., and K. Honsberger. 2022. *Expanded federal investment in home and community-based services: State approaches to serve children and youth.* https://nashp.org/expanded-federal-investment-in-home-and-community-based-services-state-approaches-to-serve-children-and-youth/ (accessed May 5, 2023).

HHS (U.S. Department of Health and Human Services). 2022. *Federal financial participation in state assistance expenditures; federal matching shares for Medicaid, the Children's Health Insurance Program, and aid to needy aged, blind, or disabled persons for October 1, 2023 through September 30, 2024.* https://www.federalregister.gov/documents/2022/12/05/2022-26390/federal-financial-participation-in-state-assistance-expenditures-federal-matching-shares-for (accessed May 5, 2023).

Himmelstein, D. U., M. Jun, R. Busse, K. Chevreul, A. Geissler, P. Jeurissen, S. Thomson, M. Vinet, and S. Woolhandler. 2014. A comparison of hospital administrative costs in eight nations: U.S, costs exceed all others by far. *Health Affairs* 33(9):1586-1594.

Hinton, E., Guth, M., Raphael, J., Haldar, S., and R. Rudowitz. 2022. *How the Pandemic Continues to Shape Medicaid Priorities: Results from an Annual Medicaid Budget Survey for State Fiscal Years 2022 and 2023.* https://files.kff.org/attachment/REPORT-How-the-Pandemic-Continues-to-Shape-Medicaid-Priorities-Results-from-an-Annual-Medicaid-Budget-Survey-for-State-Fiscal-Years-2022-and-2023.pdf (accessed July 10, 2023).

Hinton, E., and J. Raphael. 2023. *10 things to know about Medicaid managed care.* https://www.kff.org/medicaid/issue-brief/10-things-to-know-about-medicaid-managed-care/ (accessed May 5, 2023).

Holgash, K., and M. Heberlein. 2019. *Physician acceptance of new Medicaid patients.* https://www.macpac.gov/wp-content/uploads/2019/01/Physician-Acceptance-of-New-Medicaid-Patients.pdf (accessed January 4, 2023).

Itri, J. N., A. Mithqal, and A. Krishnaraj. 2017. Funds flow in the era of value-based health care. *Journal of the American College of Radiology* 14(6):818-824.

Jones, J. R., M. D. Kogan, R. M. Ghandour, and C. S. Minkovitz. 2021. Out-of-pocket health care expenditures among United States children: Parental perceptions and past-year expenditures, 2016 to 2017. *Academic Pediatrics* 21(3):480-487.

Josephson, S. A., R. L. Sacco, J. M. Czech, R. N. Maher, C. S. Knutson, and L. B. Goldstein. 2020. Funds flow in academic neurology: A potential path to financial success. *Neurology* 94(18):785-791.

KFF. 2022a. *Health insurance coverage of children 0-18 (CPS).* https://www.kff.org/other/state-indicator/health-insurance-coverage-of-children-0-18-cps/?activeTab=graph&currentTimeframe=0&startTimeframe=2&selectedDistributions=medicaid&sortModel=%7B%22colId%22:%22Location%22,%22sort%22:%22asc%22%7D (accessed January 4, 2023).

KFF. 2022b. *2022 employer health benefits survey.* https://www.kff.org/report-section/ehbs-2022-section-5-market-shares-of-health-plans/ (accessed January 4, 2023).

Klukoff, H., M. Lehan, and A. Schneider. 2023. *Medicaid managed care financial results for 2022: Another big year for the big five.* https://ccf.georgetown.edu/2023/02/22/medicaid-managed-care-financial-results-for-2022-another-big-year-for-the-big-five (accessed June 30, 2023).

Kuo, D. Z., M. Hall, R. Agrawal, E. Cohen, C. Feudtner, D. M. Goodman, J. M. Neff, and J. G. Berry. 2015. Comparison of health care spending and utilization among children with Medicaid insurance. *Pediatrics* 136(6):1521-1529.

Lakshminrusimha, S., S. Murin, J. D. Kirk, Z. Mustafa, T. R. Maurice, N. Sousa, J. Lee, and D. A. Lubarsky. 2022. "Funds flow" implementation at academic health centers: Unique challenges to pediatric departments. *The Journal of Pediatrics* 249:6-10.e14. https://doi.org/10.1016/j.jpeds.2022.01.058. Epub 2022 Feb 3. PMID: 35124013.

Lakshminrusimha, S., S. Murin, and D. A. Lubarsky. 2023. Low compensation for academic pediatric medical specialists: Role of Medicaid, productivity, work hours, and sex. *The Journal of Pediatrics* 255:1-6.

Lalezari, R. M., A. Pozen, and C. J. Dy. 2018. State variation in Medicaid reimbursements for orthopaedic surgery. *Journal of Bone and Joint Surgery* 100(3):236-242.

Larson, K., E. A. Gottschlich, W. L. Cull, and L. M. Olson. 2021. High-deductible health plans for U.S. children: Trends, health service use, and financial barriers to care. *Academic Pediatrics* 21(8):1345-1354.

Leininger, L. J., B. Saloner, and L. R. Wherry. 2015. Predicting high-cost pediatric patients: Derivation and validation of a population-based model. *Medical Care* 53(8):729-735.

Liptak, G. S., L. P. Shone, P. Auinger, A. W. Dick, S. A. Ryan, and P. G. Szilagyi. 2006. Short-term persistence of high health care costs in a nationally representative sample of children. *Pediatrics* 118(4):e1001-e1009.

Mabry, C. D., L. A. Gurien, S. D. Smith, and S. C. Mehl. 2016. Are surgeons being paid fairly by Medicaid? A national comparison of typical payments for general surgeons. *Journal of the American College of Surgeons* 222(4):387-394.

MACPAC (Medicaid and CHIP Payment and Access Commission). 2015. *Provider Networks and Access: Issues for Children's Coverage.* https://www.macpac.gov/wp-content/uploads/2015/03/Provider-Networks-and-Access-Issues-for-Children%E2%80%99s-Coverage.pdf (accessed July 10, 2023).

MACPAC. 2017a. *Medicaid payment policy for Federally Qualified Health Centers.* https://www.macpac.gov/wp-content/uploads/2017/12/Medicaid-Payment-Policy-for-Federally-Qualified-Health-Centers.pdf (accessed July 10, 2023).

MACPAC. 2017b. *State Medicaid fee-for-service physician payment policies.* https://www.macpac.gov/publication/states-medicaid-fee-for-service-physician-payment-policies (accessed January 4, 2023).

MACPAC. 2022a. *Provider payment under fee for service.* https://www.macpac.gov/subtopic/provider-payment (accessed January 4, 2023).

MACPAC. 2022b. *Annual analysis of disproportionate share hospital allotments to states.* https://www.macpac.gov/publication/annual-analysis-of-disproportionate-share-hospital-allotments-to-states-3 (accessed April 7, 2023).

MACPAC. 2022c. *Directed payments in Medicaid managed care.* https://www.macpac.gov/wp-content/uploads/2022/06/June-2022-Directed-Payments-Issue-Brief-FINAL.pdf (accessed June 30, 2023).

MACPAC. 2023a. *Matching rates.* https://www.macpac.gov/subtopic/matching-rates/ (accessed April 6, 2023).

MACPAC. 2023b. *Federal match rate exceptions.* https://www.macpac.gov/federal-match-rate-exceptions (accessed April 6, 2023).

MACPAC. 2023c. *Federal legislative milestones in Medicaid and CHIP.* https://www.macpac.gov/reference-materials/federal-legislative-milestones-in-medicaid-and-chip/ (accessed May 10, 2023).

MACPAC. 2023d. *Disproportionate share hospital payments.* https://www.macpac.gov/subtopic/disproportionate-share-hospital-payments (accessed April 7, 2023).

Manatt Health. 2023. *Proposed rules on Medicaid payments, access and quality: Implications for health care stakeholders.* https://www.manatt.com/insights/webinars/proposed-rules-on-medicaid-payments-access-and-qu (accessed June 30, 2023).

Martin, K. 2021. *Medscape pediatrician compensation report 2021.* https://www.medscape.com/slideshow/2021-compensation-pediatrician-6013859 (accessed May 5, 2023).

Massoumi, R. L., C. P. Childers, and S. L. Lee. 2021. Underrepresentation of pediatric operations in the relative value unit updating process. *Journal of Pediatric Surgery* 56(6):1101-1106.

MedPAC (Medicare Payment Advisory Committee). 2018. *June 2018 Report to the Congress: Medicare and the health care delivery system.* Washington, DC: MedPAC.

Miller, E. A. 2007. Federal administrative and judicial oversight of Medicaid: Policy legacies and tandem institutions under the Boren amendment. *Publius: The Journal of Federalism* 38(2):315-342.

Miller, S., and L. R. Wherry. 2018. The long-term effects of early life Medicaid coverage. *Journal of Human Resources*: https://doi.org/10.3368/jhr.54.3.0816.8173R1.

Miller, J. C., G. E. Andersson, M. Cohen, S. M. Cohen, S. Gibson, M. A. Hindery, M. Hooven, J. Krakower, and D. H. Browdy. 2012. Perspective: Follow the money: The implications of medical schools' funds flow models. *Academic Medicine* 87(12):1746-1751.

Ming, D. Y., K. A. Jones, M. J. White, J. E. Pritchard, B. G. Hammill, C. Bush, G. L. Jackson, and S. R. Raman. 2022. Healthcare utilization for Medicaid-insured children with medical complexity: Differences by sociodemographic characteristics. *Maternal and Child Health Journal* 26(12):2407-2418.

Moore, K. J., T. A. Felger, W. L. Larimore, and T. L. Mills. 2008. What every physician should know about the RUC. *Family Practice Management* 15(2):36.

Muhuri, P., and S. Machlin. 2017. Differences in payments for child visits to office-based physicians: Private versus Medicaid insurance, 2010 to 2015. In *Statistical brief (Medical Expenditure Panel Survey (U.S.))*. Rockville, MD: Agency for Healthcare Research and Quality.

Mulcahy, A. W., T. Gracner, and K. Finegold. 2018. Associations between the Patient Protection and Affordable Care Act Medicaid primary care payment increase and physician participation in Medicaid. *JAMA Internal Medicine* 178(8):1042-1048.

Mulcahy, A. W., K. Merrell, and A. Mehrotra. 2020. Payment for services rendered—updating Medicare's valuation of procedures. *New England Journal of Medicine* 382(4):303-306.

NASEM (National Academies of Sciences, Engineering, and Medicine). 2021. *Implementing high-quality primary care: Rebuilding the foundation of health care*. Edited by L. McCauley, R. L. Phillips, Jr., M. Meisnere, and S. K. Robinson. Washington, DC: The National Academies Press.

OECD (Organisation for Economic Co-operation and Development). 2016. *Better ways to pay for health care*. https://www.oecd.org/publications/better-ways-to-pay-for-health-care-9789264258211-en.htm (accessed May 5, 2023).

Ortaliza, J., M. McGough, E. Wager, G. Claxton, and K. Amin. 2021. *How do health expenditures vary across the population?* https://www.healthsystemtracker.org/chart-collection/health-expenditures-vary-across-population/#Proportion%20of%20individuals%20by%20health%20status,%202019 (accessed May 5, 2023).

Perkins, J. 2015. *Armstrong v. Exceptional Child Care Center: Health care providers' access to court is blocked*. https://healthlaw.org/wp-content/uploads/2015/04/2015_04_27_Armstrong_Summary_Rev.pdf (accessed May 5, 2023).

Perrin, J. M., G. M. Kenney, and S. Rosenbaum. 2020. Medicaid and child health equity. *New England Journal of Medicine* 383(27):2595-2598.

Pollitz, K. 2022. *Network adequacy standards and enforcement*. https://www.kff.org/health-reform/issue-brief/network-adequacy-standards-and-enforcement (accessed July 10, 2023).

Polsky, D., M. Richards, S. Basseyn, D. Wissoker, G. M. Kenney, S. Zuckerman, and K. V. Rhodes. 2015. Appointment availability after increases in Medicaid payments for primary care. *New England Journal of Medicine* 372(6):537-545.

Price, J., M. L. Brandt, M. L. Hudak, S. K. Berman, K. M. Carlson, A. P. Giardino, L. Hammer, K. Heggen, S. A. Pearlman, and B. G. Sood. 2020. Principles of financing the medical home for children. *Pediatrics* 145(1): e20193451.

Rueben, K. S., and M. Randall. 2017. *Balanced budget requirements*. https://www.urban.org/research/publication/balanced-budget-requirements (accessed July 17, 2023).

Rosenbaum, S. 2015. Medicaid and access to care: The CMS equal access rule. *Health Affairs Blog*.

Rosenbaum, S., Jost, T., Musimeci, M., and Somodevilla, A. 2023. A victory for Medicaid beneficiaries in Supreme Court's Talevski decision. *Health Affairs Forefront*.

Rudowitz, R. 2020. *What you need to know about the Medicaid fiscal accountability rule (MFAR)*. https://www.kff.org/medicaid/issue-brief/what-you-need-to-know-about-the-medicaid-fiscal-accountability-rule-mfar/#:~:text=States%20are%20limited%20in%20making,would%20pay%20and%20Medicaid%20payments. (accessed July 17, 2023).

Rudowitz, R., B. Corallo, and R. Garfield. 2020. *How much fiscal relief can states expect from the temporary increase in the Medicaid FMAP?* https://www.kff.org/coronavirus-covid-19/issue-brief/how-much-fiscal-relief-can-states-expect-from-the-temporary-increase-in-the-medicaid-fmap/ (accessed July 17, 2023).

Rudowitz, R., and L. Sobel. 2022. *What is at stake for Medicaid in Supreme Court case Health & Hospital Corp v. Talevski?* https://www.kff.org/policy-watch/what-is-at-stake-for-medicaid-in-supreme-court-case-health-hospital-corp-v-talevski/ (accessed April 7, 2023).

Santiago, C. C., D. C. Santiago, and R. Sebro. 2020. State variation in Medicaid and Medicare reimbursements in musculoskeletal radiology. *Clinical Imaging* 66:67-72.

Schnapp, L. M., M. J. Steiner, and S. D. Davis. 2020. Basic primer for finances in academic adult and pediatric pulmonary divisions. *Chest* 157(2):363-368.

Schneider, A. 2023. A closer look at the network adequacy provisions of CMS's proposed Medicaid managed care rule. In *Say Ahhh!*: Georgetown University Health Policy Institute Center for Children and Families.

Schneider, A., and A. Corcoran. 2022. Standards for provider network adequacy in Medicaid and the marketplaces. In *Say Ahhh!*: Georgetown University Health Policy Institute Center for Children and Families.

Sharma, R., S. Tinkler, A. Mitra, S. Pal, R. Susu-Mago, and M. Stano. 2018. State Medicaid fees and access to primary care physicians. *Health Economics* 27(3):629-636.

Singer, N. G., and K. B. Onel. 2019. Challenges to practicing pediatric rheumatology. *Rheumatic Disease Clinics* 45(1):67-78.

Smith, V. K., K. Gifford, E. Ellis, R. Rudowitz, and L. Snyder. 2010. *Hoping for economic recovery, preparing for health reform: A look at Medicaid spending, coverage and policy trends results from a 50-state Medicaid budget survey for state fiscal years 2010 and 2011*. https://www.kff.org/wp-content/uploads/2013/01/8105.pdf (accessed July 10, 2023).

Staman, J. 2011. *Medicaid reimbursement rate litigation: An overview of Douglas v. Independent Living Center of Southern California*. https://www.everycrsreport.com/files/20110718_R41923_7b27132c1be30c4e727dc85ddc64e252795fd91d.pdf (accessed May 5, 2023).

Tang, S.-F. S., M. L. Hudak, D. M. Cooley, B. N. Shenkin, and A. D. Racine. 2018. Increased Medicaid payment and participation by office-based primary care pediatricians. *Pediatrics* 141(1): e20172570.

Tseng, P., R. S. Kaplan, B. D. Richman, M. A. Shah, and K. A. Schulman. 2018. Administrative costs associated with physician billing and insurance-related activities at an academic health care system. *Journal of the American Medical Association* 319(7):691-697.

VonAchen, P., D. Gaur, W. Wickremasinghe, M. Hall, D. M. Goodman, R. Agrawal, and J. G. Berry. 2021. Assessment of underpayment for inpatient care at children's hospitals. *JAMA Pediatrics* 175(9):972-974.

Weidemann, D. K., I. Ashoor, D. Soranno, R. Sheth, C. Carter, and P. Brophy. 2022. Moving the needle toward fair compensation in pediatric nephrology. *Frontiers in Pediatrics* 10:849826. https://doi.org/10.3389/fped.2022.849826.

Weiss, A. J., L. Liang, and K. Martin. 2022. *Overview of hospital stays among children and adolescents, 2019*. https://hcup-us.ahrq.gov/reports/statbriefs/sb299-Hospital-Stays-Children-2019.jsp (accessed May 5, 2023).

West, C. P., L. N. Dyrbye, and T. D. Shanafelt. 2018. Physician burnout: Contributors, consequences and solutions. *Journal of Internal Medicine* 283(6):516-529.

Weyand, A. C., and G. L. Freed. 2020. Pediatric subspecialty workforce: Undersupply or overdemand? *Pediatric Research* 88(3):369-371.

Wherry, L. R., S. Miller, R. Kaestner, and B. D. Meyer. 2018. Childhood Medicaid coverage and later-life health care utilization. *The Review of Economics and Statistics* 100(2):287-302.

Williams, E., and M. Musumeci. 2021. *Children with special health care needs: Coverage, affordability, and HCBS access.* https://www.kff.org/medicaid/issue-brief/children-with-special-health-care-needs-coverage-affordability-and-hcbs-access (accessed January 4, 2023).

Wong, C. A., K. Kan, Z. Cidav, R. Nathenson, and D. Polsky. 2017. Pediatric and adult physician networks in Affordable Care Act marketplace plans. *Pediatrics* 139(4).

Wynn, B. O., L. F. Burgette, A. W. Mulcahy, E. N. Okeke, I. Brantley, N. Iyer, T. Ruder, and A. Mehrotra. 2015. Development of a model for the validation of work relative value units for the Medicare physician fee schedule. *RAND Health Quarterly* 5(1):5.

Zuckerman, S., K. Merrell, R. A. Berenson, S. Mitchell, D. Upadhyay, and R. Lewis. 2016. *Collecting empirical physician time data: Piloting an approach for validating work relative value units.* https://www.urban.org/sites/default/files/publication/87771/2001123-collecting-empirical-physician-time-data-piloting-approach-for-validating-work-relative-value-units_0.pdf (accessed January 4, 2023).

Zuckerman, S., L. Skopec, and J. Aarons. 2021. Medicaid physician fees remained substantially below fees paid by Medicare in 2019. *Health Affairs* 40(2):343-348.

Appendix A

Committee Member, Fellow, and Staff Biographies

COMMITTEE MEMBERS

Frederick P. Rivara, M.D., M.P.H. (*Chair*), is the holder of the Seattle Children's Guild Association Endowed Chair in Pediatric Outcomes Research, vice chair and professor of pediatrics, and adjunct professor of epidemiology at the University of Washington (UW). Dr. Rivara earned a bachelor's degree at the College of the Holy Cross in Worcester, MA, and received his M.D. from the University of Pennsylvania and an M.P.H. from the University of Washington. He completed residencies at the Children's Hospital Medical Center in Boston and the University of Washington and was a Robert Wood Johnson Clinical Scholar at the University of Washington. He is editor-in-chief of *JAMA Network Open* after serving for 17 years as editor-in-chief of *JAMA Pediatrics*.

He has received numerous honors, including the Charles C. Shepard Science Award from the Centers for Disease Control and Prevention; the American Public Health Association, Injury Control and Emergency Health Services Section Distinguished Career Award; the American Academy of Pediatrics (AAP), Section on Injury and Poison Prevention, Physician Achievement Award; the UW School of Public Health Distinguished Alumni Award; and the UW Medicine Minority Faculty Mentoring Award. Dr. Rivara was elected to the Institute of Medicine (IOM; now National Academy of Medicine [NAM]) in 2005. He was awarded the Joseph St. Geme, Jr. Leadership Award from the Federation of Pediatric Organizations in 2021.

Dr. Rivara previously was the chair of the Committee on the Biological and Psychosocial Effects of Peer Victimization: Lessons for Bullying

Prevention, IOM; chair of the Committee on Oral Health Access to Care, IOM; member of the Committee on Adolescent Health Care Services and Models of Care, IOM; and vice chair of the Committee on Sports Related Concussions in Youth, IOM.

Kelly Betts, Ed.D., APRN-NP, CPNP-PC, CNE, P-SANE, is currently the assistant dean for the University of Nebraska Medical Center (UNMC) College of Nursing in Scottsbluff, NE. She is also a practicing primary care pediatric nurse practitioner at a Federally Qualified Health Center in Gering, NE. In her clinical practice, she cares for minority and underserved children in the panhandle of rural Nebraska. Currently at UNMC, she was awarded funding for an interprofessional grant with the UNMC Dental Hygiene program to integrate oral health risk assessment into pediatric well-child visits. Dr. Betts is also trained as a Sexual Assault Nurse Examiner (SANE) and provides these services as needed to the rural counties in the Panhandle. Dr. Betts has more than 15 years of teaching nursing students at both the undergraduate and graduate levels. She received her Ed.D. from Walden University and her APRN Post-Master's Certificate as a pediatric nurse practitioner at the University of Arkansas for Medical Sciences. She is a member of Sigma Theta Tau International Nursing Society, the National Association of Pediatric Nurse Practitioners, the Nebraska Nurse Practitioner Association, and the National League for Nursing.

Kendall M. Campbell, M.D., FAAFP, is professor and chair of the Department of Family Medicine at the University of Texas Medical Branch. Prior to this appointment, he served as the senior associate dean for academic affairs and director of the Research Group for Underrepresented Minorities in Academic Medicine at the Brody School of Medicine in North Carolina. His research expertise includes issues impacting the recruitment and retention of underrepresented minority students and faculty. He is well published in this area and nationally known for his contributions. He co-founded and is a faculty member in the Society of Teachers of Family Medicine Leadership through Scholarship fellowship, a writing fellowship to promote profession advancement for early career academic family medicine physicians who are underrepresented in medicine. Dr. Campbell is a member of the NAM roundtable on health equity and was elected to NAM in 2021. He completed his medical school training at the University of Florida College of Medicine and residency training at Tallahassee Memorial Healthcare.

Kecia N. Carroll, M.D., M.P.H., is chief, Division of General Pediatrics and professor of pediatrics and environmental medicine and public health at the Icahn School of Medicine at Mount Sinai (ISMMS). She is the Black Family Chair for Pediatrics, a member of the Mount Sinai Institute for

Exposomic Research, and the Inaugural Senior Mount Sinai Biomedical Laureate in Clinical/Translational Research, a program created to foster inclusive research and mentoring environments. Dr. Carroll is a research fellowship-trained epidemiologist, clinical researcher, and board-certified pediatrician. Her current National Institutes of Health-funded research program investigates how prenatal and early life environmental exposures influence childhood asthma risk, with the long-term goals to decrease morbidity and prevent disease. Dr. Carroll serves as a co-director of the KL2 Program of the ConduITS Institute for Translational Sciences and the National Institute of Child Health and Human Development-funded T32 Research Training Program in Pediatric Exposomics at the ISMMS. She is a member of the Society for Pediatric Research and the American Pediatric Society. She obtained her undergraduate degree at Vassar College and completed medical school at Vanderbilt University School of Medicine, pediatric residency at the University of California, San Francisco, and an academic general pediatrics Fellowship at Vanderbilt.

Candice Chen, M.D., M.P.H., is an associate professor of health policy and management at the Fitzhugh Mullan Institute for Health Workforce Equity in the Milken Institute School of Public Health at The George Washington University. Her work focuses on health workforce equity, which includes diversity, social mission of health professions schools, workforce distribution, service to vulnerable populations, training for new models of care, and equity for the workforce. Her research has examined medical school outcomes in primary care, practice in underserved communities, and diversity; graduate medical education "imprinting" on the cost practice patterns of physicians; and identifying the workforce providing high-need services in reproductive health services and to Medicaid populations. Dr. Chen serves on the American Board of Pediatrics' (ABP) Research Advisory Committee and is a board member for Authority Health GME and the Accreditation Council for Graduate Medical Education, International. Dr. Chen was previously the director of the Division of Medicine and Dentistry in the Bureau of Health Workforce at the Health Resources and Services Administration, where she led programs to enhance training in primary care, oral health, and geriatrics, including graduate medical education programs in children's hospitals and teaching health centers. Dr. Chen is a board-certified pediatrician. She received her M.D. from Baylor College of Medicine and her M.P.H. from The George Washington University, with a concentration in community oriented primary care.

Christopher B. Forrest, M.D., Ph.D., is a pediatrician and health services and outcomes researcher. He is director of PEDSnet (pedsnet.org), a national pediatric learning health system with 11 children's hospital members.

PEDSnet has created a longitudinal electronic health record database for more than 12 million children, and the network conducts observational research and pediatric clinical trials across all pediatric subspecialty areas. Chris serves as the Director of the CHOP Applied Clinical Research Center, which is the institutional home for PEDSnet, and the Program Director for PEDSnet Scholars, an Agency for Healthcare Research and Patient-Centered Outcomes Research Institute funded K12 faculty development program. His research group has developed numerous pediatric patient-reported outcome measures, both child self-report and parent-proxy versions. He co-edited the new *Handbook of Life Course Health Development*, which has been downloaded more than 850,000 times from the Springer web site. Dr. Forrest received his B.A. and M.D. from Boston University and his Ph.D. in Health Policy and Management from Johns Hopkins University.

Elena Fuentes-Afflick, M.D., M.P.H., is professor of pediatrics and vice dean for Zuckerberg San Francisco General Hospital at the University of California, San Francisco. An academic generalist, Dr. Fuentes-Afflick's expertise is in the fields of perinatal epidemiology, acculturation, Latino health, professionalism, misconduct, and diversity in academic medicine. Dr. Fuentes-Afflick has served as president of the Society for Pediatric Research and the American Pediatric Society and is an elected member of the NAM and the American Academy of Arts and Sciences. Currently, she serves as Home Secretary of the NAM. She previously served on the ABP's New Subspecialties Committee (2017–2019) and the Research Advisory Committee (2018–2021). Dr. Fuentes-Afflick completed her undergraduate and medical school education at the University of Michigan and holds an M.P.H. at the University of California, Berkeley. She has served on numerous consensus committees, most recently on the underrepresentation of women and women of color in STEMM fields.

Rachel L. Garfield, M.H.S., Ph.D., is executive director of the Vermont Child Health Improvement Program (VCHIP) and associate professor in the Department of Pediatrics at the University of Vermont Larner College of Medicine. VCHIP is a maternal and child health services research and quality improvement program that aims to optimize child and family health through measurement-based efforts to enhance child health practice. Prior to her current position, Dr. Garfield was a vice president at the Kaiser Family Foundation and co-director for its Program on Medicaid and the Uninsured. Previous roles have included assistant professor in the Department of Health Policy and Management at the University of Pittsburgh Graduate School of Public Health, policy analyst in state and federal Medicaid and Children's Health Insurance Program policy, and research consultant for hospital operations and management. Dr. Garfield has more than two decades of experience in Medicaid policy research and is an expert in data analysis on insurance coverage and access to care for low-income populations. She also has expertise in behavioral health policy, particularly public financing for behavioral health services. Dr. Garfield holds a B.A. from Harvard College, an M.H.S. from the Johns Hopkins Bloomberg School of Public Health, and a Ph.D. in Health Policy from Harvard University.

Kristin Hittle Gigli, M.S.N., Ph.D., CPNP-AC, is an acute care pediatric nurse practitioner and health services researcher. She is an assistant professor of graduate nursing in the College of Nursing and Health Innovation at the University of Texas at Arlington. Her research examines roles of the hospital-based advanced practice provider workforce in providing care and health outcomes of hospitalized children. She earned her nurse practitioner degree from the University of Pennsylvania and her Ph.D. in Nursing from Vanderbilt University. She completed a postdoctoral fellowship in the Department of Critical Care Medicine CRISMA Center at the University of Pittsburgh. In addition to her research, Dr. Gigli has 15 years of experience in pediatric critical care and holds a clinical appointment in the Pediatric Intensive Care Unit at Children's Health Dallas. She is a past board member of the National Association of Pediatric Nurse Practitioners and currently a liaison to the AAP Committee on Hospital Care and the Association of Medical Schools Pediatric Department Chairs Pediatrics 2025: AMSPDC Workforce Initiative.

Javier A. Gonzalez del Rey, M.D., M.Ed., is currently a professor of pediatrics, chair of graduate medical education, Designated Institutional Officer for the Accreditation Council for Graduate Medical Education (ACGME), associate chair for education, and director of the Cincinnati Children's Pediatric Education Center at Cincinnati Children's Hospital Medical Center. He is a past president at the Association of Pediatric Program Directors, and past chair for the Executive Committee for the Section of Emergency Medicine at the AAP. He received his university and medical school education at the National University Pedro Henriquez Ureña in the Dominican Republic. He completed his pediatric residency at the University of Connecticut Pediatric Primary Care Program, and fellowship training in General Academic Pediatrics and Pediatric Emergency Medicine at the Cincinnati Children's Hospital Medical Center. He is currently certified in Pediatrics and Pediatric Emergency Medicine. He completed a master's of medical education and advanced training in quality improvement methodology (I2S2). Dr. Gonzalez del Rey's major areas of interests include resident and subspecialty medical education—pediatric emergency medicine national and for Latin America, and improvement science methodology applied to medical education and training.

Shafali Spurling Jeste, M.D., is a child neurologist with expertise in neurodevelopmental disorders (NDDs). She is chief of neurology and co-director of the Neurological Institute at Children's Hospital, Los Angeles (CHLA), and professor of pediatrics and neurology at the University of Southern California Keck School of Medicine. Her research, funded by the National Institutes of Health, the Department of Defense, and the Simons foundation, is focused on improving precision health in NDDs, through biomarkers, clinical endpoints, and scalable clinical trials. Her clinical expertise lies in the diagnosis and management of infants and children with NDDs, particularly those with complex medical needs. At CHLA and through the Child Neurology Society, she is actively engaged in efforts to expand the pediatric workforce by cultivating early clinical research careers. She is on the Board of Directors of the American Brain Foundation and the National Organization for Rare Disorders, and she is on the Programmatic Panel of the Department of Defense Tuberous Sclerosis Complex Research Program. In 2019 she was awarded the Presidential Early Career Award for Scientists and Engineers. In 2022 she was named a Woman of Influence in Health Care by the *LA Business Journal*. She earned her B.A. in Philosophy from Yale University and her M.D. from Harvard Medical School. She completed her child neurology residency and behavioral neurology fellowship at Boston Children's Hospital.

Ophir D. Klein, M.D., Ph.D., serves as the inaugural executive director of Cedars-Sinai Guerin Children's and the David and Meredith Kaplan Distinguished Chair in Children's Health. He is also adjunct professor of orofacial sciences and pediatrics at the University of California, San Francisco (UCSF), where he was previously the Larry L. Hillblom Distinguished Professor in Craniofacial Anomalies and the Charles J. Epstein Professor of Human Genetics. Until 2022, he served as director of the Institute for Human Genetics, chief of the Division of Medical Genetics, chair of the Division of Craniofacial Anomalies, and director of the Program in Craniofacial Biology at UCSF. Dr. Klein was educated at the University of California, Berkeley, where he earned a B.A. in Spanish Literature. He subsequently attended Yale University School of Medicine, where he received a Ph.D. in Genetics and an M.D. He then completed residencies at Yale-New Haven Hospital in Pediatrics and at UCSF in Clinical Genetics. Dr. Klein has received several honors, including a New Innovator Award from the National Institutes of Health and the E. Mead Johnson Award from the Society for Pediatric Research. Dr. Klein was elected to the American Society for Clinical Investigation, the Association of American Physicians, and the NAM and he is a Fellow of the American Association for the Advancement of Science. Dr. Klein's research focuses on understanding how organs form in the embryo and how they regenerate in the adult, with a particular emphasis on the processes underlying craniofacial and dental development and renewal as well as understanding how stem cells in the intestinal epithelium enable renewal and regeneration.

Victoria Fay Norwood, M.D., is the Robert J. Roberts Professor of Pediatrics at the University of Virginia (UVA), where she has practiced as a pediatric nephrologist for her entire career after earning her M.D. and completing pediatric residency training at Tulane University. She completed her pediatric nephrology fellowship at UVA and began her tenure at UVA as a physician–scientist focused on developmental nephrology. Since that time, she served as division chief of nephrology for 17 years, program director of the Peds Nephrology Fellowship for 25 years, and vice chair for academic affairs in the Department of Pediatrics. Outside of UVA she has been deeply involved in the activities of the American Society of Pediatric Nephrology, of which she was president in 2014–2016. She was the founding chair of the Council of Pediatric Subspecialties in 2007–2010 and has served on the Review Committee for Pediatrics at ACGME. Most recently, after many years and roles with the ABP, she served as chair of ABP and the ABP Foundation Board of Directors in 2020. She also serves on the Governance Committee for the American Board of Medical Specialties. Dr. Norwood received the Henry L. Barnett Award for Lifetime Achievement in Pediatric Nephrology from the Section on Nephrology of the AAP in 2020. Dr. Norwood's academic career has been and continues to be focused on issues of subspecialty pediatrics, including education, training, initial and continuing certification, credentialing, and workforce.

Eliana M. Perrin, M.D., M.P.H., is the Bloomberg Distinguished Professor of Primary Care in the Schools of Medicine and Nursing at Johns Hopkins. Previously she served as associate vice chancellor for research at the University of North Carolina (UNC), Chapel Hill; and as division chief of primary care, founding director of the Center for Childhood Obesity Research, and as one of the directors of the National Clinician Scholars Program at Duke University. She is a general pediatrician and researcher with expertise in obesity, patient-oriented prevention, health services, and health disparities and has collaborated with numerous pediatrics subspecialists. As a division chief, she supervised a faculty of about 45; oversaw a robust clinical enterprise that included three continuity clinics, a medicine-pediatrics clinic, a healthy lifestyle clinic, a child maltreatment clinic, and an adolescent medicine clinic; and bolstered interdisciplinary research and educational efforts. She is a multiple Principal Investigator (PI) of the Greenlight obesity prevention project funded by two National Institutes of Health R01s and Co-PI of a large comparative effectiveness Patient-Centered Outcomes Research Institute trial. She served as chair of the National Research Committee of the Academic Pediatrics Association, was elected to the Society of Pediatric Research and American

Pediatric Society, and is a Fellow of the AAP, where she serves on the Committee on Pediatric Research. She has mentored more than 40 trainees at all levels, including 12 prior career development awardees. She won the Hettleman Prize for Artistic and Scholarly Achievement at UNC for groundbreaking and innovative research. She earned her M.D. (Alpha Omega Alpha honors) from the University of Rochester, completed her pediatrics residency at Stanford, was a Robert Wood Johnson Clinical Scholar, and earned an M.P.H. at UNC, Chapel Hill.

Samir S. Shah, M.D., MSCE, MHM, is vice chair of clinical affairs and education at Cincinnati Children's Hospital Medical Center, where he holds the James M. Ewell Endowed Chair. He is also professor of pediatrics at the University of Cincinnati College of Medicine and editor-in-chief of the *Journal of Hospital Medicine*, an official journal of the Society of Hospital Medicine. He practices clinically as both a pediatric hospitalist and a pediatric infectious diseases physician. Dr. Shah's research focuses on improving the efficiency and effectiveness of care in the hospital setting with an emphasis on common, serious childhood infections. He co-developed an ACGME certified 3-year pediatric hospital medicine fellowship and has served as a mentor or co-mentor to seven federal K-series grant awardees. Dr. Shah has been recognized for his research and mentorship with numerous national awards, including the Excellence in Research Award (2009) and the Excellence in Teamwork in Quality Improvement Award (2014) from the Society of Hospital Medicine, the Excellence in Research Award (2020) and the Miller-Sarkin Mentorship Award (2015) from the Academic Pediatric Association, and the Pediatric Hospital Medicine Award for Excellence in Research (2015), jointly awarded by the AAP, the Academic Pediatric Association, and the Society for Hospital Medicine. In 2019, he received the Master in Hospital Medicine, a lifetime achievement award, from the Society of Hospital Medicine. Following medical school at Yale, Dr. Shah completed a pediatrics residency as well as fellowships in both Academic General Pediatrics and Pediatric Infectious Diseases at the Children's Hospital of Philadelphia. He also received an M.S. in Clinical Epidemiology from the University of Pennsylvania School of Medicine.

Christopher Stille, M.D., M.P.H., is professor of pediatrics and section head of general academic pediatrics, and the Stephen Berman, M.D., Endowed Chair in General Pediatrics at the University of Colorado School of Medicine and Children's Hospital Colorado. He leads an active group of roughly 55 pediatric faculty; practices and teaches primary care pediatrics; and conducts pediatric health services research and quality improvement focused on improving systems of care for children and youth with special health care needs (CYSHCN) in the Medical Home. He has a particular interest in improving coordination of care among primary care clinicians, subspecialists, and family members, generated by his first years in private practice, but continuing over time. He has led projects funded by the U.S. Maternal and Child Health Bureau (MCHB), the Robert Wood Johnson Foundation, the Lucile Packard Foundation for Children's Health, and local and regional funders to pursue this investigation. Since 2017, he has been principal investigator of an MCHB-funded national network to conduct health systems research for CYSHCN, CYSHCNet (www.cyshcnet.org). Much of this network's work addresses partnerships between the "medical neighborhood" and families. He is a co-chair of the Standing Committee on Patient Experience and Function of the National Quality Forum. He is membership chair and a member of the Executive Committee of the Council on Children with Disabilities of the AAP.

Bonnie T. Zima, M.D., M.P.H., is professor-in-residence, specializing in child and adolescent psychiatry, vice chair for faculty development, associate chair for academic affairs, and associate director of the University of California at Los Angeles (UCLA) Center for Health Services & Society at the UCLA-Semel Institute for Neuroscience and Human Behavior. Her research is dedicated to improving the quality of child mental health care, with priority placed on children enrolled in Medicaid-funded outpatient programs and underserved, at-risk child populations. Her research spans identification of high unmet need for mental health care among high-risk child populations, national pediatric hospitalization resource use and costs, validity of national quality measures, pediatric integrated care models, pediatric workforce development, and application of technologies and clinical informatics to improve child mental health care. Her research has received all three national research awards from the American Academy of Child and Adolescent Psychiatry (AACAP). In addition, Dr. Zima is a member of the U.S. Child and Adult Core Set Annual Review Workgroup for Center for Medicaid and Children's Health Insurance Program Services, American Psychiatric Association (APA) Council on Quality Care, Behavioral Health and Substance Abuse Steering Committee for the National Quality Forum, and AACAP Committee on Research. She is consulting editor for the *Journal of the American Academy of Child & Adolescent Psychiatry*, deputy editor for the journal of child and adolescent psychopharmacology, and Distinguished Fellow of AACAP and APA. She graduated first in medical school at Rush Medical College, and completed her general psychiatry residency, child psychiatry fellowship, and the Robert Wood Johnson Clinical Scholars Program at UCLA. She was a member of the Committee to Evaluate the Supplemental Security Income Disability Program for Children with Mental Disorders (2014–2016).

NATIONAL ACADEMY OF MEDICINE FELLOW

Julie Sees, D.O., M.B.A., is a pediatric/neuro-orthopedic surgeon with dual-fellowship training in pediatric orthopedic surgery and neuro-orthopedic surgery. She has expertise in care for children and young adults with neuromotor-orthopedic disorders. An active member of the osteopathic medical profession, Dr. Sees serves on the American Osteopathic Association Board of Trustees, American Osteopathic Academy of Orthopedics (AOAO) Board of Directors, American Osteopathic Foundation (AOF) Vice President, Delaware State Osteopathic Medical Society President, and American Academy for Cerebral Palsy and Developmental Medicine Webmaster. Dr. Sees has authored more than 75 peer-reviewed publications/chapters and made more than 200 national and international conference presentations/instructional courses, including health care delivery and international strategy. Her research and advocacy includes best practices within physician professional development, neuro-orthopedics, complex motor conditions, gait abnormalities, pediatric subspecialty care, clinician well-being, and emerging leadership in health, education, and medicine. She was the recipient of an Emerging Leader Award by the AOF and the Chicago College of Osteopathic Medicine Alumni Association, J. Richard Bowen, M.D., Teaching Award, 2 U.S. patents with Pfizer Global Research and Development, and prestigious designation as Fellow of both the AOAO and the American Orthopedic Association. Dr. Sees obtained her B.A. in Chemistry/Religious Studies as a Division I scholarly athlete from College of the Holy Cross; earned her M.D. from Midwestern University Chicago College of Osteopathic Medicine; completed her orthopedic residency at the former University of Medicine and Dentistry of New Jersey; and earned her Healthcare Executive M.B.A., summa cum laude, from Saint Joseph's University Haub School of Business. Dr. Sees is a Fellow of Osteopathic Medicine with the National Academies of Science, Engineering, and Medicine, working on the Action Collaborative for Clinician Well-Being and Resilience, Neuroscience Forum, and Pediatric Subspecialty Workforce Impact on Child Health, and medical director of Neuro-Orthopaedics/Spine Surgery for the CVS Health Medical Health Services Northeast Territory.

STAFF

Ruth Cooper, B.A., is an associate program officer with the Board on Health Care Services at the National Academies of Sciences, Engineering, and Medicine. She has worked on several National Academies projects, including studies on the organ transplantation system, space radiation and cancer risk, building data capacity for conducting patient-centered outcomes research, cancer and disability, and evidence-based opioid prescribing, as well as workshops on organ transplant and disability, companion animals as sentinels for environmental exposures, and diagnostic excellence in cardiac events, cancers, and COVID-19. She had also assisted with numerous National Cancer Policy Forum workshops ranging from the cancer workforce to health literacy. Prior to joining the National Academies, Ms. Cooper spent a year volunteering at Open Arms Home for Children in South Africa. She has previously worked at the U.S. Arctic Research Commission and participated in three Arctic field cruises. Ms. Cooper holds a B.A. from the University of Notre Dame in Neuroscience and Behavior with a minor in Mediterranean Middle Eastern studies, and is currently pursuing her Master's degree in International Science and Technology Policy at The George Washington University.

Tracy Lustig, D.P.M., M.P.H., is a senior program officer with the Board on Health Care Services at the National Academies of Sciences, Engineering, and Medicine. Dr. Lustig was trained in podiatric medicine and surgery and spent several years in private practice. In 1999 she was awarded a congressional fellowship with the American Association for the Advancement of Science and spent a year working in the office of Ron Wyden of the U.S. Senate. Dr. Lustig joined the National Academies in 2004. She was the study director for consensus studies on the geriatrics workforce, oral health, ovarian cancer research, and social isolation and loneliness, and was the co-director of a 2022 study on the quality of care in nursing homes. She has also directed workshops on the allied health workforce, the use of telehealth to serve rural populations, assistive technologies, hearing loss, and biomarkers of disability. In 2009 she staffed an Academies-wide initiative on the "Grand Challenges of an Aging Society" and subsequently helped to launch the Forum on Aging, Disability, and Independence, which she currently directs. Dr. Lustig has a doctor of podiatric medicine degree from Temple University and an M.P.H. with a concentration in health policy from The George Washington University.

Sharyl J. Nass, Ph.D., serves as senior director of the Board on Health Care Services and co-director of the National Cancer Policy Forum at the National Academies of Sciences, Engineering, and Medicine. The National Academies provide independent, objective analysis and advice to the nation to solve complex problems and inform public policy decisions related to science, technology, and medicine. To enable the best possible care for all patients, the Board undertakes scholarly analysis of the organization, financing, effectiveness, workforce, and delivery of health care, with emphasis on quality, cost, accessibility, and equity. The Forum examines policy issues pertaining to the entire continuum of cancer research and care. For more than two decades, Dr. Nass has worked on a broad range of health and science policy topics that includes the quality of health care and clinical trials, developing technologies for precision medicine, and strategies to support patient and clinician well-being. She has a Ph.D. from Georgetown University and undertook postdoctoral training at the Johns Hopkins University School of Medicine, as well as a research fellowship at the Max Planck Institute in Germany. She also holds a B.S. and an M.S. from the University of Wisconsin, Madison. She has been the recipient of the Cecil Medal for Excellence in Health Policy Research, a Distinguished Service Award from the National Academies, the Institute of Medicine staff team achievement award (as team leader), and the Health and Medicine Division Mentor Award.

Tochi Ogbu-Mbadiugha, B.S., was a senior program assistant with the National Academies of Sciences, Engineering, and Medicine (through November 2022). Prior to joining the National Academies, she assisted the legislative practice at Powers, Pyles, Sutter & Verville PC with tracking legislation relevant to the firm's health care, disability, and rehabilitation clients. She holds a B.S. in kinesiology from the University of Maryland College Park, where she completed research on the correlation between built environments and chronic disease rates among adults in urban settings.

Adaeze Okoroajuzie, B.H.S., is a senior program assistant with the Board on Health Care Services at the National Academies of Science, Engineering, and Medicine. Prior to joining the National Academies, she was the president of GlobeMed at Howard University, a grassroots organization that works directly with the Nancholi Youth Organization in Blantyre, Malawi. She is a certified birth doula, providing free doula services to young mothers through the Mary's Center doula volunteer program in Washington, DC. Through her content creator account "DazetheDoula," she creates awareness and educates her community on birth education. A recent graduate of Howard University, Ms. Okoroajuzie obtained her B.H.S., magna cum laude, with a minor in biology and maternal child health. She was a member and case writer for the National Academies DC Public Health Case Challenge in 2019, 2021, and 2022.

Isaac Suh, M.S.P.H., is a research associate in the Health and Medicine Division of the National Academies of Sciences, Engineering, and Medicine. Prior to joining the Academies, he obtained his B.S. in Global Public Health at New York University and his M.S.P.H. in Health Policy and Management at the Johns Hopkins School of Public Health, where he further specialized in risk sciences and policy.

Nikita Varman, M.P.H., was a research associate with the National Academies of Sciences, Engineering, and Medicine (through June 2022). Prior to joining the National Academies, Ms. Varman interned at Boston Children's Hospital's Office of Government Relations, where she advocated for children's health care issues at the state and federal levels, and at Medecins sans Frontieres, where she researched accessibility of hepatitis C diagnostics. She is a 2020 graduate from Boston University with an M.P.H. in public health and concentrations in health policy and law as well as community assessment, program design, implementation, and evaluation. Ms. Varman also holds a B.S. in health sciences and a B.A. in political science, cum laude, as a Posse Foundation Scholar and Scarlet Key recipient from Boston University in 2019.